Mosquito Research - Recent Advances in Pathogen Interactions, Immunity, and Vector Control Strategies

Edited by Henry Puerta-Guardo and Pablo Manrique-Saide

Published in London, United Kingdom

Mosquito Research - Recent Advances in Pathogen Interactions, Immunity, and Vector Control Strategies
http://dx.doi.org/10.5772/intechopen.98177
Edited by Henry Puerta-Guardo and Pablo Manrique-Saide

Contributors
Femi Ayoade, Tosin S. Ogunbiyi, Ahmad Zafar Baig, Huma Aslam, Aiza Zafar, Sahar Fazal, Rabbiah Manzoor Malik, Narjis Khatoon, Muneeba Ishtiaq, Emery Metelo-Matubi, Josue Zanga, Victoire Nsabatien, Fiacre Agossa, Solange Ngamukie, El Hadji Amadou Niang, Jean Maniania-Nguya-Kalenga, Mulenda Basimike, Aimé Mbala, Assad A Al-Thukair, Yasin Jamal, Alexis Nzila, Taruna Kaura, Neha Sylvia Walter, Upninder Kaur, Rakesh Sehgal, Kaushal Kumar Mahto, Pooja Prasad, Mohan Kumar, Harshita Dubey, Amar Ranjan, Rebeca Carballar-Lejarazu, Taylor Tushar, Thai Binh Pham, Anthony James, Jeyaraj John Wilson, Thangamariyappan Harimuralikrishnaa, Ponnirul Ponmanickam, Muthumadasamy Ponseetha Lakshmi, Sanchaita Rajkhowa, Himangshu Patgiri, Ankita Khataniar, Pitimoni Boro, Sushmita Baishnab, Abdiel Martin-Park, Josue Villegas-Chim, Henry Puerta-Guardo, María Eugenia Toledo-Romaní, Yamili Contreras-Perera, Azael Che-Mendoza, Jorge Palacio-Vargas, Fabian Correa-Morales, Hector Gomez-Dantés, Pablo Manrique-Saide, Norma Pavia-Ruz, Silvia Pérez-Carrillo, Daniel Adrián, Juan Navarrete-Carballo, Anuar Medina-Barreiro, Josue Herrera-Bojorquez, Miguel Xcaer, Hugo Delfin-Gonzalez, Nekpen Erhunse, Victor Okomayin, Wilber Gomez-Vargas, Giovani Esteban Zapata-Úsuga, Iram Pablo Rodriguez-Sanchez, Adriana Flores-Suarez

First published in London, United Kingdom, 2023 by IntechOpen
IntechOpen is the global imprint of INTECHOPEN LIMITED, registered in England and Wales, registration number: 11086078, 5 Princes Gate Court, London, SW7 2QJ, United Kingdom

British Library Cataloguing-in-Publication Data
A catalogue record for this book is available from the British Library

Additional hard and PDF copies can be obtained from orders@intechopen.com

Mosquito Research - Recent Advances in Pathogen Interactions, Immunity, and Vector Control Strategies
Edited by Henry Puerta-Guardo and Pablo Manrique-Saide
p. cm.
Print ISBN 978-1-80355-852-3
Online ISBN 978-1-80355-853-0
eBook (PDF) ISBN 978-1-80355-854-7

For EU product safety concerns:
IN TECH d.o.o., Prolaz Marije Krucifikse Kozulić 3, 51000 Rijeka, Croatia,
info@intechopen.com or visit our website at intechopen.com.

Meet the editors

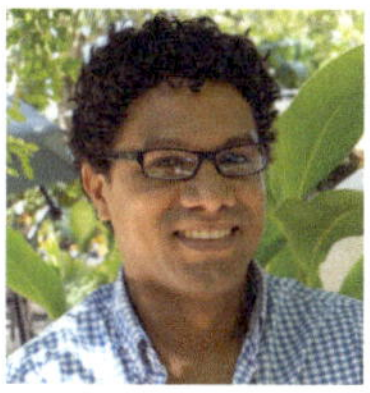

Henry Puerta-Guardo, Ph.D., is a virologist that has travelled around the Americas studying vector-borne diseases such as dengue, Zika, West Nile, and chikungunya. After living in different cities in Colombia, Venezuela, Mexico, and the United States, he has based his research studies in the city of Merida, Mexico). He is a professor and principal investigator at the Universidad Autonoma de Yucatan (UADY), Mexico, working on the understanding of the dynamics of mosquito-transmitted viruses to inform and improve vector control strategies. He is very passionate about identifying viral and host factors that contribute to virus pathogenesis and disease that would support the development of new potential prophylactics (e.g., vaccine targets) and/or therapeutics (e.g., antivirals) to combat neglected tropical diseases such as those transmitted by mosquitoes.

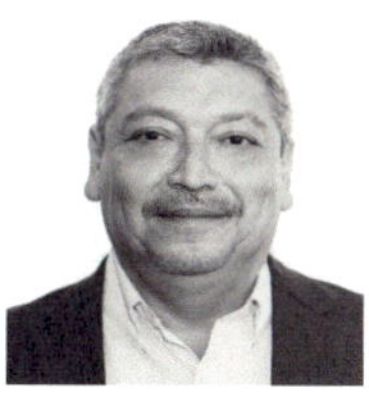

Pablo Manrique-Saide, Ph.D., is a professor and public health entomologist at the Universidad Autonoma de Yucatan (UADY), Mexico, and head of the Collaborative Unit for Entomological Bioassays (UCBE-UADY), a collaborating center of reference for the evaluation of insecticides. Key components of his research include the design of bioassays and trials for the evaluation of new vs. traditional entomological-infestation measures and control tools with an emphasis on *Ae. aegypti*, the vector of dengue, chikungunya, Zika, and Yellow Fever viruses. Dr. Manrique-Saide is also interested in how insecticide resistance can be detected and managed in the field. He has had a long career and worked collaboratively with many researchers, Latin American Ministries of Health, and international institutions. He has more than 100 peer-reviewed publications to his credit.

Contents

Preface

Mosquitoes (Diptera: Culicidae) can be vectors of human diseases such as malaria, dengue, Zika, chikungunya, yellow fever, West Nile virus, and other encephalitides, which together kill around 0.6–1.2 million people a year and put more than 80% of the population worldwide at risk of infection.

The emergence of mosquito-borne diseases (MBDs) is determined by a complex set of biological, ecological, environmental, and socio-demographic factors. The increased range and abundance of mosquito distribution and susceptibility to new pathogens are also factors resulting in increased transmission to human populations and rapid adaptation to new environmental conditions and landscapes, all of which have significant consequences in mosquito population dynamics and disease transmission.

Progress has been made in better understanding the dynamics of the interactions between mosquitoes and human-transmissible pathogens, their protective responses against invasive pathogens, the dynamics that lead to their environmental adaptation, and the potential strategies for hindering it. Despite this, there is not yet a single intervention likely to stop most MBDs. Effective vector control should be designed, structured, and delivered as Integrated Vector Management (IVM) including traditional and innovative tools and approaches with environmental management, biological control, and chemical control among other suitable cost-effective strategies that may achieve the greatest disease control benefit, minimizing the negative impact on ecosystems. However, mosquitoes continue to be the deadliest animals on Earth and public enemy number one in the fight against global infectious diseases.

This book describes recent advances in mosquito biology and ecology and their interaction with pathogens that lead to host infection. It also examines new technologies of vector control for preventing and reducing human-transmissible MBDs.

Henry Puerta-Guardo
Collaborative Unit for Entomological Bioassays,
Campus for Biological and Agricultural Sciences,
Universidad Autonoma de Yucatan,

Virology lab,
CIR-Biomedicas,
Universidad Autonoma de Yucatan,
Merida, Mexico

Pablo Manrique-Saide
Collaborative Unit for Entomological Bioassays,
Campus for Biological and Agricultural Sciences,
Universidad Autonoma de Yucatan,
Merida, Mexico

Section 1

Mosquito Biology, Ecology and Vector-Parasite Interactions

Chapter 1

Mosquito Excito-Repellency: Effects on Behavior and the Development of Insecticide Resistance

Yamili J. Contreras-Perera, Abdiel Martin-Park, Henry Puerta-Guardo, Azael Che-Mendoza, Silvia Pérez-Carrillo, Irám Pablo Rodríguez-Sánchez, Pablo Manrique-Saide and Adriana Flores-Suarez

Abstract

Mosquito's resistance to avoiding insecticide-treated surfaces ("excito-repellency") has two effects: irritation from direct contact with a treated area and repellency as an avoidance response to contact with treated surfaces. Nowadays, this behavior appears to reduce the success of mosquito control programs, particularly those based on insecticide-driven strategies. Different systems have been designed to assess the excito-repellency, evaluating numerous insecticides' irritants, deterrents, and toxic properties at different concentrations. The information provides valuable insights regarding the patterns of mosquito behavior based on their physiological conditions, such as the age of the mosquitoes and the duration of the tests. However, the physiological processes resulting from chemical stimulus contact "chemoreception") are still poorly explored and understood. This review provides an overview of insecticide effects on mosquito behavior and describes the mechanisms involved in chemical stimuli uptake, translation, and recognition.

Keywords: mosquitoes, excito-repellency, chemoreception, insecticide resistance

1. Introduction

The worldwide spread and increasing transmission of diseases such as dengue, chikungunya, and Zika transmitted by *Aedes aegypti* have made this mosquito species a primary target for the vector control programs [1]. *Ae. aegypti* control still represents the primary strategy to reduce outbreaks of these diseases. Interventions include reducing or eliminating such breeding sites during their immature aquatic phase and insecticidal control using larvicides and adulticides [2]. The natural tendency of mosquitoes to avoid insecticide-treated surfaces appears to be a general behavioral phenomenon [3]. There are two types of behavioral responses to insecticides: irritation, which is defined as an insect leaving an insecticide-treated surface after tarsal contact with it, and repellency, or spatial repellency (deterrence or avoidance), which refers to the function of a compound to influence an avoidance response movement away from a chemical stimulus through actual physical contact with it, thus diverting insects from the treated surface [4–6]. However, this behavior and the changes in the vector's resting habits and biting activity represent a challenge in the surveillance and vector control strategies [7].

Different authors have coined the term "excito-repellency" to refer to the combined effect of escape responses after the contact with the insecticide-treated area [5, 8, 9]. Likewise, studies based on the excito-repellency test system have reported that the nutritional status and physiological conditions (including age) and the duration of the tests can significantly influence the response behavior to insecticides. Therefore, chronological age, physiological status, and innate (circadian) activity patterns should be carefully considered for the proper selection of mosquitoes used in the tests [3].

The behavior of mosquitoes in response to insecticides continues to be poorly studied and understood. They do not refer to anything other than the locomotor response of mosquitoes after capturing a stimulus, either contact "irritation" or noncontact spatial repellency "deterrence" resulting from the capturing of chemical emanations "odors" by nature and/or evaporation of chemical substances [10, 11]. On the other hand, understanding mosquito behavior will enable the selection of insecticides, the operational planning of cost-effective and long-term interventions and the development of innovative surveillance and vector control tools and strategies [12, 13].

2. Vector control methods

Most of the interventions for *Aedes* mosquito control are based on adulticide and larvicide insecticides; however, this strategy alone is insufficient to reduce the mosquito populations and can induce different resistance mechanisms [2, 14]. In recent years, it has been necessary to further optimize current strategies within integrated approaches and advance the development of an alternative, an innovative design for the control [15, 16]. The integrated vector management (IVM) combines different methods for sustainable vector control; these methods are grouped into the following strategies: environmental control, mechanical/physical control, biological control, chemical control, and the use of new technologies such as the release of mosquitoes with endosymbiotic bacteria (*Wolbachia*), transgenic mosquitoes, or irradiated mosquitoes [2]. Additionally, WHO's 2017–2030 Global Vector Control Response strategy points out that vector control can be improved by educating and empowering communities to identify and eliminate breeding sites around their homes, also improving the piped water supply system, adequate management of solid waste and screened housing to reduce densities of mosquitoes biting humans indoors and thus reduce human vector contact, and personal protection by repellents application, insecticide-impregnated net and curtains [1, 2, 17].

Environmental interventions ("Immature mosquito control") are based on actions to eliminate breeding sites for these organisms, impacting adult populations. These interventions represent sustainable and safe methods as there are limited risks of environmental contamination and toxicity [18, 19]. Control of the immature stages of dengue vectors is generally conducted larval habitats using biological, chemical, environmental, or mechanical methods to maximize the reduction in vector population density [13]. The principal environmental methods are container covers with and without insecticides, waste management with and without direct garbage collection, elimination of breeding sites, drinking water supply, and urban planning [2, 19]. Similar to environmental interventions, mechanical and physical control, consists of cleaning breeding sites and physical barriers such as mosquito nets and curtains [15].

The biological control interventions to control mosquitos are based on pathogens and mosquito symbionts. Regarding successful experiences of biological control, some examples of interventions regarding the vertical or community-based introduction of Cyclopoid copepods (*Mesocyclops longisetus*) and one with fish of different species have been reported for the control of dengue vector populations [20–22]. However, their implementation and sustainability function depends on breeding sites and their ultimate productivity. Regarding biorational management, different formulations based on *Bacillus thuringiensis* var. *israelensis* (Bti) are efficient as bio-larvicides for malaria and dengue vectors [23, 24]. On the other hand, the use of innovative technologies based on interventions with "modified mosquitoes," either genetically by dominant lethal genes (RISL) or immunity genes (RNAi), by irradiation as sterile insect technique (SIT) or biologically as incompatible insect technique IIT, the SIT and IIT strategies are not classified as genetically modified [25].

Chemical control is an essential element in vector control strategies worldwide and can be implemented under two approaches: 1) to reduce density/increase vector mortality by adulticides and larvicides application and 2) to reduce human vector contact by insecticide-treated materials (ITMs) such as long-lasting insecticide nets (LLINs), traditional nets, and personal repellents [2]. Vector control programs have favored insecticides to control adults, mainly based on ultralow-volume (ULV) space application for outdoors in open spaces due to the ease of covering large areas in the shortest possible time and thermal fog indoors [26–28]. Aerial ultralow-volume (AULV) applications are also being tested in México [29]. Targeted indoor residual spraying (IRS, TIRS) is another control method with evidence of efficacy in México [30].

The most common insecticide products to control malaria and any other mosquito vector transmission combine two different modes of action: 1) conventional insecticide activity that kills mosquitoes exposed to the insecticide, and 2) deterring mosquitoes away from humans [17]. Space spraying of insecticides is still considered to be a valuable tool to control the vectors of human diseases [31]. S-methoprene, pyriproxyfen, temephos, and Bti are among larvicidal and pupicidal agents recommended and approved by the World Health Organization (WHO) to treat *Ae. aegypti* larval environments. Temephos is the most extensively used larvicide for *Ae. aegypti* control [13]. Personal protection in the form of repellent application with DEET (N, N-diethyl-3-methylbenzamide) at a concentration of 25% can provide protection against *Ae. aegypti* [32].

Insecticide-treated materials (ITMs) can provide bite protection by killing or repelling vectors [6]. The use of nets impregnated with long-lasting insecticides used as pavilions or mosquito nets is currently one of the most promoted strategies to reduce the transmission of arboviral or parasitic diseases [17, 33]. Long-lasting insecticidal nets (LLINs) are materials pretreated with insecticides designed to prolong their useful life. Studies in several Latin American countries indicate that using LLINs fixed on doors and windows and insecticide-treated screening (ITS) are innovative approaches to control vector mosquito populations, and they may be promising in reducing the transmission of diseases such as dengue [34–37]. The efficacy of these interventions is reflected in reduced vector-human interaction and sustained indoor adult vector densities as blood-fed and arbovirus-positive *Ae. aegypti* females [38, 39], either due to its effects of repellency and excito-repellency or due to its toxic action, causing the death of the vector, in addition to acting as a physical barrier [40, 41]. Furthermore, its use in the form of mosquito nets permanently installed on doors and windows could solve one of the main problems associated with interventions using LLINs: the decrease in coverage over time (due to disuse or misuse of the LLIN by the community), limiting its effectiveness [35].

Spatial repellents (SRs) are products containing volatile chemicals that disperse in the air under ambient conditions. Besides, the term "spatial repellency" is used here to refer to a range of insect behaviors induced by airborne chemicals that result in a reduction in human-vector contact and, therefore, personal protection [42, 43]. The behaviors can include movement away from a chemical stimulus, interference with host detection (attraction inhibition), and feeding response [43]. In clinical trials, SR products reduced malaria and *Aedes*-borne virus infection through mechanisms of reduced human-vector interaction, being and are effective against insecticide-susceptible and resistant mosquito vectors [44]. Lethal ovitraps are small to medium-sized plastic cups or buckets with an oviposition substrate (usually cloth or paper-based) treated with a residual insecticide or an adhesive that may be used indoors or outdoors to reduce *Ae. aegypti* populations [13].

3. Effect of insecticides on mosquito behavior

For example, indoor residual spraying against malaria vectors depends on whether mosquitoes rest indoors (i.e., endophilic behavior); likewise, the optimum effectiveness of insecticide-treated nets presumably depends on vectors biting at hours when most people are in bed. Prospects for genetic control by sterile males or genes rendering mosquitoes harmless to humans will depend on competitive mating behavior [45]. Some works have provided evidence for the existence of behavioral modification because of widespread IRS or ITN use [46]. The behavioral responses of mosquitoes to insecticide products must be determinate to understand the main mechanisms involved in their effectiveness; this task is vital not only for success in chemical control strategies used in vector control programs but also for the development of new insecticides and the design of innovative control strategies [6, 12, 47]. The devices developed to analyze the behavior of mosquitoes evaluate three main components of chemical action: 1) contact irritation (excito-repellency), 2) spatial repellency, and 3) toxicity [8, 47–49].

Malaithong et al. [11] criticize the subjective way of using terms such as avoidance, excitation, irritability, deterrence, and excito-repellency by different authors in a system based on "success-repellency" tests, to refer to locomotor response behavior caused by contact with insecticides. The experts point out that this test system distinguishes two main locomotor responses: 1) stimulation of the musculoskeletal apparatus "excitation," "irritation" as a result of tarsal contact with a treated surface and 2) noncontact spatial repellency "deterrence" as a result of chemical emanations, that is, the capture of "odors" in the evaporation phase of chemical compounds at a distance, that is, the capture of "odors" in the evaporation phase of chemical compounds at a distance, without the need to make contact with the treated area and emphasizes the need for a clearer understanding of the behavior, stimuli, effects, and mechanisms involved in the response locomotive of mosquitoes against different xenobiotics.

Kongmee [50] reported no repellency effect without contact generated by insecticides in a study with anophelines based on excite-repellency tests with two pyrethroids; nevertheless, deltamethrin produced a high irritating effect, while bifenthrin exhibited low levels. At operational field doses of alpha-cypermethrin, low noncontact repellency was observed in three mosquito populations; thus, spatial repellency may play a minor role in escaping vectors from treated surfaces, with contact irritation being the most important main effect on *Ae. aegypti* populations [11]. Mongkalangoon et al. [51], in a study of irritability and repellency to synthetic pyrethroids, found a strong repellent effect of cyphenothrin in all doses evaluated compared with deltamethrin and d-tetramethrin; however, the irritant effect on contact was similar in the three insecticides evaluated. On the other hand, the presence of insecticide resistance by kdr and ace1 mutations can modify the mosquito response to DEET and natural repellents. These findings were validated for two resistant *Anopheles gambie* strains (KdrKis and AcerKis) in that the mutation can increase or decrease the effectiveness of DEET and natural compounds [52]. Cross-resistance has also been reported in the pyrethroid-resistant (PR) Puerto Rico strain of *Ae. aegypti*. All repellents tested in the study were less effective against the PR strain. Furthermore, the reduced susceptibility to these repellents may reflect a fitness cost caused by the PR strain's kdr mutation. As a result, it is critical to understand the secondary effects of pesticide resistance evolution in mosquitos, as well as the importance of developing alternative resistance-control strategies [53].

4. Sensory receptor and stimulus uptake

The functions of insect chemoreceptors have primarily been studied using antennae (olfactory receptors) and mouthparts (gustatory receptors) through specialized structures called sensilla, which comprise neurons and non-neuronal support cells, extracellular lymph fluid, and a precisely shaped cuticle [54]. Other appendages with chemoreceptive sensilla include the leg tarsi and the anterior wing margin. Their specific roles in chemoreception and mosquito behavior remain largely unknown [55]. This review provides a brief description and illustration of the sensilla and its function in chemical stimulus, transduction, recognition, and understanding in insect behavior.

4.1 Sensilla

Modified cuticular structures are the basic sensory unit in insects; they are made up of four components: sensory neurons, a thermogenic cell (socket), a trichogenous cell that gives rise to the hair, and a thecogenous cell that surrounds and protects the axon terminal and provides it with ions and nutrients (**Figure 1C**), sensory neurons are bipolar, extending their dendrites from the cuticular portion and their axons toward the central nervous system (CNS). Due to their external morphology, they can be classified into trichoid, basiconic, placoid, styloconic, coeloconic, and bell-shaped [58].

These structures, which are found on the surface of mosquito antennae and maxillary palps (olfactory sensilla), as well as mouthparts, tarsi, and wings (gustatory sensilla), play a major role in host detection and other sensory-mediated behaviors. (**Figure 1A**) [56, 59, 60]. In mosquitoes, the trichoid sensilla is the most common and abundant sensory structure. A single pore is typically observed at the distal end of a blunt tip. (**Figure 1C**) [60]. Bohbot et al. (2014) described the basiconica, chaetica, and campaniformia sensilla in *Ae. aegypti* and identified also in *Culex pipiens* with other classifications such as coeloconica, ampullacea, squamiformia, and styloconica. (**Figure 1B**) [59, 61]. Similar types of sensilla were observed on *An. kochi* antennae (ampullacea, chaetica, trichodea, basiconica, and coeloconica) [62]. Likewise, according to the type of stimulus they receive, these structures can be classified as: odorant receptors (chemoreceptors), gustatory receptors, ionotropic receptors, and olfactory receptors [56].

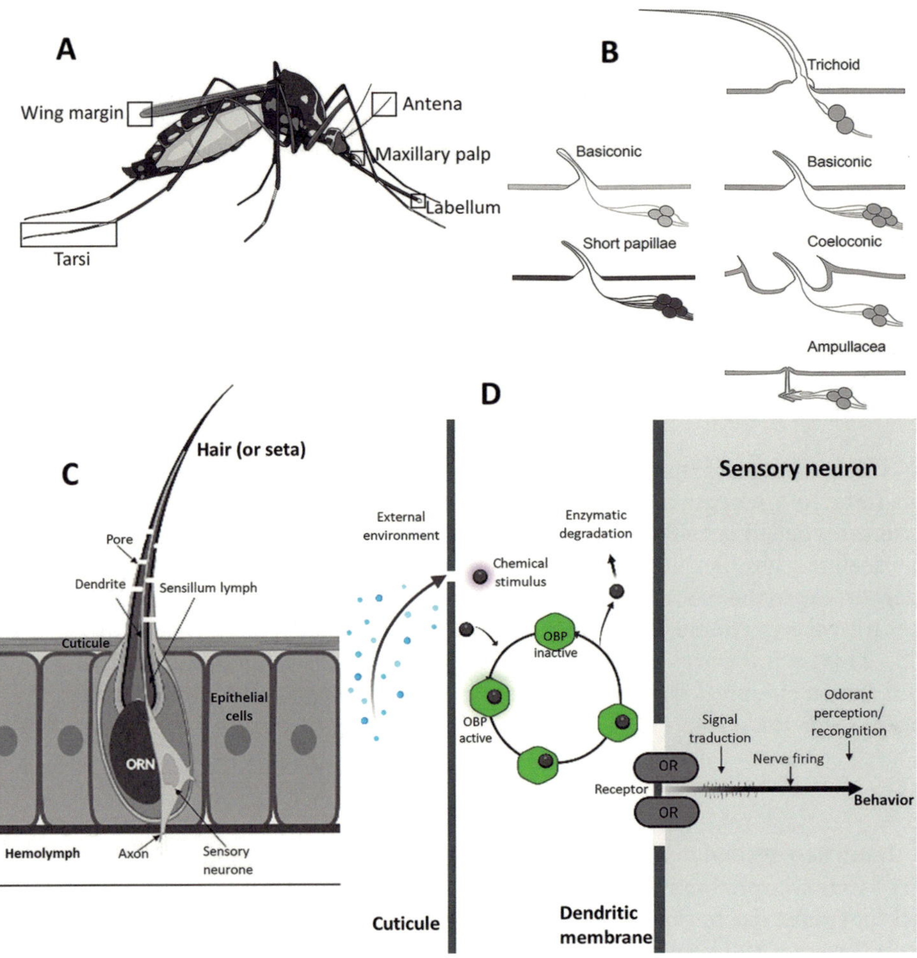

Figure 1.
Sensory receptors in mosquitoes, the sensilla and the stimulus. A) Sensory receptors on appendages based on Sparks et al. [56], B) different types of sensilla ae. Aegypti adapted from Jonathan Bohbot's lab (https://jonathanbohbot.weebly.com/the-mosquito-nose.html) [57], C) schematic organization of the trichoid sensilla (ORN: Olfactory receptor neuron), D) chemical stimulus, signal transduction, and recognition (OBP: Odorant-binding proteins) (A, C and D figures created with BioRender.com).

4.2 Chemoreceptors

Highly sensitive units can react to an external stimulus, mainly of "gustatory" character in the mouthparts, legs, and ovipositor, or olfactory character, mainly in the antennae and palps. Zwonitzer (1962) [63] within this classification includes those known as "general chemical sensitivity", which in turn respond to volatile materials classified as "distance chemical receptors" that are moderately sensitive. The categorization also comprises the receptors that are stimulated by nonvolatile substances ("chemoreceptors senses"), and those that are relatively insensitive and lead to protective responses defined as "general chemical senses." Chemoreception is the ability to perceive specific chemical stimuli. It is one of the most evolutionarily ancient forms of interaction between living organisms and their environment; this physiological process occurs because of the contact with a chemical stimulus and presents a broad spectrum of sensations [64, 65].

4.3 Stimulus reception

The chemical signals produced by semiochemicals and chemical substances reach the sensilla and penetrate the cuticle through pores; these substances are hydrophobic and cannot pass through the fluid. Lymphatic (aqueous medium) is achieved thanks to odorant-binding proteins (OBPs) that encapsulate them and direct them to the surface of the sensory cell where a structural change of charges in the membrane causes the stimulus to be expelled on the nerve receptor (**Figure 1D**) [58].

4.4 Chemical-sensory transduction

Once the union between the stimulus and the receptor has occurred (stimulus-receptor complex), the event must be communicated to other parts of the sensory cell to ensure the final message through the effect of action potentials transmitted to the brain. The amplification involves a series of membrane-bound intracellular molecules, usually calcium; at least one ion channel detects the increase in calcium and opens, thus triggering membrane depolarization [58].

4.5 Recognition and meaning in behavior

The sensory system acts as a filter allowing the insect to capture stimuli and to differentiate one stimulus from another. Therefore, receptor proteins and translation-associated molecules possess high specificity and sensitivity [66]. Several works have been published regarding the recognition by mosquitoes of emanations such as CO_2 and lactic acid on human skin; these works also show that high concentrations of these compounds can have a deterrent effect on mosquitoes [67, 68].

In female and male *Ae. aegypti*, chemoreceptors have been reported in the labella, tarsi, and at least in the first third of the legs; these receptors are curved setae present in the labella, and possibly they are those found in the tarsi. With these receptors, the mosquitoes can distinguish between acceptable and unacceptable solutions [69]. The presence of chemoreceptors in antennae has also been reported, it consists of sensilla classified as basiconic sensilla, and it is found in the ninth antennal segment [70]. However, multilayered molecular and cellular mechanisms determine the selectivity, sensitivity, and dynamic modulation of responses in insects [54]. Several studies on the development of attractants based on host-seeking behavior in mosquitoes have also provided important data to understand mosquito uptake of stimuli and different behavior patterns [71].

5. Effect of the physiological status of mosquitoes on the efficacy of insecticides

Different studies have compared the behavioral response of mosquitoes under different physiological conditions, including age. Experiments were carried out on *Ae. aegyti* females with four different physiological conditions: parous, without copulating, copulating (nulliparous), and fed to repletion. The results show that females without copulating and nulliparous females had higher responses of irritation and repellency than parid or newly fed females [3]. Polsomboon et al. [72] evaluated the relationship of the same physiological conditions in two pyrethroids; all the assessed females, regardless of their physiological state, were susceptible to deltamethrin and resistant to DDT; and two of the test groups from the same populations (without mating and nulliparous) showed higher mortality to DDT compared with parid females and recently fed females. Because blood can serve as an additional glycogen and protein storage, mosquitoes that were not mating or feeding showed reduced vigor in both insecticide tests.

Oliver & Brooke [73] were the first to demonstrate the expression of resistance to insecticides because of multiple blood feedings; they also point out the variability of the expression levels of detoxification enzymes as a function of age that presented a decrease in these due to aging. This could be because blood feeding can modify the expression of genes that affect the action of detoxifying enzymes. This expression is more evident during the first, second, and third days following a single blood feeding showing a dependence on sex [74].

This association seems to influence mosquito susceptibility or resistance to insecticides in terms of mosquito parasitism. According to Agnew et al. [75], parasitism can act as a source modifying the costs of resistance to organophosphate insecticides and as qualitatively different interactions (increasing or decreasing relative fitness in resistant individuals) that occur depending on the type of resistance involved.

In several insect groups and disease vectors across the world, "physiological" resistance, metabolic, and target site modifications to insecticides have been well documented [76], including highly physiologically insecticide-resistant mosquitoes. It also implies the application of chemical products at higher concentrations, which is neither practically feasible nor cost-effective [12].

6. Conclusions

Although the behavioral responses of mosquito vectors to insecticides differ based on the type of product and concentration, it is also true that the product's properties (irritant-repellent) can help to reduce human-vector interaction. The behavioral response of avoiding the treated surface seeks to integrate products with such properties to reduce the transmission of pathogens because they reduce the opportunity for blood feeding. Understanding mosquito behavior, including oviposition site selection, dispersal behavior, and competitive mating, can allow the development of innovative mosquito surveillance and control strategies to control these important and deadly insects better. On the other hand, molecular and structural studies and the signaling pathways of these receptors must be studied better to understand their function and role in resistance development.

Conflict of interest

"The authors declare no conflict of interest."

Author details

Yamili J. Contreras-Perera[1*], Abdiel Martin-Park[1], Henry Puerta-Guardo[1], Azael Che-Mendoza[1], Silvia Pérez-Carrillo[1], Irám Pablo Rodríguez-Sánchez[2], Pablo Manrique-Saide[1] and Adriana Flores-Suarez[2]

1 Autonomous University of Yucatan, Mérida, Yucatán, México

2 Autonomous University of Nuevo León, San Nicolas de los Garza, Nuevo León, Mexico

*Address all correspondence to: yamjaz_85@hotmail.com

References

[1] World Health Organization. UNICEF/UNDP/World Bank/WHO Special Programme for Research and Training in Tropical Diseases. Global vector control response 2017-2030. France: World Health Organization; 2017. Available from: https://apps.who.int/iris/handle/10665/259205. Licensee: CC BY-NC-SA 3.0 IGO

[2] Pan American Health Organization. Handbook for Integrated Vector Management in the Americas. Washington, D.C.: PAHO; 2019

[3] Chareonviriyaphap T, Kongmee M, Bangs MJ, Sathantriphop S, Meunworn V, Parbaripai A, et al. Influence of nutritional and physiological status on behavioral responses of *Aedes aegypti* (Diptera: Culicidae) to deltamethrin and cypermethrin. Journal of Vector Ecology. 2006;**31**:89-101. DOI: 10.3376/1081-1710(2006)31[89,ionaps]2.0.co;2

[4] Dethier VG, Browne BL, Smith CN. The designation of Chemicals in Terms of the responses they elicit from insects. Journal of Economic Entomology. 1960;**53**:134-136. DOI: 10.1093/jee/53.1.134

[5] Roberts DR, Chareonviriyaphap T, Harlan HH, Hshieh P. Methods of testing and analyzing excito-repellency responses of malaria vectors to insecticides. Journal of the American Mosquito Control Association. 1997;**13**:13-17

[6] Achee NL, Sardelis MR, Dusfour I, Chauhan KR, Grieco JP. Characterization of spatial repellent, contact irritant, and toxicant chemical actions of standard vector control compounds. Journal of the American Mosquito Control Association. 2009;**25**:156-167. DOI: 10.2987/08-5831.1

[7] Zhou G, Yu L, Wang X, Zhong D, Lee MC, Kibret S, et al. Behavioral response of insecticide-resistant mosquitoes against spatial repellent: A modified self-propelled particle model simulation. PLoS One. 2020;**15**:e0244447. DOI: 10.1371/journal.pone.0244447

[8] Chareonviriyaphap T, Prabaripai A, Sungvornyothrin S. An improved excito-repellency test chamber for mosquito behavioral tests. Journal of Vector Ecology. 2002;**27**:250-252

[9] Grieco JP, Achee NL, Chareonviriyaphap T, Suwonkerd W, Chauhan K, Sardelis MR, et al. A new classification system for the actions of IRS chemicals traditionally used for malaria control. PLoS One. 2007;**2**:e716. DOI: 10.1371/journal.pone.0000716

[10] Miller JR, Siegert PY, Amimo FA, Walker ED. Designation of chemicals in terms of the locomotor responses they elicit from insects: An update of Dethier et al. (1960). Journal of Economic Entomology. 2009;**102**:2056-2060. DOI: 10.1603/029.102.0606

[11] Malaithong N, Tisgratog R, Tainchum K, Prabaripai A, Juntarajumnong W, Bangs MJ, et al. Locomotor behavioral responses of *Anopheles minimus* and *Anopheles harrisoni* to alpha-Cypermethrin in Thailand. Journal of the American Mosquito Control Association. 2011;**27**:217-226. DOI: 10.2987/11-6132.1

[12] Day J. Mosquito oviposition behavior and vector control. Insects. 2016;7:65. DOI: 10.3390/insects7040065

[13] Ritchie S, Devine G, Vazquez-Prokopec G, Lenhart A, Manrique-Saide P, Scott TW. Insecticide-based approaches for dengue vector control. In: Koenraadt C, Spitzen J, Takken W, editors. Innovative Strategies for Vector Control. Wageningen: Wageningen Academic Publishers; 2021. pp. 59-89. DOI: 10.3920/978-90-8686-895-7_4

[14] Dusfour I, Vontas J, David JP, Weetman D, Fonseca DM, Corbel V, et al. Management of insecticide resistance in the major *Aedes vectors* of arboviruses: Advances and challenges. PLoS Neglected Tropical Diseases. 2019;**13**:e0007615. DOI: 10.1371/journal.pntd.0007615

[15] Achee NL, Grieco JP, Vatandoost H, Seixas G, Pinto J, Ching-Ng L, et al. Alternative strategies for mosquito-borne arbovirus control. PLoS Neglected Tropical Diseases. 2019;**13**:e0006822. DOI: 10.1371/journal.pntd.0006822

[16] Jones RT, Ant TH, Cameron MM, Logan JG. Novel control strategies for mosquito-borne diseases. Philosophical Transactions B Royal Society B. 2021;**376**:20190802. DOI: 10.1098/rstb.2019.0802

[17] Killeen GF, Smith TA. Exploring the contributions of bed nets, cattle, insecticides and excitorepellency to malaria control: A deterministic model of mosquito host-seeking behaviour and mortality. Transactions of the Royal Society of Tropical Medicine and Hygiene. 2007;**101**:867-880. DOI: 10.1016/j.trstmh.2007.04.022

[18] Manrique-Saide P, Davies CR, Coleman PG, Rebollar-Tellez E, Che-Medoza A, Dzul-Manzanilla F, et al. Pupal surveys for *Aedes aegypti* surveillance and potential targeted control in residential areas of Mérida, México. Pupal surveys for *Aedes aegypti* surveillance and potential targeted control in residential areas of Mérida, México. Journal of the American Mosquito Control Association. 2008;**24**:289-298. DOI: 10.2987/5578.1

[19] Buhler C, Winkler V, Runge-Ranzinger S, Boyce R, Horstick O. Environmental methods for dengue vector control - A systematic review and meta-analysis. PLoS Neglected Tropical Diseases. 2019;**13**:e0007420. DOI: 10.1371/journal.pntd.0007420

[20] Gorrochotegui-Escalante N, Fernandez-Salas I, Gomez-Dantes H. Field evaluation of *Mesocyclops longisetus* (Copepoda: Cyclopoidea) for the control of larval *Aedes aegypti* (Diptera Culicidae) in northeastern Mexico. Journal of Medical Entomology. 1998;**35**:699-703. DOI: 10.1093/jmedent/35.5.699

[21] Suárez-Rubio M, Suárez ME. The use of the copepod *Mesocyclops longisetus* as a biological control agent for *Aedes aegypti* in Cali, Colombia. J ournal of the American Mosquito Control Association. 2004;**20**:401-404

[22] Morales-Pérez A, Nava-Aguilera E, Legorreta-Soberanis J, Cortés-Guzmán AJ, Balanzar-Martínez A, Harris E, et al. Where we put little fish in the water there are no mosquitoes: A cross-sectional study on biological control of the *Aedes aegypti* vector in 90 coastal-region communities of Guerrero, Mexico. BMC Public Health. 2017;**17**:433. DOI: 10.1186/s12889-017-4302-z

[23] Naz S, Maqbool A, Ahmad MUD, Anjum AA. Toxins of bacillus thuringiensis var. israelensis for control of malaria vector *Anopheles stephensi* under laboratory and semi field conditions. International Journal of Agriculture and Biology. 2014;**16**:966-970

[24] Boyce R, Lenhart A, Kroeger A, Velayudhan R, Roberts B, Horstick O. *Bacillus thuringiensis israelensis* (Bti) for the control of dengue vectors: Systematic literature review. Tropical Medicine & International Health. 2013;**18**:564-577. DOI: 10.1111/tmi.12087 Epub 2013 Mar 26

[25] WHO & IAEA. Guidance Framework for Testing the Sterile Insect Technique as a Vector Control Tool against *Aedes*-Borne Diseases. Geneva: World Health Organization and the International Atomic Energy Agency; 2020 Licence: CC BY-NC SA 3.0 IGO

[26] Arrendondo-Jimenez JI, Rivero NE. Space treatments of insecticide for control of dengue virus vector *Aedes aegypti* in southern Mexico. I. Baseline penetration trials in open field and houses. Journal of the American Mosquito Control Association. 2006;**22**:301-305. DOI: 10.2987/8756-971X(2006)22[301,STOIFC]2.0.CO;2

[27] Farooq M, Cilek JE, Sumners E, Briley AKC, Weston J, Richardson AG, et al. Potential of outdoor ultra-low-volume aerosol and thermal fog to suppress the dengue vector, *Aedes aegypti*, inside dwellings. Journal of the American Mosquito Control Association. 2020;**36**:189-196. DOI: 10.2987/20-6922.1

[28] Ordoñez-González JG, Cisneros-Vázquez LA, Danis-Lozano R, Valdez-Delgado KM, Fernández-Salas I, Penilla-Navarro RP, et al. Nebulización térmica intradomiciliar de la mezcla de flupyradifurona y transflutrina en mosquitos *Aedes aegypti* susceptibles y resistentes a piretroides en el Sur de México [indoor thermal fogging of the mixture of flupyradifurone and transflutrin on *Aedes aegypti* mosquitoes susceptible and resistant to pyrethroids in southern Mexico]. Salud Publica de Mexico. 2020;**62**:432-438

[29] Correa-Morales F, Dzul-Manzanilla F, Bibiano-Marín W, Vadillo-Sánchez J, Medina-Barreiro A, Martin-Park A, et al. Entomological efficacy of aerial ultra-low volume insecticide applications against *Aedes aegypti* (Diptera: Culicidae) in Mexico. Journal of Medical Entomology. 2019;**56**:1331-1337. DOI: 10.1093/jme/tjz066

[30] Vazquez-Prokopec GM, Montgomery BL, Horne P, Clennon JA, Ritchie SA. Combining contact tracing with targeted indoor residual spraying significantly reduces dengue transmission. Science Advances. 2017;**3**:e1602024. DOI: 10.1126/sciadv.1602024

[31] Van den Berg H, Velayudhan R, Yadav RS. Management of insecticides for use in disease vector control: Lessons from six countries in Asia and the Middle East. PLoS Neglected Tropical Disease. 2021;**15**:e0009358. DOI: 10.1371/journal.pntd.0009358

[32] Uc-Puc V, Herrera-Bojórquez J, Carmona-Carballo C, Che-Mendoza A, Medina Barreiro A, Chablé-Santos J, et al. Efectividad de repelentes comerciales disponibles contra el mosquito *Aedes aegypti* (L.) vector del virus de dengue y Chikungunya en Yucatán, México. Salud Pública de México. 2016;**58**:472-475. DOI: 10.21149/spm.v58i4.8030

[33] Ansari MA, Razdan RK. Relative efficacy of insecticide treated mosquito nets (Diptera: Culicidae) under field conditions. Journal of Medical Entomology. 2000;**37**:201-204. DOI: 10.1603/0022-2585-37.1.201

[34] Rizzo N, Gramajo R, Escobar MC, Arana B, Kroeger A, Manrique-Saide P,

et al. Dengue vector management using insecticide treated materials and targeted interventions on productive breeding-sites in Guatemala. BMC Public Health. 2012;**12**:931. DOI: 10.1186/1471-2458-12-931

[35] Quintero J, Brochero H, Manrique-Saide P, Barrera-Pérez M, Basso C, Romero S, et al. Ecological, biological and social dimensions of dengue vector breeding in five urban settings of Latin America: A multi-country study. BMC Infectious Diseases. 2014;**38**:1-13. DOI: 10.1186/1471-2334-14-38

[36] Manrique-Saide P, Che-Mendoza A, Herrera-Bojórquez J, Villegas-Chim J, Guillermo-May G, Medina Barreiro A, et al. Insecticide-treated house screens to reduce infestations of dengue vectors. In: Aparecida Sperança M editor. Dengue-Immunopathology and Control Strategies. London: IntechOpen; 2017. pp. 93-107. DOI: 10.5772/67934

[37] Che-Mendoza A, Medina-Barreiro A, Koyoc-CardenaE,Uc-PucV,Contreras-PereraY, Herrera-Bojorquez J, et al. House screening with insecticide-treated netting provides sustained reductions in domestic populations of *Aedes aegypti* in Merida, Mexico. Plos Neglected Tropical Diseases. 2018;**12**:e0006283. DOI: 10.1371/journal.pntd.0006283

[38] Manrique-Saide P, Che-Mendoza A, Herrera-Bojórquez J, Villegas-Chim J, Guillermo-May G, Medina Barreiro A, et al. Insecticide-treated house screens to reduce infestations of dengue vectors. En: Aparecida Sperança M editor. Dengue-immunopathology and control. Strategies. 2017:93-107. DOI: 10.5772/67934

[39] Manrique-Saide P, Herrera-Bojórquez J, Villegas-Chim J, Puerta-Guardo H, Ayora-Talavera G, Parra-Cardeña M, et al. Protective effect of house screening against indoor *Aedes aegypti* in Mérida, Mexico: A cluster randomised controlled trial. Tropical Medicine & International Health. 2021;**26**:1677-1688. DOI: 10.1111/tmi.13680

[40] Rafinejad J, Vatandoost H, Nikpoor F, Abai MR, Duchen SM, S and Rafia F. Effect of washing on the bioefficacy of insecticide-treated nets (ITNs) and long-lasting insecticidal nets (LLINs) against main malaria vector *Anopheles stephensi* by three bioassay methods. Journal of Vector Borne Diseases. 2008;**45**:143-150. DOI: DOI

[41] Darriet F, Robert V, Vien N, Carnevale P, Organization WH. Evaluation of the Efficacy of Permethrin Impregnated Intact and Perforated Mosquito Nets Against Vectors of Malaria [internet]. Available from: https://apps.who.int/iris/handle/10665/65908 [Accessed: May 18, 2022]

[42] World Health Organization & WHO Pesticide Evaluation Scheme. Guidelines for Efficacy Testing of Spatial Repellents [Internet]. Available from: https://apps.who.int/iris/handle/10665/78142 [Accessed: May 19, 2022]

[43] Norris EJ, Coats JR. Current and future repellent technologies: The potential of spatial repellents and their place in mosquito-borne disease control. International Journal of Environmental Research and Public Health. 2017;**14**:124. DOI: 10.3390/ijerph14020124

[44] Achee NL, Grieco JP. Current status of spatial repellents in the global vector control community. In: Corona C, Debboun M, Coats J, editors. Advances in Arthropod Repellents. Cambridge: Academic Press; 2022. pp. 267-278. DOI: 10.1016/ B978-0-323-85411-5.00009-1

[45] Pates H, Curtis C. Mosquito behavior and vector control. Annual Review

of Entomology. 2005;**50**:53-70. DOI: 10.1146/annurev.ento.50.071803.130439

[46] Durnez L, Coosemans L. Residual transmission of malaria: An old issue for new approaches. In: Sylvie M editor. *Anopheles* Mosquitoes: New Insights into Malaria Vectors. London: IntechOpen; 2013. pp. 671-704. DOI: 10.5772/55925

[47] Grieco JP, Achee NL, Sardelis MR, Chauhan KR, Roberts DR. A novel high-throughput screening system to evaluate the behavioral response of adult mosquitoes to chemicals. Journal of the American Mosquito Control Association. 2005;**21**:404-411. DOI: 10.2987/8756-971X (2006)21[404, ANHSST]2.0.CO;2

[48] Tanasinchayakul S, Polsomboon S, Prabaripai A, Chareonviriyaphap T. An automated, field-compatible device for excito-repellency assays in mosquitoes. Journal of Vector Ecology. 2006;**31**:210-212. DOI: 10.3376/1081-1710(2006)31[210, AAFDFE]2.0.CO;2

[49] Morimoto Y, Kawada H, Kuramoto KY, Mitsuhashi T, Saitoh T, Minakawa N. New mosquito repellency bioassay for evaluation of repellents and pyrethroids using an attractive blood-feeding device. Parasites & Vectors. 2021;**14**:151. DOI: 10.1186/s13071-021-04656-y

[50] Kongmee M, Boonyuan W, Achee NL, Prabaripai A, Lerdthusnee K, Chareonviriyaphap T. Irritant and repellent responses of *Anopheles harrisoni* and *Anopheles minimus* upon exposure to Bifenthrin or Deltamethrin using an Excito-repellency system and a live host. Journal of the American Mosquito Control Association. 2012;**28**:20-29. DOI: 10.2987/11-6197.1

[51] Mongkalangoon P, Grieco JP, Achee NL, Suwonkerd W, Chareonviriyaphap T. Irritability and repellency of synthetic Pyrethroids on an *Aedes aegypti* population from Thailand. Journal of Vector Ecology. 2009;**34**:217-224. DOI: 10.1111/j.1948-7134.2009.00029.x

[52] Deletre E, Martin T, Duménil C, Chandre F. Insecticide resistance modifies mosquito response to DEET and natural repellents. Parasites Vectors. 2019;**12**:89. DOI: 10.1186/s13071-019-3343-9

[53] Yang L, Norris EJ, Jiang S, Bernier UR, Linthicum KJ, Bloomquist JR. Reduced effectiveness of repellents in a pyrethroid-resistant strain of *Aedes aegypti* (Diptera: Culicidae) and its correlation with olfactory sensitivity. Pest Management Science. 2020;**76**: 118-124. DOI: 10.1002/ps.5562

[54] Schmidt HR, Benton R. Molecular mechanisms of olfactory detection in insects: Beyond receptors. Open Biology. 2020;**10**:200252. DOI: 10.1098/rsob.200252

[55] Yang L, Agramonte N, Linthicum KJ, Bloomquist JR. A survey of chemoreceptive responses on different mosquito appendages. Journal of Medical Entomology. 2020;**58**:475-479. DOI: 10.1093/jme/tjaa154

[56] Sparks JT, Bohbot JD, Dickens JC. Olfactory disruption: Toward controlling important insect vectors of disease. Progress Molecular Biology Translational Science. 2015;**130**:81-108. DOI: 10.1016/bs.pmbts.2014.11.004

[57] Bohbot J. The Mosquito Nose [Internet]. Available from: https://jonathanbohbot.weebly.com/the-mosquito-nose.html [Accessed: May 16, 2022]

[58] Klowden MJ. Physiological Systems in Insects. 3era ed. USA: Academia Press; 2007. p. 696

[59] Bohbot JD, Sparks JT, Dickens JC. The maxillary palp of *Aedes aegypti*,

a model of multisensory integration. Insect Biochemistry and Molecular Biology. 2014;**48**:29-39. DOI: 10.1016/j.ibmb.2014.02.007

[60] Baik LS, Carlson JR. The mosquito taste system and disease control. Proceedings of the National Academy of Sciences. 2020;**117**:32848-32856. DOI: 10.1073/pnas.2013076117

[61] Ibrahim HAM, Sawires SG, Hamza AF. Morphological characterization and distribution of antennal sensilla of irradiated female mosquito, *Culex pipiens* (Diptera: Culicidae) with gamma radiation. Journal of Radiation Research and Applied Scienses. 2018;**11**:291-298

[62] Jatuwattana W, Saeung A, Taai K, Srisuka W, Thongsahuan S, Aupalee K, et al. Systematic studies of *anopheles* (Cellia) *Kochi* (Diptera: Culicidae): Morphology, cytogenetics, cross-mating experiments, molecular evidence and susceptibility level to infection with nocturnally subperiodic Brugia malayi. Acta Tropica. 2020;**205**:105300. DOI: 10.1016/j.actatropica.2019.105300

[63] Zwonitzer RL. The Morphology and Histology of the Labellar Contact Chemoreceptors of the Female Mosquito *Culiseta inornata* (Williston) [Dissertation/Thesis]. Laramie: University of Wyoming; 1962

[64] Zwonitzer RL. An Electrophysiological Study of the Labellar Contact Chemoreceptors of the Female Mosquito, *Culiseta inornata* (Williston) [Dissertation/Thesis]. Laramie: University of Wyoming; 1969

[65] Sokolinskaya EL, Kolesov DV, Lukyanov KA, Bogdanov AM. Molecular principles of insect chemoreception. Acta Naturae. 2020;**12**:81-91. DOI: 10.32607/actanaturae.11038

[66] Szyszka P, Stierle JS, Biergans S, Galizia CG. The speed of smell: Odor-object segregation within milliseconds. PLoS One. 2012;**7**:e36096. DOI: 10.1371/journal.pone.0036096

[67] Shirai Y, Kamimura K, Seki T, Morohashi M. L-lactic acid as a mosquito (Diptera: Culicidae) repellent on human and mouse skin. Journal of Medical Entomology. 2001;**38**:51-54. DOI: 10.1603/0022-2585-38.1.51

[68] Turner SL, Li N, Guda T, Githure J, Cardé RT, Ray A. Ultra-prolonged activation of CO2-sensing neurons disorients mosquitoes. Nature. 2011;**474**:87-91. DOI: 10.1038/nature10081

[69] Frings H, Hamrum CL. The contact chemoreceptors of adult yellow fever mosquitoes, *Aedes ægypti*. Journal of the New York Entomological Society. 1950;**58**:133-142

[70] Davis EE. Identification of antennal chemoreceptors of the mosquito, *Aedes aegypti*: A correction. Experientia. 1974;**30**:1282-1283. DOI: 10.1007/BF01945187

[71] Mathew N, Ayyanar E, ShanmugaveluS,MuthuswamyK.Mosquito attractant blends to trap host seeking *Aedes aegypti*. Parasitology Research. 2013;**112**:1305-1312. DOI: 10.1007/s00436-012-3266-2

[72] Polsomboon S, Poolprasert P, Bangs MJ, Suwonkerd W, Grieco JP, Achee NL, et al. Effects of physiological conditioning on behavioral avoidance by using a single age group of *Aedes aegypti* exposed to Deltamethrin and DDT. Journal of Medical Entomology. 2008;**45**:251-259. DOI: 10.1093/jmedent/45.2.251

[73] Oliver SV, Brooke BD. The effect of multiple blood-feeding on the

longevity and insecticide resistant phenotype in the major malaria vector *anopheles arabiensis* (Diptera: Culicidae). Parasites Vectors. 2014;**7**:390. DOI: 10.1186/1756-3305-7-390

[74] Marinotti O, Calvo E, Nguyen QK, Dissanayake S, Ribeiro JM, James AA. Genome-wide analysis of gene expression in adult *Anopheles gambiae*. Insect Molecular Biology. 2006;**15**:1-12. DOI: 10.1111/j.1365-2583.2006.00610.x

[75] Agnew P, Berticat C, Bedhomme S, Sidobre C, Michalakis Y. Parasitism increases and decreases the costs of insecticide resistance in mosquitoes. Evolution. 2004;**58**:579-586

[76] Chareonviriyaphap T, Bangs MJ, Suwonkerd W, Kongmee M, Corbel V, Ngoen-Klan R. Review of insecticide resistance and behavioral avoidance of vectors of human diseases in Thailand. Parasites Vectors. 2013;**6**:280. DOI: 10.1186/1756-3305-6-280

Chapter 2

Vector-Parasite Interactions and Malaria Transmission

Nekpen Erhunse and Victor Okomayin

Abstract

Malaria remains one of the world's most devastating vector-borne diseases. During the complex sexual development of the malaria parasite in the mosquito, it is faced with physical and physiological barriers which it must surmount before it can be transmitted to a human host. Proof-of-concept studies using RNAi have unearthed several parasite molecules which are important for countering the immunity of its vector. Understanding the counter-adaptations between the parasite and its vector could inform novel public health intervention strategies. For instance, it could guide the transgenic construction of resistant mosquitoes in which mosquito factors that restrict the parasite growth have been enhanced and/or factors promoting parasite growth deleted so as to make them refractory to malaria parasite infection. Such strategies, when deemed feasible, could be combined with conventional vector control methods as well as treatment of infection with effective malaria therapy, to actualize the malaria eradication goal.

Keywords: malaria transmission, vector-parasite interactions, transmission-blocking strategies, genetics-based tools, malaria eradication

1. Introduction

Malaria is one of the world's deadliest parasitic diseases affecting hundreds of millions of people worldwide. In 2020, the World Health Organization (WHO) reported an estimate of 241 million cases as compared to 227 million cases in 2019, with the number of deaths standing at 627,000 [1]. Due to the spread of insecticide-resistant mosquitoes as well as the development of *Plasmodium falciparum* resistant strains, control strategies are no longer as effective as they should. Thus, novel innovative strategies are required to combat this disease. A better understanding of the interactions between the mosquito and the malaria parasite may inform the development of new tools to control the disease. Transmission intervention by way of vaccines or transgenic mosquitoes may offer additional control strategies. Their development will, however, require the identification of valid molecular targets. The effective transmission of malaria requires specific compatibility between vector and parasite genotypes. Even within the susceptible *Anopheles gambiae* species (the most effective vector of the human malaria parasite), while some are resistant to infection, others, though unable to eliminate the infection, are capable of drastically reducing pathogen numbers [2, 3]. The mosquito molecules which interact with the malaria parasite to cause refractoriness in resistant strains have the potential to serve as targets for the development of novel transmission-blocking intervention strategies [4].

2. Malaria parasite life cycle stages

The female anopheles mosquito requires blood to nourish her eggs. As she sucks her victim's blood, she secretes saliva and, if infected, injects sporozoites into the subcutaneous layer of the skin of her victim. The sporozoite travel to the liver where it invades hepatocytes. Here, it replicates asexually (mitotically) producing thousands of merozoites over a period of 6–15 days without causing any symptoms. Thereafter, the merozoites are released from the hepatocytes in the form of vesicles (merozomes). The vesicles disintegrate, releasing merozoites into the bloodstream to begin the erythrocytic stage of the disease. Within RBCs, parasites develop through ring, trophozoite, and schizont stages producing approximately 16 daughter merozoite per schizont. The schizont then ruptures in near synchrony with each other (unlike other human malaria parasites, *P. falciparum* does not exhibit distinct paroxysms) releasing hemozoin (malaria pigment) into the bloodstream of the victim which is responsible for the intermittent fever that accompanies the disease. The released merozoites invade new cells to initiate a new erythrocytic cycle. This cycle can go on and on resulting in host death from anemia unless the individual gets treated by an effective antimalarial therapy or the parasite gets killed by the immune system of the host. With each replication, some merozoites, instead of producing daughter merozoites, develop into male (microgametocyte) and female (macrogametocyte) gametocytes. Once gametocytes are picked up by a mosquito, transmission is initiated. The increased pH, lowered temperature as well as the presence of xanthurenic acid in the mosquito stomach, trigger the formation of the male and female gametes which fuse to form zygotes thereby initiating the sexual cycle [5]. The fusion of the gametes results in the formation of actively moving ookinete that migrates through the mosquito midgut to form oocytes containing thousands of sporozoites. The oocysts eventually burst to release these sporozoites which travel to the salivary gland of the mosquito for onward transmission.

3. Vector-malaria parasite interactions

3.1 Mosquito immune defenses

While the male anopheles mosquito feeds exclusively on plant nectar, in addition to feeding on plant nectar, the female anopheles mosquito requires blood to nourish and develop her eggs. During blood feeding, she's exposed to malaria parasites (gametocytes), which must complete its complex developmental life cycle inside a mosquito host. The mosquito vector risks infection when there is physical injury to its cuticle or following cuticular degradation by the parasite. However, infection can be limited or reduced by mounting immune (innate and humoral) responses mediated by pattern recognition receptors and factors that trigger parasite killing via lysis, melanization (deposition of melanin on the surface of invading pathogens), and hemocyte-mediated phagocytosis. Further, many other mosquito molecules have also been reported to limit infection in the primary mosquito compartments which pathogens inhabit i.e. the midgut, the hemocoel, and the salivary glands.

3.1.1 Midgut

Upon ingestion of erythrocytes, cibarial armatures which mosquitoes use for RBC lysis are the first barriers faced by pathogens before they reach the midgut. Although the cibarial armature is effective in limiting infection by large metazoan parasites, it is not very effective at destroying protozoan parasites such as the malaria parasite [6, 7]. Transformation of ookinete to oocyst in the midgut is drastically reduced following lytic and melanization events. A number of molecules have been found to either facilitate or inhibit the parasite development within the midgut. They include the protein alanyl aminopeptidase N (AnAPN1); a surface recognition molecule which acts as a receptor for the malaria parasite in the mosquito midgut [8], a thioester-containing protein (TEP1), and leucine-rich repeat immune protein, (LRIM1) which recognizes the invading ookinetes at the basal lamina which surrounds the mosquito midgut and trigger immune responses [9, 10]. On the other hand, molecules such as C-type lectin 4 (CTL4), caspar, and cactus have been reported to negatively regulate the immune response of the mosquito, as silencing of these proteins resulted in decreased oocyst count [11, 12]. In *A. gambiae* midgut, (CTL4) and C-type lectin mannose-binding 2 (CTLMA2) negatively regulates the melanization of *Plasmodium berghei* ookinetes [13]. Further, the Serine protease inhibitor serpin 2 (SRPN2) also facilitates midgut invasion through inhibition of lysis and melanization [14, 15].

3.1.2 Hemocoel

The hemocoel is a nutrient-rich medium containing immune surveillance cells known as hemocytes. Hemocytes can be grouped into two sub-populations; granulocytes and oenocytoid. The granulocyte sub-population is capable of phagocytosing pathogens. Thioester-containing proteins (TEPs) are hemolymph proteins involved in the killing of *Plasmodium* ookinetes. The most studied (TEP) is the hemocyte-produced phagocytosis enhancer (TEP1). (TEP1) gets activated by complexing with the leucine-rich repeat containing proteins (LRIM1) and (APL1C) after which it opsonizes ookinetes for destruction by phagocytes [16]. Genetic variations in (TEP1) and (APL1C) are reported to affect mosquito immune competence against the parasite [3, 17].

Oenocytoids constitute the remaining population of the hemocytes. They are known to secrete enzymes of the melanization pathway (such as phenoloxidase and phenylalanine hydroxylase) used by mosquito to kill pathogens. Although the mechanism of pathogen killing by melanization remains unclear, it has been suggested that killing could either be the result of oxidative stress generated by unstable intermediates during melanogenesis or the result of starvation since melanization isolates the pathogen from the nutrient-rich hemocoel [18, 19]. In a literature search, Sreenivasamurthy et al. [20] identified a total of 22 molecules which play a role in melanization of ookinetes within the mosquito midgut.

3.1.3 Salivary gland

Sporozoites that successfully break through the mosquito immune defense system in the midgut lamina migrate to the salivary gland via the hemolymph. This they must do for transmission to occur. About 80–90% of sporozoites are reportedly lost during migration through the hemolymph. The mechanism by which this occurs is however not fully understood [21]. The invasion of the mosquito's salivary gland has been reported to be triggered by effective and specific associations of sporozoite surface antigens such as thrombospondin-related anonymous protein (TRAP), with receptors such as saglin present on the salivary glands of the mosquito [14]. Using knockdown assays, Cui et al. [22] showed that four genes {AGAP006268 (peritrophin), AGAP002848 (Niemann-Pick Type C-2) (NPC-2), AGAP006972 (keratin-associated protein 16–1), and AGAP002851 (NPC-2)} play a crucial role in protecting the mosquito from parasite invasion whereas three other genes {AGAP008138 (uncharacterized), FREP1 (*fibrinogen-related protein 1*), and HPX15 (Heme peroxidase)} facilitated *P. falciparum* transmission to mosquitoes.

3.2 Parasite strategies for evading mosquito immune defenses

3.2.1 Midgut invasion

The malaria parasite must evolve mechanisms to evade the barriers put in place by the mosquito for successful completion of its life cycle which is an absolute requirement for parasite survival and effective transmission. A *Plasmodium falciparum* surface protein Pfs47 protects the parasite from the immune system of the mosquito in the midgut [23]. The result of the study by Molina-Cruz et al. [23] suggest that *Plasmodium falciparum* Pfs47 haplotypes dictate vector compatibility. The researchers demonstrated that *A. gambiae* fails to mount a proper immune response against several *P.falciparum* lines including NF54 and GB4 partly because of Pfs47 which mediates immune evasion by disrupting JNK/caspase-mediated apoptosis in the mosquito midgut [24]. Whereas, evasion of the complement-like response in *Anopheles coluzzii,* (a dominant species of the *An. gambiae* complex in West Africa) is mediated by the protein Plasmodium Infection of the Mosquito Midgut Screen 43 (PIMMS43) which is present on the surface of ookinete and sporozoite [25].

3.2.2 Salivary gland invasion

Once sporozoites are released from the oocyst, they migrate to the salivary gland via the hemocoel [21]. Salivary gland invasion is a key step in the life cycle of the parasite since changes that take place on the sporozoites surface proteins in the salivary gland enable them to invade the salivary gland of the mosquito and also to be successfully transmitted. The proteins, *Plasmodium* responsive salivary 1 (PRS1), epithelial serine protease (ESP), peptide-O-xylosyltransferase 1 (OXT1), and a serine protease inhibitor (SRPN6) have been shown to play crucial roles in parasite invasion of both midgut and salivary glands. While (SRPN6) limits salivary gland invasion by *Plasmodium* sporozoites [26], knocking down PRS1, ESP, retinoid and fatty-acid binding glycoprotein (RFABG) and (OXT1) have been reported to decrease oocyst and sporozoite numbers [27–30]. Further, malaria parasites carrying mutations in conserved region II of the circumsporozoite protein (CSP) are unable to escape the oocyst [31]. Deletion of TRAP and LIMP (a highly conserved protein in *Plasmodium* parasites) severely impairs gliding motility which is important for salivary gland invasion [32, 33]. Whereas, although deletion of rhoptry neck protein 2 (RON) does not affect parasite's gliding motility, salivary gland invasion is abolished [34].

4. Past, present, and future of transmission-blocking intervention strategies

Over the last two decades, the use of long-lasting insecticide-treated nets (LLINs) and indoor residual spraying (IRS) have been major contributors to gains in malaria eradication efforts [35–38]. Even with the routine use of these key malaria interventions as well as effective malaria treatment with artemisinin-based combination therapies (ACTs), malaria-related mortality and morbidity remain unacceptably high with about half a million people losing their lives to the disease annually. Further, the development of resistance by the vector to insecticides as well as generation of parasite resistance to antimalarial drugs highlights the need for sustaining current gains and developing additional innovative control measures. Novel transmission-blocking intervention by vaccines or genetically engineered mosquitoes may provide a promising approach.

In 2013, the Malaria Vaccine Initiative (MVI) was rolled out. One of its key goals is the development of vaccines capable of interrupting transmission. Transmission- blocking vaccines (TBVs) are the result of efforts put in place by researchers to understand the interaction between the parasite and mosquito. Some TBVs are currently undergoing trials for efficacy and other key measures of success (**Table 1**). Alanyl aminopeptidase

Vaccine candidate	Target	Stage of development/ClinicalTrials.gov identifier number	Reference
AnANP1	Midgut	Preclinical	[8]
FREP1	Midgut	Preclinical	[39]
Carboxypeptidase	Midgut	Preclinical	[40]
Calreticulin	Midgut	Preclinical	[41]
Croquemort SCRBQ2	Midgut	Preclinical	[42]
Myosin	Midgut	Preclinical	[43]
PfHAP2	Zygote	Preclinical	[44]
Pfs25	Midgut	Phase I (NCT01867463; NCT00295581)	[45]
Pfs28	Ookinete	Preclinical	[46, 47]
Pfs47	Midgut	Preclinical	[48]
Pfs48/45	Gametocytes & gametes	Preclinical	[49, 50]
Pfs230	Gametocytes & gametes	Phase I (NCT02942277)	[51]
Pfs2400	Gametocytes & gametes	Preclinical	[52]
Pvs25	Gametocytes, gametes, zygote & ookinete	Phase I (NCT00295581)	[53]
Pvs48/45	Gametocytes & gametes	Preclinical	[48]

Table 1.
Transmission-blocking vaccine candidates.

N (AnAPN1) is the leading midgut TBV immunogen [8]. (AnAPN1) is highly immunogenic and conserved between different anophelines. This makes it very attractive for vaccine development as vaccines prepared with this antigen should be active against all human malaria vectors hence saving the resources needed to develop specific targets for different Anopheles/Plasmodium species combinations [54]. Other midgut candidate molecules include carboxypeptidase [40], calreticulin [41], Croquemort SCRBQ2 [42] and myosin [43]. Candidate parasite molecules include those found on the surface of gametocytes and gametes (Pfs 2400, Pfs230, Pfs48/45) as well as zygotes and ookinetes (Pfs25, Pfs28) [55]. Vaccine against Pvs25 and Pfs25, which blocks *P. vivax* and *P.falciparum* respectively, are currently the leading molecule for a TBV [45, 56].

More recently, scientists have shifted attention from regular vector-control strategies (LLINs and IRS) to engaging advanced molecular tools such as CRISPR-cas9 to re-program the vector genome so as to make them refractory to the parasite (**Figure 1**). Gene drives skew the pattern of inheritance of genes creating mosquitoes that will either reduce mosquito populations or make mosquitoes less likely to spread the malaria parasite. Using such gene-drive systems in the laboratory, researchers have been able to transfer antimalarial effector genes to mosquitoes [57, 58]. Intriguing using similar allelic drive system in a *Drosophila melanogasta* model, Kaduskar et al. [59] were successful at reversing the most widely spread insecticide resistance mutation in anophelines (L1014F) (a mutation in the

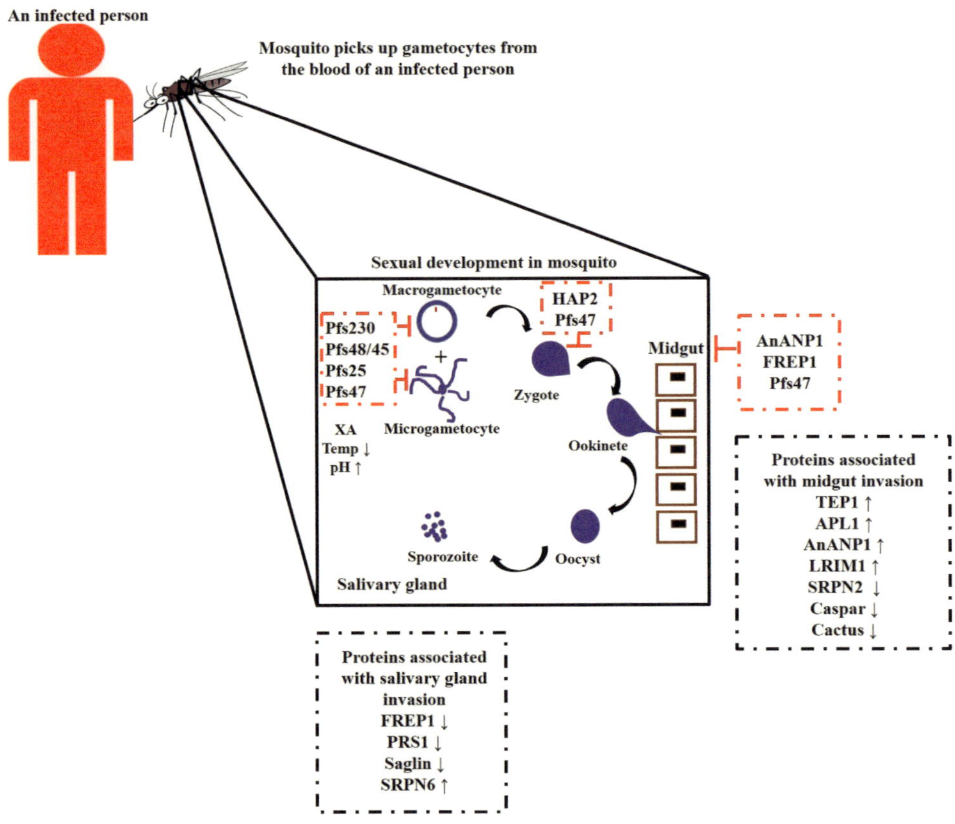

Figure 1.
Breaking the cycle of malaria transmission.

voltage-gated sodium channels of mosquitoes which make them resistant to pyrethroids) to susceptible wild-type genes (1014 L). The report of these researchers opens new vistas for vector control as it demonstrated that not only can insecticide resistance (IR) be reversed but that there is a relative negative fitness cost for the (L1014F) insecticide-conferring mutation as compared to the wild-type allelic variant. Thus, offering the opportunity to synergize the use of a gene drive that confers a bias inheritance of the preferred wild-type allelic variant with regular vector control methods. They went on to suggest that the identification of target site variants that would make the vector hypersensitive to insecticides will hold an even better promise. Further, they suggested the possibility of combining such gene drives for reversing insecticide resistance with other systems promoting refractoriness in mosquitoes [59].

Mosquito picks up gametocytes from the blood of an infected person. The sexual cycle is initiated due to the presence of xanthurenic acid (XA) as well as

Strategy	Pros	Cons
TBVs	It can reduce child mortality in areas of malaria endemicity	Extremely long duration for vaccine preparation
	It can slow down the spread of mutant parasites thereby prolonging the efficacy of antimalarial drugs.	Lack of industrial partners which has hampered the progress of development [61].
	It can be combined with other multi-stage vaccines and contribute immensely to actualizing the eradication goal	Due to their mechanism of action, acceptability may be an issue. Although a recent survey in Bo, Sierra Leone reported that 96% of adults in that region will be willing to take TBVs [62], it remains to be seen if this will be the case when TBVs are eventually ready for use.
Gene drive	It can reduce or eliminate malaria by interrupting the transmission chain.	Safety concerns. The impact of gene drives on ecological habitat and the world at large is unknown. There is a possibility of off-targets that could cause serious harm to other organisms and even humans.
	Reduced use of insecticides thereby saving endangered species such as butterflies.	Ethical concerns of elimination of an entire population [63].
	Mosquitoes can be controlled in a more effective manner other than the conventional use of insecticides to which mosquitoes often become resistant.	Genetically modified mosquitoes could spread across borders creating more legal issues [64].
	It may reduce the economic and human cost of managing malaria.	Affordability. Many malaria endemic countries may be unable to afford it.
	It may be more long-lasing than conventional vector control methods since gene-drives can continue to spread through multiple generations without the need to re-introduce them	Cost-effectiveness. Although gene drive was seen to be the most cost-effective tool for the elimination of malaria in the Democratic republic of Congo using a mathematical model [65], some school of thoughts believe investing more money on health systems would be more beneficial and less risky than developing a gene drive technology for malaria.

Table 2.
Pros and cons of transmission-blocking intervention strategies.

the low temperature and high pH of the mosquito stomach. The parasite then progresses through different stages and eventually forms sporozoites which are infective to humans. As depicted in the image above, parasite development can be interrupted at any stage of its sexual cycle either by using TBVs (candidate molecules are in boxes bordered by red broken lines) or genetic-based tools could be used to alter the expression levels of proteins crucial for mosquito infection (see boxes with broken black lines). Such tools capable of breaking the transmission chain could be incorporated as part of an integrated antimalarial strategy to eradicate the disease.

Although successful transgenic manipulation of mosquitoes has been achieved in the laboratories, their relative negative fitness in relation to wild-type populations is an important limitation for their relevance for large-scale use. For example, in a mark-release-recapture study in Burkina Faso recently, hemizygous genetically-modified (GM) sterile and non-transgenic sibling males of *Anopheles coluzzii* were released into a field in a controlled study. Recovered carriers of the GM trait had lower survival and were less mobile than their wild-type siblings [60]. Another shortcoming to the use of genetic-based vector control tools is that employing methods such as transposon-mediated transformation which modify only one allele of the desired gene, would spread the desired trait only to half of the offspring, and would eventually get eliminated in the wild population. This can however be overcome by employing gene drive systems such as CRISPR nuclease Cas9 which are capable of copying themselves to both gene alleles that will be inherited by all offspring, and thus spread more efficiently through a wild population [59]. Despite their great promise, scientists are wary of gene drive because they could cause irreparable damage since they permanently alter an entire population (**Table 2**). Further, issues bothering on their safety, governance, affordability, and cost-effectiveness need to be addressed (**Table 2**).

5. Conclusion and future perspectives

The prolonged and repeated use of insecticides of a limited chemical class is a major contributor for the acquisition of resistance mutations in insecticide-target genes in insects. On the part of the malaria parasite, it also constantly evades antimalarial drugs by generating resistance mutations. Hence, the need to identify additional control measures that TBVs and genetics-based vector control tools may offer. Broad-spectrum malaria transmission-blocking vaccine antigens such as FREP1 [66] and (AnAPN1) offer attractive targets for the development of TBVs. However, due to the lack of industrial partners, the development and production of TBVs have stalled [61].

To generate transgenic mosquitoes, mosquito proteins that cause complete refractoriness in the vector upon silencing may be the target of choice. An ideal target molecule would be one that does not impose a relative negative fitness cost on the insect and one which could be used in combination with others targeting different stages of the parasite life cycle [67]. However, a major challenge with genome editing techniques is devising means to safely drive effector genes into mosquito populations in the field without causing harm to other organisms, including humans. Once safety concerns are addressed, such tools could be integrated with traditional vector control strategies, in addition to effective malaria treatment and good sanitation practices for the actualization of the eradication goal.

Author's contribution

NE conceptualized the write-up. VO contributed to writing. NE contributed to writing, review and editing. Both authors have read and agreed to the final version of the manuscript.

Conflict of interests

Authors declare no conflict of interests exists.

Author details

Nekpen Erhunse* and Victor Okomayin
Faculty of Life Sciences, Department of Biochemistry, University of Benin, Benin City, Nigeria

*Address all correspondence to: nekpen.erhunse@uniben.edu

References

[1] World Health Organization. World Malaria Report: 20 years of global progress and challenges. 2020

[2] Niaré O, Markianos K, Volz J, et al. Genetic loci affecting resistance to human malaria parasites in a West African mosquito vector population. Science. 2002;**298**(5591):213-216

[3] Riehle MM, Markianos K, Niaré O, et al. Natural malaria infection in Anopheles gambiae is regulated by a single genomic control region. Science. 2006;**312**(5773):577-579

[4] Simões ML, Caragata EP, Dimopoulos G. Diverse host and restriction factors regulate mosquito–pathogen interactions. Trends in Parasitology. 2018;**34**(7):603-616. DOI: doi.org/10.1016/j.pt.2018.04.011

[5] Billker O, Lindo V, Panico M, Etienne AE, Dell A, Rogers M, et al. Identification of xanthurenic acid as the putative inducer of malaria development in the mosquito. Nature. 1998;**392**:289-292

[6] Abraham EG, Jacobs-Lorena M. Mosquito midgut barriers to malaria parasite development. Insect Biochemistry and Molecular Biology. 2004;**34**(7):667-671

[7] McGreevy PB, Bryan JH, Oothuman P, et al. The lethal effects of the cibarial and pharyngeal armatures of mosquitoes on microfilariae. Transactions of the Royal Society of Tropical Medicine and Hygiene. 1978;**72**(4):361-368

[8] Atkinson SC, Armistead JS, Mathias DK, Sandeu MM, Tao D, Borhani-Dizaji N, et al. Structural analysis of Anopheles midgut aminopeptidase N reveals a novel malaria transmission-blocking vaccine B-cell epitope. Nature Structural & Molecular Biology. 2015;**22**(7):532-539. DOI: 10.1038/nsmb.3048

[9] Fraiture M, Baxter RHG, Steinert S, et al. Two mosquito LRR proteins function as complement control factors in the TEP1-mediated killing of Plasmodium. Cell Host & Microbe. 2009;**5**(3):273-284

[10] Povelones M, Waterhouse RM, Kafatos FC, et al. Leucine-rich repeat protein complex activates mosquito complement in defense against Plasmodium parasites. Science. 2009;**324**(5924):258-261

[11] Garver LS, Dong Y, Dimopoulos G. Caspar controls resistance to Plasmodium falciparum in diverse anopheline species. PLOS Pathogens 2009;**5**(3):e1000335

[12] Volz J, Müller HM, Zdanowicz A, et al. A genetic module regulates the melanization response of Anopheles to Plasmodium. Cellular Microbiology. 2006;**8**(9):1392-1405

[13] Osta MA, Christophides GK, Kafatos FC. Effects of mosquito genes on *Plasmodium* development. Science. 2004;**303**(5666):2030-2032

[14] Abraham EG et al. An immune-responsive serpin, SRPN6, mediates mosquito defense against malaria parasites. Proceedings of the National Academy Science USA. 2005;**102**:16327-16332

[15] Michel K, Budd A, Pinto S, Toby J, Gibson TJ, Kafatos FC. *Anopheles gambiae* SRPN2 facilitates midgut invasion by

the malaria parasite *Plasmodium berghei*. EMBO. 2005;**6**:891-889

[16] Levashina EA, Moita LF, Blandin SA, et al. Conserved role of a complement-like protein in phagocytosis revealed by dsRNA knockout in cultured cells of the mosquito *Anopheles gambiae*. Cell. 2001;**104**(5):709-718

[17] Blandin SA, Wang-Sattler R, Lamacchia M, et al. Dissecting the genetic basis of resistance to malaria parasites in *Anopheles gambiae*. Science. 2009;**326**(5949):147-150

[18] Chen CC, Chen CS. Brugia pahangi: Effects of melanization on the uptake of nutrients by microfilariae in vitro. Experimental Parasitology 1995;**81**(1):72-78

[19] Nappi AJ, Christensen BM. Melanogenesis and associated cytotoxic reactions: applications to insect innate immunity. Insect Biochemistry and Molecular Biology. 2005;**35**(5):443-459

[20] Sreenivasamurthy SK, Dey G, Ramu M, Kumar M, Gupta MK, Mohanty AK, et al. A compendium of molecules involved in vector-pathogen interactions pertaining to malaria. Malaria Journal. 2013;**12**:216

[21] Hillyer JF, Barreau C, Vernick KD. Efficiency of salivary gland invasion by malaria sporozoites is controlled by rapid sporozoite destruction in the mosquito haemocoel. International Journal for Parasitology. 2007;**37**(6):673-681

[22] Cui Y, Niu G, Li VV, Wang X, Li J. Analysis of blood-induced *Anopheles gambiae* midgut proteins and sexual stage *Plasmodium falciparum* interaction reveals mosquito genes important for malaria transmission. Scientific Reports. 2020;**10**:14316

[23] Molina-Cruza A, Canepaa GE, Silva TLA, Williams AE, Nagyal S, Yenkoidiok-Douti L, et al. *Plasmodium falciparum* evades immunity of anopheline mosquitoes by interacting with a Pfs47 midgut receptor. PNAS. 2020;**117**(5):2597-2605

[24] Ramphul UN, Garver LS, Molina-Cruz A, Canepa GE, Barillas-Mury C. *Plasmodium falciparum* evades mosquito immunity by disrupting JNK-mediated apoptosis of invaded midgut cells. Proceedings of the National Academy of Science USA. 2015;**112**:1273-1280

[25] Ukegbua CV, Giorgallia M, Tapanellia S, Ronaa LDP, Jayea A, Wyera C, et al. PIMMS43 is required for malaria parasite immune evasion and sporogonic development in the mosquito vector. PNAS. 2020;**117**(13):7363-7373

[26] Pinto SB, Kafatos FC, Michel K. The parasite invasion marker SRPN6 reduces sporozoite numbers in salivary glands of *Anopheles gambiae*. Cellular Microbiology. 2008;**10**:891-898

[27] Armistead JS, Wilson IB, van Kuppevelt TH, Dinglasan RR. A role for heparan sulfate proteoglycans in *Plasmodium falciparum* sporozoite invasion of anopheline mosquito salivary glands. The Biochemical Journal. 2011;**438**:475-483

[28] Chertemps T, Mitri C, Perrot S, Sautereau J, Jacques JC, Thiery I, et al. *Anopheles gambiae* PRS1 modulates *Plasmodium* development at both midgut and salivary gland steps. PLoS One. 2010;**5**:e11538

[29] Ramakrishnan C, Rademacher A, Soichot J, Costa G, Waters AP, Janse CJ, et al. Salivary gland-specific *P. berghei* reporter lines enable rapid evaluation of tissue-specific sporozoite loads in mosquitoes. PLoS One. 2012;7:e36376

[30] Rodrigues J, Oliveira GA, Kotsyfakis M, Dixit R, Molina-Cruz A, Jochim R, et al. An epithelial serine protease, AgESP, is required for *Plasmodium* invasion in the mosquito *Anopheles gambiae*. PLoS One. 2012;7:e35210

[31] Wang Q, Fujioka H, Nussenzweig V. Exit of plasmodium sporozoites from oocysts is an active process that involves the circumsporozoite protein. PLoS Pathogens. 2005;**1**:e9. DOI: 10.1371/journal.ppat.0010009

[32] Santos JM, Egarter S, Zuzarte-Luís V, Kumar H, Moreau CA, Kehrer J, et al. Malaria parasite LIMP protein regulates sporozoite gliding motility and infectivity in mosquito and mammalian hosts. eLife. 2017;**6**:e24109. DOI: 10.7554/eLife.24109

[33] Sultan AA, Thathy V, Frevert U, Robson KJH, Crisanti A, Nussenzweig V, et al. TRAP is necessary for gliding motility and infectivity of Plasmodium sporozoites. Cell. 1997;**90**:511-522. DOI: 10.1016/S0092-8674(00)80511-5

[34] Ishino T, Murata E, Tokunaga N, Baba M, Tachibana M, Thongkukiatkul A, et al. Rhoptry neck protein 2 expressed in *Plasmodium* sporozoites plays a crucial role during invasion of mosquito salivary glands. Cellular Microbiology. 2019;**21**:e12964. DOI: 10.1111/cmi.12964

[35] Hemingway J, Shretta R, Wells TNC, Bell D, Djimdé AA, Achee N, et al. Tools and strategies for malaria control and elimination: What do we need to achieve a grand convergence in malaria? PLoS Biology. 2016;**14**:e1002380

[36] Mnzava AP, Knox B, Temu EA, Trett A, Fornadel C, Hemingway J, et al. Implementation of the global plan for insecticide resistance management in malaria vectors: Progress, challenges and the way forward. Malaria Journal. 2015;**14**:173

[37] Ranson H, Lissenden N. Insecticide resistance in African Anopheles mosquitoes: A worsening situation that needs urgent action to maintain malaria control. Trends in Parasitology. 2016;**32**:187-196

[38] World Health Organization; Global Malaria Programme. Global Plan for Insecticide Resistance Management in Malaria Vectors'. Geneva PP - Geneva: World Health Organization; 2012. Available from: https://apps.who.int/iris/handle/10665/44846.

[39] Niu G, Franc A, Zhang G, Roobsoong W, Nguitragool W, Wang X, et al. The fibrinogen-like domain of FREP1 protein is a broad-spectrum malaria transmission-blocking vaccine antigen. The Journal of Biological Chemistry. 2017;**292**(28):11960-11969. DOI: 10.1074/jbc.M116.773564

[40] Raz A, Djadid ND, Zakeri S. Molecular characterization of the carboxypeptidase B1 of *Anopheles stephensi* and its evaluation as a target for transmission-blocking vaccines. Infection and Immunity. 2013;**81**(6):2206-2216

[41] Dizaji NB, Basseri HR, Naddaf SR, Heidari M. Molecular characterization of calreticulin from *Anopheles stephensi* midgut cells and functional assay of the recombinant calreticulin with *Plasmodium berghei* ookinetes. Gene. 2014;**550**(2):245-252

[42] González-Lázaro M, Dinglasan RR, Hernández-Hernández F, Rodríguez MH, Laclaustra M, Jacobs-Lorena M, et al. Anopheles gambiae Croquemort SCRBQ2, expression profile in the mosquito and its potential interaction with the malaria parasite *Plasmodium*

berghei. Insect Biochemistry and Molecular Biology. 2009;**39**(5-6):395-402. DOI: 10.1016/j.ibmb.2009.03.008

[43] Lecona-Valera AN, Tao D, Rodriguez MH, Lopez T, Dinglasan RR, Rodriguez MC. An antibody against an *Anopheles albimanus* midgut myosin reduces *Plasmodium berghei* oocyst development. Parasites & Vectors. 2016;**9**(274):1-11

[44] Miura K, Takashima E, Deng B, Tullo G, Diouf A, Moretz SE, et al. Functional comparison of Plasmodium falciparum transmission-blocking vaccine candidates by the standard membrane-feeding assay. Infection and Immunity. 2013;**81**(12):4377-4382. DOI: 10.1128/IAI.01056-13

[45] Wu Y, Ellis RD, Shaffer D, Fontes E, Malkin EM, Mahanty S, et al. Phase 1 trial of malaria transmission blocking vaccine candidates Pfs25 and Pvs25 formulated with montanide ISA 51. PLoS One. 2008;**3**(7):e2636

[46] Duffy PE, Kaslow DC. A novel malaria protein, Pfs28, and Pfs25 are genetically linked and synergistic as falciparum malaria transmission-blocking vaccines. Infection and Immunity. 1997;**65**(3):1109-1113

[47] Qian F, Aebig JA, Reiter K, Barnafo E, Zhang Y, Shimp RL Jr, et al. Enhanced antibody responses to *Plasmodium falciparum* Pfs28 induced in mice by conjugation to ExoProtein A of *Pseudomonas aeruginosa* with an improved procedure. Microbes and Infection. 2009;**11**(3):408-412. DOI: 10.1016/j.micinf.2008.12.009

[48] Tachibana M, Suwanabun N, Kaneko O, Iriko H, Otsuki H, Sattabongkot J, et al. *Plasmodium vivax* gametocyte proteins, Pvs48/45 and Pvs47, induce transmission-reducing antibodies by DNA immunization. Vaccine. 2015;**33**(16):1901-1908. DOI: 10.1016/j.vaccine.2015.03.008

[49] Merino KM, Bansal GP, Kumar N. Reduced immunogenicity of *Plasmodium falciparum* gamete surface antigen (Pfs48/45) in mice after disruption of disulphide bonds: Evaluating effect of interferon-γ-inducible lysosomal thiol reductase. Immunology. 2016;**148**(4):433-447. DOI: 10.1111/imm.12621

[50] Pritsch M, Ben-Khaled N, Chaloupka M, Kobold S, Berens-Riha N, Peter A, et al. Comparison of Intranasal Outer Membrane Vesicles with Cholera Toxin and Injected MF59C.1 as Adjuvants for Malaria Transmission Blocking Antigens AnAPN1 and Pfs48/45. Journal of Immunology Research. 2016;**2016**:3576028. DOI: 10.1155/2016/3576028

[51] Farrance CE, Chichester JA, Musiychuk K, Shamloul M, Rhee A, Manceva SD, et al. Antibodies to plant-produced Plasmodium falciparum sexual stage protein Pfs25 exhibit transmission blocking activity. Human Vaccines. 2011;**7**(Suppl):191-198. DOI: 10.4161/hv.7.0.14588

[52] Feng Z, Hoffmann RN, Nussenzweig RS, Tsuji M, Fujioka H, Aikawa M, et al. Pfs2400 can mediate antibody-dependent malaria transmission inhibition and may be the *Plasmodium falciparum* 11.1 gene product. The Journal of Experimental Medicine. 1993;**177**(2):273-281. DOI: 10.1084/jem.177.2.273

[53] Malkin EM, Durbin AP, Diemert DJ, Sattabongkot J, Wu Y, Miura K, et al. Phase 1 vaccine trial of Pvs25H: A transmission blocking vaccine for *Plasmodium vivax* malaria. Vaccine. 2005;**23**(24):3131-3138. DOI: 10.1016/j.vaccine.2004.12.019

[54] Armistead JS, Morlais I, Mathias DK, Jardim JG, Jo J, Fridman A, et al. Antibodies to a single, conserved epitope in Anopheles APN1 inhibit universal transmission of *Plasmodium falciparum* and *Plasmodium vivax* malaria. Infection and Immunity. 2014;**82**(2):818-829

[55] Acquah FK, Adjah J, Williamson KC, Amoah LE. Transmission-blocking vaccines: Old friends and new prospects. Infection and Immunity. 2019;**87**(6):e00775-e00718

[56] Reyes-Sandoval A, Bachmann MF. *Plasmodium vivax* malaria vaccines. Human Vaccines & Immunotherapeutics. 2013;**9**(12):2558-2565

[57] Adolfi A, Gantz VM, Jasinskiene N, Lee H, Hwang K, Terradas G, et al. Efficient population modification gene-drive rescue system in the malaria mosquito *Anopheles stephensi*. Nature Communications. 2020;**11**:5553

[58] Carballar-Lejarazú R, Ogaugwu C, Tushar T, Kelsey A, Pham TB, Murphy J, et al. Next-generation gene drive for population modification of the malaria vector mosquito, *Anopheles gambiae*. Proceedings of the National Academy of Science USA. 2020;**117**(37):22805-22814. DOI: 10.1073/pnas.2010214117

[59] Kaduskar B, Kushwah RBS, Auradkar A, Guichard A, Li M, Bennett JB, et al. Reversing insecticide resistance with allelic-drive in Drosophila melanogaster. Nature Communications. 2022;**13**(291):1-8. DOI: doi.org/10.1038/s41467-021-27654-1

[60] Yao FA, Millogo A, Epopa PS, North A, Noulin F, Dao K, et al. Mark-release-recapture experiment in Burkina Faso demonstrates reduced fitness and dispersal of genetically-modified sterile malaria mosquitoes. Nature Communications. 2022;**13**(796):1-11. DOI: doi.org/10.1038/s41467-022-28419-0

[61] Carter R, Mendis KN, Miller LH, Molineaux L, Saul A. Malaria transmission-blocking vaccines-how can their development be supported. Nature Medicine. 2000;**6**:241-244

[62] McCoy KD, Weldon CT, Ansumana R, Lamin JM, Stenger DA, Ryan SJ, et al. Are malaria transmission-blocking vaccines acceptable to high burden communities? Results from a mixed methods study in Bo, Sierra Leone. Malaria Journal. 2021;**20**:183

[63] Wise IJ, Borry P. An ethical overview of the CRISPR-based elimination of *Anopheles gambiae* to combat malaria. Journal of Bioethical Inquiry. 2021. pp. 1-10. DOI: 10.1007/s11673-022-10172-0

[64] Brossard D, Belluck P, Gould F, Wirz CD. Promises and perils of gene drives: Navigating the communication of complex, post-normal science. PNAS. 2018;**116**(16):7692-7697

[65] Metchanun N, Borgemeister C, Amzati G, von Braun J, Nikolov M, Selvaraj P, et al. Modeling impact and cost-effectiveness of driving-Y gene drives for malaria elimination in the Democratic Republic of the Congo. Evolutionary Applications. 2021;**15**:132-148. DOI: 10.1111/eva.13331

[66] Zhang G, Niu G, Franca CM, Dong Y, Wang X, Noah S, et al. Anopheles midgut FREP1 mediates *Plasmodium* invasion. The Journal of Biological Chemistry. 2015;**290**:16490-16501

[67] Gonçalves D, Hunziker P. Transmission-blocking strategies: The roadmap from laboratory bench to the community. Malaria Journal. 2016;**15**:95

Chapter 3

Systems Biology Approaches towards Immunity against *Plasmodium*

Himangshu Patgiri, Ankita Khataniar, Pitimoni Boro, Sushmita Baishnab and Sanchaita Rajkhowa

Abstract

Malaria is one of the most devastating infectious diseases known to humans. It is caused by unicellular protozoan parasites belonging to the genus *Plasmodium*. Till date, over 200 species of *Plasmodium* have been formally described, and each species infects a certain range of hosts. However, the human infection is limited to only five of the species, of which *P. falciparum* is the most responsible. Due to the emergence of parasite resistance to frontline chemotherapies and mosquito resistance to current insecticides which threaten the control programmes, new antimalarial therapeutics or approaches capable of predicting useful models of how different cells of the innate immune system function, is the need of the hour. Systems Immunology is a relatively recent discipline under Systems Biology to understand the structure and function of the immune system and how the components of the immune system work together as a whole. Thus, this chapter aims to give insight into the approaches of Systems Biology for investigating the immune factors that are formed during *Plasmodium falciparum* infection in the human body. Here, the numerous experimental and computational works with the ongoing methodologies using Systems Biology approaches along with the interactions of host and pathogen will be discussed.

Keywords: omics, *Plasmodium falciparum*, systems immunology, Systems Biology

1. Introduction

Plasmodium falciparum is a protozoan parasite that causes malaria in humans and is transmitted through an insect vector, the female *Anopheles* mosquito. The species' malaria (also called malignant malaria or *falciparum* malaria) is the most deadly type of malaria with the highest incidence of complication and mortality rates. Malaria is a world-wide infectious illness that continues to be a leading source of morbidity and mortality in developing countries. Malaria is an ancient disease, with references to what was nearly actually a protozoan ailment believed to be malaria, appearing in a Chinese document from around 2700 BC, clay tablets from Mesopotamia from 2000 BC, Egyptian papyri from 1570 BC, and Hindu scriptures from the sixth century BC. For over 2500 years the thought that malaria fevers were caused by miasmas rising from marshes for many years and it is usually believed that held that the word malaria comes from the Italian *mal'aria,* which spoiled air; however, this is controversial. The origins of the *Plasmodium* parasites infecting humans have long been a source of fascination. Ancient scriptures from China, India, the Middle East, Africa, and the European continent, contain descriptions of malaria-like illnesses indicating that humans have been fighting *Plasmodium* infections throughout our recorded history [1, 2]. Scientific studies were only possible after the discovery of the parasites themselves by Charles Louis Alphonse Laveran in 1880 and the incrimination of mosquitoes as vectors, first for avian malaria by Ronald Ross in 1897 and then for human malaria by Amico Bignami, Angelo Celli, Camillo Golgi, Ettore Marchiafava, Giovanni Battista Grassi and Giuseppe Bastianelli between 1898 and 1900.

Malaria is a world-wide infectious disease that continues to be a major cause of morbidity and mortality in developing countries. Malaria is found in more than 90 countries and affects over 40% of the world's population. Out of four species of malaria, *Plasmodium falciparum* is the lethal one. *P. falciparum* is responsible for more than 90% of the global malaria death and hence continues to be a major public health concern on a global scale. According to WHO, World Malaria report 2020, there are 241 million cases of malaria world-wide, resulting in 627,000 fatalities world-wide. In non-malarial nations such as North America and Europe, there are a considerable number of instances of imported malaria and local transmission following importation [2].

Variants in the human genome linked with resistance to *Plasmodium* infection and malaria-related illness are thought to be thousands of years old [3]. One long-held theory proposed that humans and chimpanzees both acquired *P. falciparum*-like infections from their common ancestor and that these parasites co-evolved for millions of years with their respective host species. *P. vivax,* on the other hand, is thought to have emerged hundreds of thousands of years ago, when the cross-species transmission of a parasite from a macaque occurred in South-eastern Asia [4, 5]. However, both of these notions have recently been debunked following the characterisation of a large number of new *Plasmodium* parasites from African apes. *P. falciparum* infection is now known to be relatively new for humans, having emerged after the acquisition of a parasite from a gorilla, most likely within the last 10,000 years [6, 7]. Characterisation of the numerous ape *Laverania* spp. discovered a parasite lineage in western gorillas with parasites that were nearly identical to *P. falciparum* [5, 7]. This was first misinterpreted that gorillas can be infected by human parasites [5]. However, after analysing the mtDNA sequences from significant numbers of additional wild-living gorillas, it was discovered that all extant *P. falciparum* strains from humans fall within the radius of these gorilla parasites [7]. *P. praefalciparum* is the name given to this gorilla parasite lineage to indicate its role in the origin of *P. falciparum*.

When compared to viruses and bacteria, eukaryotic protozoans present a larger genome and have a complex biology, which hinders the development of vaccines. Even though malaria is a curable disease, there are currently no established vaccines. Quinine and artemisinin, both extracted from the bark of the Peruvian Cinchona Succirubra tree and the Chinese herb *Artemisia annua*, are now the most potent antimalarials available. Artemisinin-based Combination Therapies (ACTs), which have just recently been accepted as a last option in the fight against malaria, are already being tested by ACT-resistant strains in Southeast Asia. With parasite resistance to all current antimalarial medications spreading, successful control and eradication will need the development of new tools and cost-effective antimalarial tactics [8]. The complex biology of *Plasmodium* poses a hindrance in the detailed understanding of

DOI: http://dx.doi.org/10.5772/intechopen.104614

the mechanisms that control malarial infection, thus giving rise to technical challenges in the eradication of malaria. New approaches to elucidate key host–parasite interactions, and predict how the parasites will respond in various biological settings, could dramatically enhance the efficacy of intervention strategies [9]. Advances in the field of Systems Biology are well poised to meet these challenges.

2. Immune response to *Plasmodium falciparum* using systems biology approaches

The immune response involves components from both innate and adaptive immune system molecules. During *Plasmodium* infection, an innate immune response is generated as the first line of defence, followed by an adaptive immunological response that comprises T-cells, B-cells, and antibodies. The sporozoites remain active for several hours after being inoculated into the host's skin. Systems Immunology is a part of Systems Biology that aims to better understand the structure and function of the immune system, and how its various components interact [10]. In contrast to a reductionist approach focused on limited subsets of a class of biomolecules, Systems Biology approaches encompass the study of biological systems through a near-comprehensive investigation of specific classes of biomolecules. Because of the complexity of the system under consideration and the vast information created by experimental approaches connected with Systems Biology, computational modelling and analysis are also essential parts of Systems Biology [11]. **Figure 1** illustrates the life cycle of *P. falciparum* alongwith the immune responses to *P. falciparum* and how Systems Biology can be incorporated into it.

Beyond the aforementioned computational models and analysis, Systems Biology ideally involves mechanistic mathematical models of a system, allowing biological understanding and the ability to forecast system behaviour [12]. In the realm of malaria research, mathematical modelling is most typically employed in population modelling to track and predict malaria transmission via host- parasite populations.

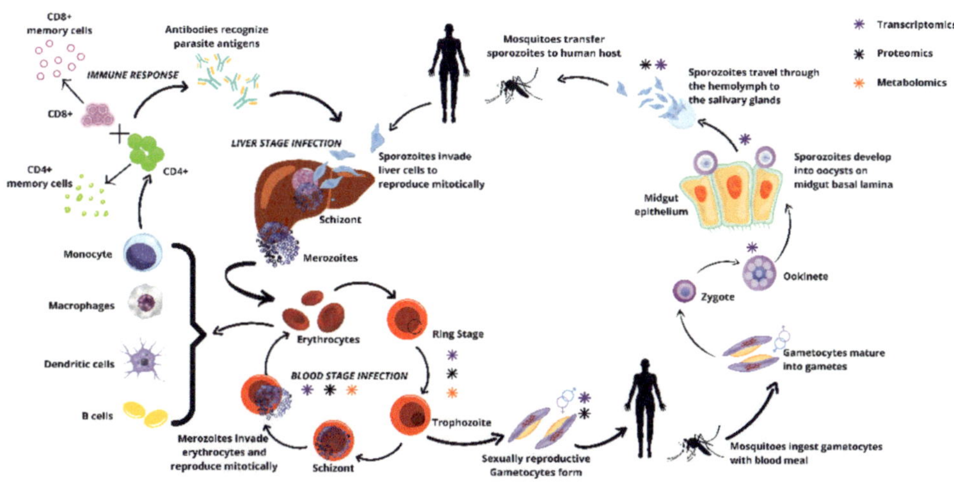

Figure 1.
Life cycle of P. falciparum *and the different stages of immune responses to it. The different systems biology approaches, i.e. Transcriptomics, proteomics and metabolomics, to study the different stages of the life cycle has been shown using asterics.*

Using modelling approaches and mathematical modelling at system-scale data, specific phases of the immune response along with the distribution and timing of parasite sequestration in different tissues of the body have been recently studied in malaria host-pathogen interactions effectively and also in other diseases, such as cancer. As a matter of fact, prevalence of system-scale data has been generated in-vitro rather than in-vivo in the literature to date [13–16].

The advanced analytical approaches are required to generate the large, systems-scale experimental datasets that are distinctive of Systems Biology, which is frequently referred to as "Omics" collectively and generically. Omics datasets, a biological system of transitions from one state to another, are the starting point for Systems Biology. They are systematic and complete identifications and quantifications of molecules. Several researchers have generated Omics data during the malaria life cycle transitions. Omics data include genomics, transcriptomics, proteomics, metabolomics, and translational repression/de-repression of transcripts as the parasite transitions throughout the malaria life cycle stages [17]. Transcriptomics implies the use of RNA-sequencing and microarrays for the investigation of gene expression at the systems level. Protein levels, proteomics, and metabolites levels for metabolomics are typically measured using mass spectrometry or nuclear magnetic resonance spectroscopy, respectively. Omics technologies are being increasingly employed to investigate how *Plasmodium* parasites impact their hosts and how the parasite affects the host environment [13]. The range of computational approaches used to analyse and understand such large datasets is crucial to turning them into biological knowledge. Computational methodologies such as network modelling, ontology analysis, and phenotypic association are utilised to analyse and interpret these data in addition to classic statistical analyses. The use of a structural or graphical model to depict relationships between constituent pieces of a dataset is known as network modelling. These connections could arise from the experimental dataset itself, such as a substantial correlation or mutual information between two measured variables, or from other sources, such as sequence data or previously published links. Individual measured variables are associated with groups, sets, or classes to which they belong, and statistical trends, such as enrichment in significantly changing variables for each class, are assessed based on the dataset. Identification of correlations between abundances of a biomolecule, such as a protein or RNA product, and a trait of interest in order to determine which biomolecules may impact the characteristics is referred to as phenotype association. These computational techniques, when combined, can lead to a systems-scale knowledge of host–parasite relationships, which will be critical for disrupting them through the development of novel treatments and vaccines in the battle against malaria.

Recent research shows that the immune response of the host may potentially play a role in the pathogenesis of the illness in humans. Human investigations of the immune response to malaria parasites have yielded a lot of information about the cells and cytokines involved in the pathophysiology of survival and death in severe infections [18, 19]. This chapter will look at a variety of experimental and computational activities that are currently being done utilising Systems Biology techniques, as well as the methodology that is being used.

3. Experimental approaches

To solve biological questions, Systems Biology techniques use both experimental and computational frameworks. We discussed the newly evaluated continuing techniques of omics datasets in this chapter in order to better understand the mechanisms of underlying illnesses and to learn more about target medications for enhanced malaria therapeutics. Genes, mRNAs, proteins, and metabolites supply a wealth of information through omics technology. The omics revolution has accelerated the data-intensive approach to biology, which stresses large-scale, aggregate investigations employing high-throughput methods. Despite the fact that these treatments were time-consuming and costly, they were now inexpensive and widely available because of technological advancements. During the experimental strategies, a variety of methodologies are used. Microarray Techniques, Shotgun Proteomics (LC-MS), Conditional Gene Knockout, Conditional Knockdown of Translation and Conditional Knockdown of Protein Function may be summarized.

3.1 Microarray technique

Microarray techniques are the developing techniques to study gene expression all at once. Transcriptomics studies involve microarray techniques to study gene expression and are also involved in immune response and play a significant role. Transcriptomics is a commonly used approach in malaria for omics studies used by collecting blood samples [13, 18, 19]. In 2003, the first high-resolution *P. falciparum* blood-stage transcriptome was published for studying various gene expressions to achieve diverse parasite phenotypes, immune evasion, adaptations, reproduction, and transmission. To study more about the *Plasmodium falciparum* gene functions, shotgun DNA microarray is implied. The shotgun DNA microarray by Rhian *et al.* studies variation of gene expression during the parasite life cycle, and the array is probed with differently labelled cDNAs prepared from the total RNA isolated cells from the defined developmental stage. Yatsushiro *et al.*, put forward a cell microarray chip system for rapid and accurate diagnosis for malaria, which included a push column for recovery of erythrocytes and a fluorescence detector [20]. The malarial shotgun microarray is constructed by printing PCR-amplified inserts from the *P. falciparum* library. The shotgun microarray is useful for analysing malarial transcriptomics programs for comparing gene expression of *Plasmodium*. But to date, in *P. falciparum,* only a few proteins have been identified in the sexual stage of the life-cycle [21]. Microarray techniques have answered many fundamental questions but due to limited cost and comparatively large amount of biological materials required, which is limited in clinical isolates [19].

3.2 Shotgun proteomics

Shotgun proteomics refers to bottom-up proteomics techniques to identify proteins that are detected during the malaria life cycle using Liquid Chromatography (LC) coupled to tandem Mass spectrometry (MS). Proteomics studies involve understanding multiprotein systems in an organism for identifying, characterising, or quantifying proteins in the field of Systems Biology. In this LC–MS method, the peptides are loaded onto the reserved phase column using C18 and then separated according to hydrophobicity through the mobile phase medium, which consists of water and elongated percentage acetonitrile. In this method, at first, the proteins are extracted from a given sample, followed by removal of contaminants and protein of no interest, followed by digestion of proteins into peptides, followed by separation of post digestions to obtain a more homogeneous mixture of peptides, and lastly analysis by MS [22, 23]. A study by Briquet *et al.*, using shotgun proteomics tools, has explored the nuclear proteins of *P. falciparum* extracted from erythrocytes [24]. To identify novel drug targets, there is a significant challenge which lies in identifying genes that are probably essential to parasite viability. Despite the progress in proteomics techniques, these techniques remain limited in the clinical field due to the time-consuming and huge cost of equipment.

3.3 Conditional gene knockout

The *P. falciparum* genome is haploid for the majority of its life cycle, thus preventing the generation of random mutants except under exceptional circumstances. This prevents the use of random mutagenesis screens to identify biological mechanisms behind the parasitic pathways in most cases. *Plasmodium* is evolutionarily distant from model organisms that have been thoroughly studied. A large percentage of parasitic genes lack homology outside of the phylum, thus suggesting that while some protein functions are conserved, the complex biological machinery of the life cycle of *Plasmodium* spp. prevents direct comparison with the established biological function of conserved proteins from work on model systems [25]. The development of conditional gene or protein expression systems that allow disruption of the spatio-temporal protein function has aided in transcending the roadblocks set by the biology of the parasite. The ability to conditionally disrupt essential protein function is critical for understanding parasite biology and identifying new drug targets. This was further advanced by the important technological tool of CRISPR/Cas-9 gene editing that enabled the implementation of these conditional tools to be widely applied in *Plasmodium falciparum*. Conditional gene/protein systems are present at various levels of the genomic system. This allows researchers to modify the parasitic genome. Modifications include disruption of translation or direct inhibition of protein function by adding or removing small molecules. While some systems have been adapted for use from other organisms, e.g., the Cre recombinase, few systems like the *Pf*DOZI-TetR aptamer system have been developed specifically for *P. falciparum*. These systems have been widely used to study the clinical manifestations caused by the blood stages of *P. falciparum*, albeit a few exceptions.

Conditional gene knockout involves the perturbation of transcription by completely removing DNA sequences by activating a site-specific recombinase expressed in the parasite. A major advantage of this approach is that translation can be completely prevented in the parasites that excise the DNA, although the knockout may not be 100% penetrant within the population. The use of site-specific recombinases in *P. falciparum* has become a powerful tool to study the function of essential genes in the parasite in the last few decades. Two site-specific recombinases, Cre and Flippase recombination enzyme (FLP), have been successfully utilised to modify the parasitic genome [26]. The DiCre system is another tool that has been put forward to conditionally knockout genes. This system was adapted for *P. falciparum* blood stages to introduce conditional control over DNA excision. The majority of current conditional systems have been adapted to *Plasmodium falciparum* strains that are not mosquito-infectious. This makes it impossible to study protein function during the parasite's transmission stages. To overcome this challenge, a DiCre-expressing line was recently generated using the mosquito-infective *P. falciparum* NF54 strain. The DiCre-expressing parasites have been recently used to characterise the entire FIKK kinase family in the asexual stage, identifying essential kinases for virulence, growth, and host cell remodelling [27].

3.4 Conditional knockdown of translation

Introducing protein knockdown by targeting mRNA translation has been a valuable strategy for studying protein functions in many organisms. This involves the introduction of double-stranded RNA into cells, which binds homologous mRNA within the cell, leading to the degradation of the RNA transcripts. However, *Plasmodium* parasites lack a functional RNAi pathway, leading to the development of other RNA-based knockdown systems for use in the parasites. The *glmS* and PfDOZI-TetR systems are mRNA-targeting knockdown systems that have been used to study the *P. falciparum* blood stages. The *glmS* ribozyme sequence is inserted into the gene of interest after the stop codon. The transcribed mRNA containing the ribozyme is activated by glucosamine-6-phosphate to cleave its associated mRNA, thus leading to transcript instability and degradation. Modifying the parasite genome to introduce the ribozyme is a relatively uncomplicated protocol, with the simultaneous introduction of an epitope tag sequence at the end of the ORF, a stop codon, then the ribozyme sequence, being a common approach. The culture medium is supplemented with glucosamine to activate the ribozyme in *P. falciparum*. The parasite converts glucosamine to glucosamine-6-phosphate. An advantage of this system is the availability of an inactive "M9" version of the ribozyme containing a single point mutation rendering it incapable of cleaving mRNA. One significant concern associated with the *glmS* system is whether the knockdown achieved will result in a definite observable phenotype. For example, the use of the *glmS* system to determine the essentiality of the proteases *Pf*PMV and *Pf*ClpP showed no growth defects after the knockout of the respective proteases. Both *Pf*PMV and *Pf*ClpP proteases have been reported to be essential via different methods. These observations suggest that while the *glmS* system has been extensively utilised to study parasite biology, it may prove insufficient to establish the utility of high expression protein systems [28].

Another conditional approach for controlling protein expression via translation is *Pf*DOZI-TetR. Although its mode of function and use is more complex than the above-mentioned glmS system, the *Pf*DOZI-TetR system has become a go-to in studying asexual parasite biology. Following the stop codon of the gene of interest, ten copies of a TetR-binding aptamer sequence are introduced in this conditional system [29]. The TetR protein, which is linked to *Pf*DOZI, a protein that localises to mRNA sequestration sites known as P-bodies, recognises the aptamers in the mRNA. *Pf*DOZ-TetRI binds to the mRNA, causing it to relocalize to P-bodies and suppress translation. The *Pf*DOZI-TetR regulatory fusion protein is introduced into the parasite genome using CRISPR/Cas-9 technology, which includes a linearized repair template with homology regions to the gene of interest, a drug selection marker, 10x aptamer sequences, an epitope tag, and a cassette to express the *Pf*DOZI-TetR regulatory fusion protein. Tang and colleagues utilised the *Pf*DOZI-TetR system to validate results from a forward genetic screen aimed at uncovering genes essential for apicoplast biogenesis. Their work demonstrates the importance of having conditional knockdown tools for researching druggable pathways in the parasites [25].

An important feature of the *glmS* system is its ease of use, simple molecular cloning, and addition of a molecule to induce knockdown. However, research shows that the *Pf*DOZI-TetR approach accomplished a better knockdown than the glmS technique when used to study *Pf*ClpP or the apicoplast resident protease. This demonstrates that the same protein may respond distinctly to different conditional systems. Unlike the more direct molecular cloning used to make glmS mutant parasites, the plasmids used to make *Pf*DOZI-TetR mutants are significantly bigger, making them more susceptible to recombination. However, this particular issue may be combated by growing bacteria containing the plasmids at 30°C. It has been reported that the loss of aptamer copies can also occur in clonal parasites that originally possessed all ten aptamer copies, leading to loss of knockdown efficiency. In light of this, a newer, optimised version of the TetR system has been developed that is less prone to loss of the aptamer copies via recombination [30]. Another negative feature of the *glmS* system is that the drug used to induce knockdown, glucosamine, can be toxic to the parasites at certain concentration levels. However, both systems continue to be widely used to research *P. falciparum* biology [31].

3.5 Conditional knockdown of protein function

Knockdown atprotein level is advantageous because the protein of interest is directly targeted instead of target transcription or translation. The FK506 binding protein destabilisation domain (FKBP-DD) is one of the first systems adapted to modify the protein levels in *P. falciparum*. FKBP-DD can be appended to the N or carboxyl terminus of the protein of interest to initiate its degradation via the proteasome [32]. Another similar protein degradation system was applied to *P. falciparum* through the use of dihydrofolate reductase (DHFR) domain derived from *Escherichia coli*. The DHFR degradation domain (DDD), contains mutations that cause the unfolding of the domain. This unfolded domain is then targeted for degradation in the absence of trimethoprim (TMP). This technique was first employed in *P. falciparum* asexual parasites to demonstrate the ability to degrade yellow fluorescent protein-tagged with the degradation domain and to establish the requirement of the proteasome subunit RPN6 [33]. The TMP concentrations involved in stabilising the DDD domain are lethal to the parasite. To combat this particular problem, DDD-mediated protein knockdowns are performed in a TMP-resistant parasite line that has the human DHFR cassette integrated into the nonessential gene, plasmepsin I. This system has also been widely used to study chaperone functions in the asexual stages of *P. falciparum*. DDD tagging of a cytoplasmic chaperone (HSP110) reveals that chaperones are not targeted for degradation in the absence of TMP. Instead, inhibition was achieved through the chaperone binding to the unfolded domain, thereby preventing interactions with client proteins [34]. However, there are drawbacks to both the FKBP-DD and DDD methods. Both necessitate the addition of domains to the protein's N-terminus or carboxyl terminus, which may affect the protein's function or localization. Furthermore, both systems necessitate the ongoing supply of a stabilising ligand, such as TMP or Shld1, to the parasite in order to sustain steady expression of the protein of interest. Shld1 is toxic to asexual parasite development at high concentrations, while TMP is lethal to parasites unless used in a parasite line that expresses the hDHFR gene [35].

One other option which does not utilise an unfolded domain is the knock sideways (KS) system. This system relies on subcellular relocalisation of the protein of interest to disable the protein functionality. A KS system was recently established in *P. falciparum*, using the rapamycin-dimerizable domains FRB and FKBP. In a parasite line expressing a "mislocalizer" fusion protein, the protein of interest is fused to two copies of the FKBP domain. This mislocalizer is made up of the FRB domain, which has been engineered to localise to the nucleus and/or the plasma membrane, causing the protein of interest to relocalize to one of these places when rapamycin is added. As with the previously discussed degradation based system, the KS system likely has similar limitations. One such limitation being that the the protein of interest must be amenable to fusion with larger domains. Also, it must have access to the mislocalizer protein. Exported proteins may be expected to have limited utility. This may be countered by expressing and exporting a new mislocalizer protein in addition to the previously exported proteins [36].

4. Need for new antimalarial strategies

Artemisinin-based combination treatments (ACTs), which have only lately been chosen as the last choice in the fight against malaria, are already being challenged by ACT-resistant strains discovered in Southeast Asia. With parasite resistance to all currently available antimalarial medications spreading, successful control and eradication will require the development of more efficient tools and cost-effective antimalarial methods.

Chloroquine-resistant transporter (crt), Multidrug-resistant protein (mdr1), Kelch13(k13), Bifunctional dihydrofolate reductase (dhfr), Dihydropteroate synthetase(dhps), and cytochrome b are the drug resistance genes of *P. falciparum*. Drug resistance is mostly linked to single nucleotide polymorphisms. To discover the probable genetic alterations that result in drug resistance, next-generation sequencing technologies such as end-to-end Illumina targeted amplicon deep sequencing (TADS), and Malaria Resistance Surveillance (MaRS) was created [37].

5. Methods to identify the drug resistant gene of *P. falciparum*

Over the last few decades, a number of molecular genotyping approaches for tracking antibiotic resistance in clinical isolates have been developed and implemented. RFLP analysis [38], molecular beacons [39], real-time PCR [40, 41], dot blot probe hybridization [42], and single-nucleotide primer extension [43] are all examples of traditional approaches. High-resolution DNA melting (HRM) [44, 45], and SNP-based custom genotyping assay [46, 47], TaqMan allelic discrimination assay [48], mass spectrometry-based SNP genotyping [49], ligase detection reaction fluorescent microsphere (LDR-FM) assay [50], and loop-mediated isothermal amplification (LAMP) [51] are some of the more recent high-throughput methods. While these techniques allow for the detection of known drug resistance alleles of a given gene, they do not allow the discovery of novel genetic polymorphisms involved in drug resistance [52].

5.1 Genomics study

Sanger sequencing and Next-generation sequencing (NGS) are the methods that allow fragment sequencing, where NGS is appropriate for high throughput methodologies.

5.1.1 Genomics study

Sanger sequencing, or the chain termination method, is used to sequence DNA regions up to 900 base pairs in length. Fred Sanger, a British biochemist, and his collaborators invented Sanger sequencing in 1977. Sanger sequencing is still widely used for the sequencing of individual pieces of DNA, such as fragments used in DNA cloning or generated through a polymerase chain reaction. Sanger sequencing is still commonly used for sequencing specific pieces of DNA, such as fragments used in DNA cloning or created through polymerase chain reaction (PCR), despite the fact that genomes are now generally sequenced using alternative faster and less expensive methods. Compared to the Sanger sequencing approach, NGS detected a much larger number of mutant alleles. Sanger's method of DNA sequencing is less sensitive than NGS [53].

5.1.2 Next-generation sequencing

Next-generation sequencing (NGS) is a massively parallel sequencing technology with extremely high throughput, scalability, and speed. This approach has been applied to determine the order of nucleotides in entire genomes or individual DNA or RNA segments. NGS has changed biological sciences, allowing labs to conduct a wide range of experiments and investigate biological systems on a scale that was previously unattainable. The methods for fragment sequencing are Sanger sequencing and next-generation sequencing (NGS), with NGS being more ideal for high-throughput procedures. Targeted Amplicon Deep Sequencing (TADS) and Malaria Resistance Surveillance (MaRS) are two of the most sensitive NGS-based technologies of relevance for antimalarial drug resistance surveillance [38]. The Roche 454, the Applied Biosystems SOLiD, and eventually the Illumina® (formerly known as Solexa) Genome Analyser and Hi-Seq platforms have been commercialised in the last few five years. Illumina® sequencers can presently produce up to 2 billion reads each run, with a recommended read length of 35–100 bp [54]. This value is constantly increasing due to steady advances in reagents and consumables.

6. Protein–protein interaction study

Artemisinin-resistant malaria parasites are emerging, as evidenced by prior reports of resistance to other antimalarial medicines. A greater understanding of the parasite's biology is essential for unravelling the mechanisms behind the emergence of drug-resistant strains and identifying better pharmacological targets. In the late 1990s, a ground-breaking effort to sequence the genome of *P. falciparum* was launched. *P. falciparum* 3D7's 22.8 megabase genome was sequenced and annotated in 2002 [17, 55]. Compared to other known eukaryotic species, the malaria proteome is projected to contain fewer enzymes and transporters and more proteins related to cell adhesion and immune system evasion. Along with publishing the genome, the first high-throughput proteomics experiments, which provided a life cycle stage-specific perspective of the malaria proteome [56, 57], marked another major step forward in malaria genetics. Understanding an organism at the molecular level is difficult due to the highly dynamic nature of cellular machinery and the complicated interactions that all proteins have with one another. The first-generation malaria protein interaction network was revealed using high-throughput yeast two-hybrid (Y2H) systems [58].

Other high-throughput methods for inferring cellular networks, such as RNA expression profiles, genetic interaction data, and mass spectrometry analysis of protein complexes, have intrinsic limits that affect the network's coverage and accuracy. However, combining these disparate pieces of evidence into a single PPI

Dataset used for integration	Integrative algorithm	Data source for validation	Algorithm	Nodes (protein)	Edges (Interaction)	Publication
Phylogenetic profiles, Rosetta stone fusion protein dataset, Microarray expression datasets	Bayesian approach	Gene ontology (GO assignment) KEGG database	High confidence links (confidence score > 14)	3667	388,969	Date et al. [65]
Orthologs datasets, Y2H dataset, Pfam DDI dataset	Hypergeometric distribution	Microarray expression datasets, GO functional annotation	Markov-Cluster algorithm	2321	19,979	Wuchty et al. [66]
Orthologs datasets (Chaperones only), Y2H dataset				212 (chaperones)	344	Pavithra et al. [68]
Orthologs datasets, Y2H dataset		Yeast protein complexes, microarray expression datasets	Clique-percolation algorithm	1872	4918	Wuchty et al. [64]
Y2H dataset, Microarray expression datasets (Stage specific), Orthologs datasets, Metabolic pathways	Bayesian approach	GO functional annotation				Mitrofanova et al. [69]
Y2H dataset, Microarray expression datasets	Weighted Interaction Grap	GO functional annotation	Linear time algorithm			Oyelade et al. [70]

Table 1.
An outline of the malaria PPI network's computational inference and analysis to date. (microarray expression datasets — Transcriptome data; Y2H dataset — Yeast two-hybrid generated interaction).

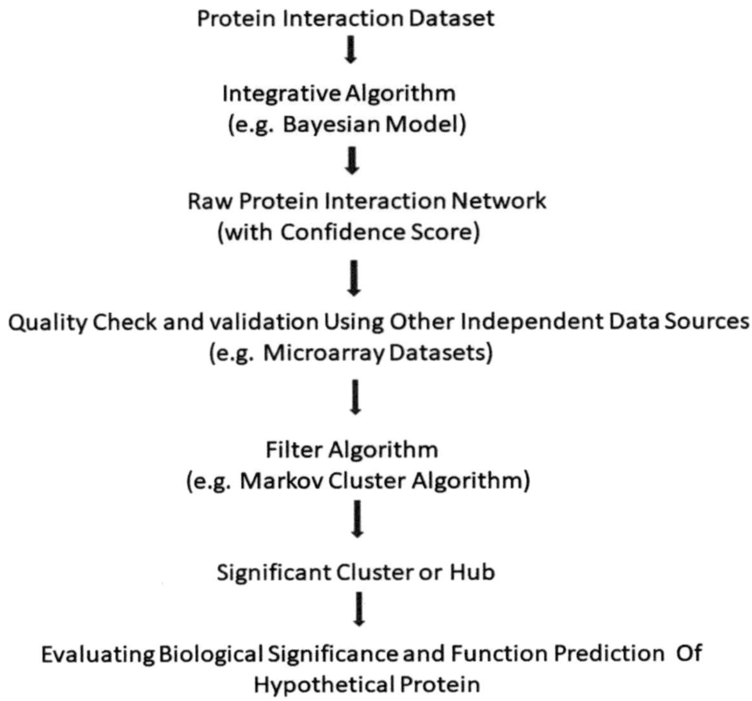

Figure 2.
Methods to construct PPI network of P. falciparum.

network improves accuracy and coverage. Such integrations can be done in software, and they have been used to predict the PPI network in yeast [59, 60]. A Y2H data collection [58], microarray expression profiles [61, 62], and more recently, an RNA-Seq dataset [63] are the experimentally determined datasets available for building malaria protein interaction networks (**Table 1**). Various computationally created datasets, such as the ortholog dataset [64], phylogenetic profiles [65], and P*fam* domain-domain interactions (DDI) dataset [66], have been utilised to supplement these datasets. These derived datasets are based on homology searches, with the only difference being the data range for which the search is conducted. Interlogs and protein–protein interactions are predicted using these databases. These datasets are collected from independent sources, and the linkages are measured by combining different parameters. Integrating the various parameters would necessitate a data integration Framework or algorithm. For example, a Bayesian framework is an integrative algorithm. **Figure 2** depicts the methods used to construct PPI network of *P. falciparum*.

Agamah *et al.,* curated data of pathogen and host selective genes, protein–protein interaction datasets, and data from literature and databases to perform network-based analysis of human host and *P. falciparum*. The study revealed 8 hub protein targets essential for parasite and human host-directed malaria drug therapy. In a semantic similarity approach, 26 potential repurposable anti-inflammatory drugs inhibiting residual malaria infection were put forward that can be appropriated for malaria treatment. Further analysis of host–pathogen network shortest paths enabled the prediction of immune-related biological processes and pathways impaired by *P. falciparum* to increase its survivability within the host [67].

7. Combined computer-aided drug designing (CADD) and virtual screening

Computer-aided drug discovery (CADD) can be described as utilising computer technology and software to elevate drug discovery efforts. It is also known as *in silico* drug discovery and is the application of computational methods to guide and systemise the process of drug discovery and its various stages. The two most commonly reported computational approaches to drug discovery are structure-based methods (primarily molecular docking studies) and ligand-based approaches such as ligand-based pharmacophore methods and three-dimensional quantitative structure–activity relationship (3D QSAR) models. Many therapeutically relevant malarial proteins have been identified and characterised, from receptors and transporters involved in membrane transport and signalling to enzymes used in biosynthesis. Many structure-based antimalarial drug development studies have been predicated on this diversity of protein targets [68].

Structure-based drug discovery (SBDD) searches for novel compounds that work against a specific target using information from the target's structure. The crystal structure of the drug target, preferably co-crystallised with a known ligand, can be used to extract the 3D structural information. It aids in the discovery of new ligands by identifying them from virtual chemical libraries or directing the design of novel compounds. The most commonly used SBDD approach is molecular docking, whereby computer software simulates ligand-target binding and predicts binding conformations and molecular interactions between ligands and target macromolecules. In the absence of a 3D crystal structure or a realistic homology model of the therapeutic target is unavailable, a ligand-based drug design (LBDD) technique can be useful. In research when the active inhibitors/ligands are known, ligand-based approaches are a potential alternative. Ligand-based pharmacophores are constructed using molecular descriptors of known active ligands. These models identify the ligand characteristics that are required for ligand-target compatibility, such as H-bond acceptors/donors, hydrophobicity, ionizable groups, and so on, making it easier to run comparison searches of huge compound datasets [68].

Drug development attempts for antiplasmodial drugs commonly use structure-based virtual screening techniques. Dahlgren et al. used structure-based screening of the Maybridge and ZINC drug-like databases to find four small-molecule inhibitors of *Plasmodium falciparum* macrophage migratory inhibitory factor (*Pf*MIF; PDB: 2WKF) [69]. In another study by Carrasco et al., 4 active compounds were identified against the chloroquine-resistant W2 strain *of P. falciparum.* For their study, they used the structure-based virtual screening a drug-like database included in the MOE package [70]. Similarly, a potential antiplasmodial against the *Plasmodium falciparum* FKBD35 protein was identified by Harikishore *et al*. by screening the database, ChemDiv, applying the same approaches. A structure-based pharmacophore model was developed 1st which was based on the *P. falciparum* FKBD35-FK506 X-ray crystal structure. As a result of pharmacophore-based screening of the ChemDiv library, a condensed library of 13,000 compounds was presented. ADME (absorption, distribution, metabolism, and excretion) filters were used to refine the library, yielding 2600 compounds. In docking investigations of the focused library into the active site of *P. falciparum* FKBP35, the docking software GOLD was used [71].

Lima *et al*. utilised a combi-QSAR approach, combining 2D- and 3D-QSAR models, in a virtual screening study of the ChemBridge database for a selection of new antimalarial virtual hits. This was followed by in vitro experimental tests of the potential *Pf*dUTPase inhibitors against chloroquine-sensitive and multidrug-resistant strains of *P. falciparum*, in an effort to identify new potential and selective antimalarial hits [72].

CADD approaches represent the best opportunity so far to enhance productivity pipelines not only in malaria, but also in various other diseases [73]. CADD is a very appealing venture for improved and efficient drug discovery for not only tropical infections but also for non-tropical diseases, due to the easy availability of many diverse chemical libraries in pharmaceutical companies, virtual discovery organisations, and academic institutions, as well as the increased genomic information that facilitates computational predictions [74–76].

8. Conclusions

Malaria is one of the deadliest infectious diseases in the world with no certified vaccine against malaria pathogens. Artemisinin and quinine are two most efficacious drugs that prevail. Unfortunately, ACT (Artemisinin-based combination therapies) resistant strain has been discovered in Southeast Asia. *P. falciparum* has developed drug resistance through single nucleotide polymorphism (SNP) in its genome. Traditional methods have been utilised to identify SNPs, however, with the advancement of NGS technologies, new possibilities were being opened up in the malarial research development as well as in the primary and applied field. As the new genomic data revealed a large number of processes, which can transform it into new therapeutic strategies. New quantitative analysis methods are continually being developed and tested for the most accurate analytical approach in the case of the *Plasmodium* genome. Studies in genomics and Systems Biology have made a huge contribution towards a better understanding of the *P. falciparum* parasite. Most significantly, they have built an impressive pipeline of novel therapeutic targets and several potent vaccine candidates. Along with the malarial parasite, the genomic study has also contributed to the genetic factor of humans that have a significant vulnerability and response against both malaria and its potent drug or vaccines. Beyond new drug and vaccine candidates, genomics has also contributed towards the drug mechanism of action. Thus, integration of both the genomic and system can lead to a better eradication of malaria strategies.

Acknowledgements

SR would like to acknowledge Dibrugarh University for providing computational facilities and financial support. The authors would also like to acknowledge Mr. Abhichandan Das for helping with the preparation of the chapter.

Conflict of interest

The authors declare no conflict of interest.

Author details

Himangshu Patgiri, Ankita Khataniar, Pitimoni Boro, Sushmita Baishnab and Sanchaita Rajkhowa*
Centre for Biotechnology and Bioinformatics, Dibrugarh University, Dibrugarh, Assam, India

*Address all correspondence to: s_rajkhowa@dibru.ac.in

References

[1] Loy DE, Liu W, Li Y, Learn GH, Plenderleith LJ, Sundararaman SA, et al. Out of Africa: Origins and evolution of the human malaria parasites *plasmodium falciparum* and *plasmodium vivax*. International Journal for Parasitology. 2017;**47**:87-97

[2] Carter R, Mendis KN. Evolutionary and historical aspects of the burden of malaria. Clinical Microbiology Reviews. 2002;**15**(4):564-594. Available from: https://pubmed.ncbi.nlm.nih.gov/12364370/

[3] Hedrick PW. Population genetics of malaria resistance in humans. Heredity. 2011;**107**(4):283-304. Available from: https://pubmed.ncbi.nlm.nih.gov/21427751/

[4] Escalante AA, Ayala FJ. Phylogeny of the malarial genus *plasmodium*, derived from rRNA gene sequences (*plasmodium falciparum*/host switch/small subunit rRNA/human malaria). 1st ed. Proceedings of the National Academy of Sciences of the United States of America. 1994 Nov 22;**91**(24):11373-11377

[5] Branch OH, Sutton PL, Barnes C, Castro JC, Hussin J, Awadalla P, et al. *Plasmodium falciparum* genetic diversity maintained and amplified over 5 years of a low transmission endemic in the Peruvian Amazon. Molecular Biology and Evolution. 2011;**28**(7):1973. Available from: /pmc/articles/PMC3112368/

[6] Prugnolle F, Durand P, Neel C, Ollomo B, Ayala FJ, Arnathau C, et al. African great apes are natural hosts of multiple related malaria species, including *plasmodium falciparum*. Proceedings of the National Academy of Sciences of the United States of America. 2010;**107**(4):1458-1463. Available from: https://pubmed.ncbi.nlm.nih.gov/20133889/

[7] Sundararaman SA, Plenderleith LJ, Liu W, Loy DE, Learn GH, Li Y, et al. Genomes of cryptic chimpanzee *plasmodium* species reveal key evolutionary events leading to human malaria. Nature Communications. 2016;**7**:11078. Available from: /pmc/articles/PMC4804174/

[8] Le Roch KG, Chung DWD, Ponts N. Genomics and integrated systems biology in *plasmodium falciparum*: A path to malaria control and eradication. Parasite Immunology. 2012;**34**(2-3):50. Available from: /pmc/articles/PMC3265687/

[9] Das A, Pathak U, Rajkhowa S, Jha AN. *Plasmodium Falciparum*: Experimental and Theoretical Approaches in Last 20 Years. London, UK: IntechOpen; 2021. Available from: https://www.intechopen.com/chapters/75466. DOI: 10.5772/intechopen.96529

[10] Malaguarnera L, Musumeci S. The immune response to *Plasmodium falciparum* malaria. The Lancet Infectious Diseases. 2002;**2**(8):472-478. Available from: https://pubmed.ncbi.nlm.nih.gov/12150846/

[11] Loiseau C, Cooper MM, Doolan DL. Deciphering host immunity to malaria using systems immunology. Immunological Reviews. 2020;**293**(1):115-143

[12] Rajkhowa S, Hazarika Z, Jha AN. Systems biology and bioinformatics approaches in leishmaniasis. Applications of Nanobiotechnology for Neglected Tropical Diseases. 2021:509-548

[13] Smith ML, Styczynski MP. Systems biology-based investigation of host-*plasmodium* interactions. Trends in Parasitology. 2018;**34**(7):617-632.

Available from: https://pubmed.ncbi.nlm.nih.gov/29779985/

[14] Zuck M, Austin LS, Danziger SA, Aitchison JD, Kaushansky A. The promise of systems biology approaches for revealing host pathogen interactions in malaria. Frontiers in Microbiology. 2017;**8**(NOV):2183

[15] Subudhi AK, Boopathi PA, Middha S, Acharya J, Rao SN, Mugasimangalam RC, et al. A cross strain *plasmodium falciparum* microarray optimized for the transcriptome analysis of *plasmodium falciparum* patient derived isolates. Genomics Data. 2016;**9**:118. Available from: /pmc/articles/PMC4961827/

[16] Davis MM, Tato CM, Furman D. Systems immunology: Just getting started. Nature Immunology. 2017;**18**(7):725-732. Available from: https://pubmed.ncbi.nlm.nih.gov/28632713/

[17] Gardner MJ, Hall N, Fung E, White O, Berriman M, Hyman RW, et al. Genome sequence of the human malaria parasite *plasmodium falciparum*. Nature. 2002;**419**(6906):498-511. Available from: https://www.nature.com/articles/nature01097

[18] Dhillon BK, Smith M, Baghela A, Lee AHY, Hancock REW. Systems biology approaches to understanding the human immune system. Frontiers in Immunology. 2020;**11**:1683. Available from: https://pubmed.ncbi.nlm.nih.gov/32849587/

[19] Winzeler EA. Applied systems biology and malaria. Nature Reviews. Microbiology. 2006;**4**(2):145-151. Available from: https://www.nature.com/articles/nrmicro1327

[20] Yatsushiro S, Yamamoto T, Yamamura S, Abe K, Obana E, Nogami T, et al. Application of a cell microarray chip system for accurate, highly sensitive, and rapid diagnosis for malaria in Uganda. Scientific Reports. 2016;**6**:30136. Available from: /pmc/articles/PMC4995311/

[21] Hayward RE, DeRisi JL, Alfadhli S, Kaslow DC, Brown PO, Rathod PK. Shotgun DNA microarrays and stage-specific gene expression in *plasmodium falciparum* malaria. Molecular Microbiology. 2000;**35**(1):6-14. Available from: https://pubmed.ncbi.nlm.nih.gov/10632873/

[22] Karpievitch YV, Polpitiya AD, Anderson GA, Smith RD, Dabney AR. Liquid chromatography mass spectrometry-based proteomics: Biological and technological aspects. The Annals of Applied Statistics. 2010;**4**(4):1797-1823. Available from: https://pubmed.ncbi.nlm.nih.gov/21593992/

[23] Swearingen KE, Lindner SE. *Plasmodium* parasites viewed through proteomics. Trends in Parasitology. 2018;**34**(11):945-960. Available from: https://pubmed.ncbi.nlm.nih.gov/30146456/

[24] Briquet S, Ourimi A, Pionneau C, Bernardes J, Carbone A, Chardonnet S, et al. Identification of *plasmodium falciparum* nuclear proteins by mass spectrometry and proposed protein annotation. PLoS One. 2018;**13**(10):e0205596. Available from: /pmc/articles/PMC6209197/

[25] Tang Y, Meister TR, Walczak M, Pulkoski-Gross MJ, Hari SB, Sauer RT, et al. A mutagenesis screen for essential plastid biogenesis genes in human malaria parasites. PLoS Biology. 2019;**17**(2):e3000136. Available from: https://journals.plos.org/plosbiology/article?id=10.1371/journal.pbio.3000136

[26] O'Neill MT, Phuong T, Healer J, Richard D, Cowman AF. Gene deletion from *plasmodium falciparum* using FLP and Cre recombinases: Implications for applied site-specific recombination. International Journal for Parasitology. 2011;**41**(1):117-123. Available from: https://pubmed.ncbi.nlm.nih.gov/20816845/

[27] Kudyba HM, Cobb DW, Vega-Rodríguez J, Muralidharan V. Some conditions apply: Systems for studying *plasmodium falciparum* protein function. PLoS Pathogens. 2021;**17**(4):e1009442. Available from: /pmc/articles/PMC8062007/

[28] Prommana P, Uthaipibull C, Wongsombat C, Kamchonwongpaisan S, Yuthavong Y, Knuepfer E, et al. Inducible knockdown of *plasmodium* gene expression using the glmS ribozyme. PLoS One. 2013;**8**(8):e73783. Available from: https://journals.plos.org/plosone/article?id=10.1371/journal.pone.0073783

[29] Belmont BJ, Niles JC. Engineering a direct and inducible protein-RNA interaction to regulate RNA biology. ACS Chemical Biology. 2010;**5**(9):851-861. Available from: https://pubmed.ncbi.nlm.nih.gov/20545348/

[30] Rajaram K, Liu HB, Prigge ST. Redesigned TetR-Aptamer system to control gene expression in *plasmodium falciparum*. mSphere. 2020;**5**(4):e00457-20. Available from: https://journals.asm.org/doi/abs/10.1128/mSphere.00457-20

[31] Sleebs BE, Lopaticki S, Marapana DS, O'Neill MT, Rajasekaran P, Gazdik M, et al. Inhibition of Plasmepsin V activity demonstrates its essential role in protein export, *Pf*EMP1 display, and survival of malaria parasites. PLoS Biology. 2014;**12**(7):e1001897. Available from: https://journals.plos.org/plosbiology/article?id=10.1371/journal.pbio.1001897

[32] Armstrong CM, Goldberg DE. An FKBP destabilization domain modulates protein levels in *Plasmodium falciparum*. Nature Methods. 2007;**4**(12):1007-1009. Available from: https://pubmed.ncbi.nlm.nih.gov/17994030/

[33] Muralidharan V, Oksman A, Iwamoto M, Wandless TJ, Goldberg DE. Asparagine repeat function in a *plasmodium falciparum* protein assessed via a regulatable fluorescent affinity tag. Proceedings of the National Academy of Sciences of the United States of America. 2011;**108**(11):4411-4416. Available from: https://www.pnas.org/content/108/11/4411

[34] Muralidharan V, Oksman A, Pal P, Lindquist S, Goldberg DE. *Plasmodium falciparum* heat shock protein 110 stabilizes the asparagine repeat-rich parasite proteome during malarial fevers. Nature Communications. 2012;**3**:1310. Available from: https://pubmed.ncbi.nlm.nih.gov/23250440/

[35] de Azevedo MF, Gilson PR, Gabriel HB, Simões RF, Angrisano F, Baum J, et al. Systematic analysis of FKBP inducible degradation domain tagging strategies for the human malaria parasite *plasmodium falciparum*. PLoS One. 2012;**7**(7):e40981. Available from: https://pubmed.ncbi.nlm.nih.gov/22815885/

[36] Birnbaum J, Flemming S, Reichard N, Soares AB, Mesén-Ramírez P, Jonscher E, et al. A genetic system to study *plasmodium falciparum* protein function. Nature Methods. 2017;**14**(4):450-456. Available from: https://pubmed.ncbi.nlm.nih.gov/28288121/

[37] Talundzic E, Ravishankar S, Kelley J, Patel D, Plucinski M, Schmedes S, et al. Next-generation sequencing and bioinformatics protocol for malaria

drug resistance marker surveillance. Antimicrobial Agents and Chemotherapy. 2018;**62**(4):e02474-17. Available from: https://pubmed.ncbi.nlm.nih.gov/29439965/

[38] Duraisingh MT, Curtis J, Warhurst DC. *Plasmodium falciparum*: Detection of polymorphisms in the dihydrofolate reductase and dihydropteroate synthetase genes by PCR and restriction digestion. Experimental Parasitology. 1998;**89**(1):1-8. Available from: https://pubmed.ncbi.nlm.nih.gov/9603482/

[39] Durand R, Eslahpazire J, Jafari S, Delabre JF, Marmorat-Khuong A, Di Piazza JP, et al. Use of molecular beacons to detect an antifolate resistance-associated mutation in *plasmodium falciparum*. Antimicrobial Agents and Chemotherapy. 2000;**44**(12):3461-3464. Available from: https://journals.asm.org/doi/abs/10.1128/AAC.44.12.3461-3464.2000

[40] Wilson PE, Alker AP, Meshnick SR. Real-time PCR methods for monitoring antimalarial drug resistance. Trends in Parasitology. 2005;**21**(6):278-283. Available from: https://pubmed.ncbi.nlm.nih.gov/15922249/

[41] Alker AP, Mwapasa V, Purfield A, Rogerson SJ, Molyneux ME, Kamwendo DD, et al. Mutations associated with sulfadoxine-pyrimethamine and chlorproguanil resistance in *plasmodium falciparum* isolates from Blantyre, Malawi. Antimicrobial Agents and Chemotherapy. 2005;**49**(9):3919-3921. Available from: https://europepmc.org/articles/PMC1195417

[42] Ranford-Cartwright LC, Johnston KL, Abdel-Muhsin AM, Khan BK, Babiker HA. Critical comparison of molecular genotyping methods for detection of drug-resistant *plasmodium falciparum*. Transactions of the Royal Society of Tropical Medicine and Hygiene. 2002;**96**(5):568-572. Available from: https://pubmed.ncbi.nlm.nih.gov/12474492/

[43] Nair S, Brockman A, Paiphun L, Nosten F, Anderson TJC. Rapid genotyping of loci involved in antifolate drug resistance in *plasmodium falciparum* by primer extension. International Journal for Parasitology. 2002;**32**(7):852-858. Available from: https://pubmed.ncbi.nlm.nih.gov/12062556/

[44] Cruz RE, Shokoples SE, Manage DP, Yanow SK. High-throughput genotyping of single nucleotide polymorphisms in the *plasmodium falciparum* dhfr gene by asymmetric PCR and melt-curve analysis. Journal of Clinical Microbiology. 2010;**48**(9):3081-3087. Available from: https://journals.asm.org/doi/abs/10.1128/JCM.00634-10

[45] Daniels R, Ndiaye D, Wall M, McKinney J, Séne PD, Sabeti PC, et al. Rapid, field-deployable method for genotyping and discovery of single-nucleotide polymorphisms associated with drug resistance in *plasmodium falciparum*. Antimicrobial Agents and Chemotherapy. 2012;**56**(6):2976. Available from: /pmc/articles/PMC3370755/

[46] Daniels R, Volkman SK, Milner DA, Mahesh N, Neafsey DE, Park DJ, et al. A general SNP-based molecular barcode for *plasmodium falciparum* identification and tracking. Malaria Journal. 2008;**7**(1):1-11. Available from: https://malariajournal.biomedcentral.com/articles/10.1186/1475-2875-7-223

[47] Campino S, Auburn S, Kivinen K, Zongo I, Ouedraogo JB, Mangano V, et al. Population genetic analysis of *plasmodium falciparum* parasites using

a customized Illumina GoldenGate genotyping assay. PLoS One. 2011;**6**(6): e20251. Available from: https://pubmed.ncbi.nlm.nih.gov/21673999/

[48] Kamau E, Alemayehu S, Feghali KC, Tolbert LS, Ogutu B, Ockenhouse CF. Development of a TaqMan allelic discrimination assay for detection of single nucleotides polymorphisms associated with anti-malarial drug resistance. Malaria Journal. 2012;**11**(1):1-12. Available from: https://malariajournal.biomedcentral.com/articles/10.1186/1475-2875-11-23

[49] Ali IM, Evehe MSB, Netongo PM, Atogho-Tiedeu B, Akindeh-Nji M, Ngora H, et al. Host candidate gene polymorphisms and associated clearance of *P. falciparum* amodiaquine and fansidar resistance mutants in children less than 5 years in Cameroon. Pathogens and Global Health. 2014;**108**(7):323-333. Available from: https://pubmed.ncbi.nlm.nih.gov/25388906/

[50] Nankoberanyi S, Mbogo GW, Leclair NP, Conrad MD, Tumwebaze P, Tukwasibwe S, et al. Validation of the ligase detection reaction fluorescent microsphere assay for the detection of *plasmodium falciparum* resistance mediating polymorphisms in Uganda. Malaria Journal. 2014;**13**(1):1-5. Available from: https://malariajournal.biomedcentral.com/articles/10.1186/1475-2875-13-95

[51] Aydin-Schmidt B, Xu W, González IJ, Polley SD, Bell D, Shakely D, et al. Loop mediated isothermal amplification (LAMP) accurately detects malaria DNA from filter paper blood samples of low density parasitaemias. PLoS One. 2014;**9**(8):e103905. Available from: https://pubmed.ncbi.nlm.nih.gov/25105591/

[52] Rao PN, Uplekar S, Kayal S, Mallick PK, Bandyopadhyay N, Kale S, et al. A method for amplicon deep sequencing of drug resistance genes in *plasmodium falciparum* clinical isolates from India. Journal of Clinical Microbiology. 2016;**54**(6):1500-1511. Available from: https://pubmed.ncbi.nlm.nih.gov/27008882/

[53] Sharma D, Lather M, Dykes CL, Dang AS, Adak T, Singh OP. Disagreement in genotyping results of drug resistance alleles of the *plasmodium falciparum* dihydrofolate reductase (Pfdhfr) gene by allele-specific PCR (ASPCR) assays and sanger sequencing. Parasitology Research. 2016;**115**(1):323-328. Available from: https://pubmed.ncbi.nlm.nih.gov/26407876/

[54] Liu L, Li Y, Li S, Hu N, He Y, Pong R, et al. Comparison of next-generation sequencing systems. Journal of Biomedicine & Biotechnology. 2012;**2012**:251364. Available from: https://pubmed.ncbi.nlm.nih.gov/22829749/

[55] Ramaprasad A, Pain A, Ravasi T. Defining the protein interaction network of human malaria parasite *plasmodium falciparum*. Genomics. 2012;**99**(2):69-75. Available from: https://pubmed.ncbi.nlm.nih.gov/22178265/

[56] Lasonder E, Ishihama Y, Andersen JS, Vermunt AMW, Pain A, Sauerwein RW, et al. Analysis of the *plasmodium falciparum* proteome by high-accuracy mass spectrometry. Nature. 2002;**419**(6906):537-542. Available from: https://pubmed.ncbi.nlm.nih.gov/12368870/

[57] Florens L, Washburn MP, Raine JD, Anthony RM, Grainger M, Haynes JD, et al. A proteomic view of the *plasmodium falciparum* life cycle. Nature. 2002;**419**(6906):520-526. Available from: https://pubmed.ncbi.nlm.nih.gov/12368866/

[58] LaCount DJ, Vignali M, Chettier R, Phansalkar A, Bell R, Hesselberth JR, et al. A protein interaction network of the malaria parasite *plasmodium falciparum*. Nature. 2005;**438**(7064):103-107. Available from: https://pubmed.ncbi.nlm.nih.gov/16267556/

[59] von Mering C, Krause R, Snel B, Cornell M, Oliver SG, Fields S, et al. Comparative assessment of large-scale data sets of protein-protein interactions. Nature. 2002;**417**(6887):399-403. Available from: https://pubmed.ncbi.nlm.nih.gov/12000970/

[60] Lee I, Date SV, Adai AT, Marcotte EM. A probabilistic functional network of yeast genes. Science. 2004;**306**(5701):1555-1558. Available from: https://pubmed.ncbi.nlm.nih.gov/15567862/

[61] Le Roch KG, Zhou Y, Blair PL, Grainger M, Moch JK, Haynes JD, et al. Discovery of gene function by expression profiling of the malaria parasite life cycle. Science. 2003;**301**(5639):1503-1508. Available from: https://pubmed.ncbi.nlm.nih.gov/12893887/

[62] Bozdech Z, Llinás M, Pulliam BL, Wong ED, Zhu J, DeRisi JL. The transcriptome of the intraerythrocytic developmental cycle of *plasmodium falciparum*. PLoS Biology. 2003;**1**(1):E5. Available from: https://pubmed.ncbi.nlm.nih.gov/12929205/

[63] Otto TD, Wilinski D, Assefa S, Keane TM, Sarry LR, Böhme U, et al. New insights into the blood-stage transcriptome of *plasmodium falciparum* using RNA-Seq. Molecular Microbiology. 2010;**76**(1):12-24. Available from: https://pubmed.ncbi.nlm.nih.gov/20141604/

[64] Wuchty S, Adams JH, Ferdig MT. A comprehensive *plasmodium falciparum* protein interaction map reveals a distinct architecture of a core interactome. Proteomics. 2009;**9**(7):1841-1849. Available from: https://pubmed.ncbi.nlm.nih.gov/19333996/

[65] Date SV, Stoeckert CJ. Computational modeling of the *plasmodium falciparum* interactome reveals protein functionon a genome-wide scale. Genome Research. 2006;**16**(4):542. Available from: /pmc/articles/PMC1457034/

[66] Wuchty S, Ipsaro JJ. A draft of protein interactions in the malaria parasite *P. falciparum*. Journal of Proteome Research. 2007;**6**(4):1461-1470. Available from: https://pubmed.ncbi.nlm.nih.gov/17300188/

[67] Agamah FE, Damena D, Skelton M, Ghansah A, Mazandu GK, Chimusa ER. Network-driven analysis of human–*plasmodium falciparum* interactome: Processes for malaria drug discovery and extracting in silico targets. Malaria Journal. 2021;**20**(1):1-20. Available from: https://malariajournal.biomedcentral.com/articles/10.1186/s12936-021-03955-0

[68] Pavithra SR, Kumar R, Tatu U. Systems analysis of chaperone networks in the malarial parasite *plasmodium falciparum*. PLoS Computational Biology. 2007;**3**(9):e168. Available from: https://journals.plos.org/ploscompbiol/article?id=10.1371/journal.pcbi.0030168

[69] Mitrofanova A, Kleinberg S, Carlton J, Kasif S, Mishra B. Predicting malaria interactome classifications from time-course transcriptomic data along the intraerythrocytic developmental cycle. Artificial Intelligence in Medicine. 2010;**49**(3):167-176. Available from: https://nyuscholars.nyu.edu/en/publications/predicting-malaria-interactome-classifications-from-time-course-t

[70] Oyelade J, Ewejobi I, Brors B, Eils R, Adebiyi E. Computational identification of signalling pathways in *plasmodium falciparum*. Infection, Genetics and Evolution. 2011;**11**(4):755-764. Available from: https://pubmed.ncbi.nlm.nih.gov/21112415/

[71] Hung CL, Chen CC. Computational approaches for drug discovery. Drug Development Research. 2014;**75**(6):412-418. Available from: https://pubmed.ncbi.nlm.nih.gov/25195585/

[72] Dahlgren MK, Garcia AB, Hare AA, Tirado-Rives J, Leng L, Bucala R, et al. Virtual screening and optimization yield low-nanomolar inhibitors of the tautomerase activity of *plasmodium falciparum* macrophage migration inhibitory factor. Journal of Medicinal Chemistry. 2012;**55**(22):10148-10159. Available from: https://pubmed.ncbi.nlm.nih.gov/23067344/

[73] Carrasco MP, Gut J, Rodrigues T, Ribeiro MHL, Lopes F, Rosenthal PJ, et al. Exploring the molecular basis of Qo bc1 complex inhibitors activity to find novel Antimalarials hits. Molecular Informatics. 2013;**32**(7):659-670. Available from: https://pubmed.ncbi.nlm.nih.gov/27481771/

[74] Harikishore A, Niang M, Rajan S, Preiser PR, Yoon HS. Small molecule *plasmodium* FKBP35 inhibitor as a potential antimalaria agent. Scientific Reports. 2013;**3**(1):1-8. Available from: https://www.nature.com/articles/srep02501

[75] Lima MNN, Melo-Filho CC, Cassiano GC, Neves BJ, Alves VM, Braga RC, et al. QSAR-driven design and discovery of novel compounds with antiplasmodial and transmission blocking activities. Frontiers in Pharmacology. 2018;**9**(MAR):146

[76] Rajkhowa S, Jha AN, Deka RC. Anti-tubercular drug development: Computational strategies to identify potential compounds. Journal of Molecular Graphics & Modelling. 2015;**62**:56-68

Chapter 4

Role of Mosquito Microbiome in Insecticide Resistance

Sahar Fazal, Rabbiah Manzoor Malik, Ahmad Zafar Baig, Narjis Khatoon, Huma Aslam, Aiza Zafar and Muneeba Ishtiaq

Abstract

The gut microbiota of insects is one of the unexplored areas. The association with these microbiomes plays a vital role in supporting their survival and combat with ecological challenges. Mosquito is one of the focal attention insects among the Arthopods, being the vector of many pathogenic diseases including dengue and malaria. A variety of strategies have been designed and implemented to fight against these vectors including obnoxious use of insecticides. Indiscriminate use of insecticides has led to development of resistance against broad range of insecticides. Crucial role of bacteria in insecticide resistance has been under discussion. Many studies focus on the insecticide resistance due to gut microbiome. Thus, the role of gut microbiome is an important area for designing new vector control strategies and their role in improvement of a healthy environment.

Keywords: mosquito, microbiome, microbiome diversity, insecticide resistance, gut microbiota, Anopheles, metagenome

1. Introduction

The medical importance of mosquito can be estimated from this fact that almost 300–500 million people are affected from malaria annually, from which 1 million people lost their lives with the maximum numbers of mortalities in infants and young children. The region mostly affected by malaria is Sub-Saharan African region. In the recent years, dengue virus has expanded its range to 50–100 million population annually with thousands of mortalities due to severe form, i.e., dengue hemorrhage fever. In the past few decades, a new endemic emerged in East Africa and America by West Nile virus named Chikungunya, which caused many deaths in the region [1]. Mosquitoes (family *Culicidae*) have great medical importance due to their property as vector for medically important diseases of human. The wide range of disease spread is due to the dual property of mosquito as it can be biological vector as well as can be the mechanical vector [2, 3]. It is known that half of the world population is at risk of getting mosquito vectored disease such as Malaria, Dengue, Chikungunya, West Nile Virus, and Japanese encephalitis [4]. According a World Health Organization (WHO) report published in 2010, about 247 million world's population became ill due to mosquito and around 1 million people got the disease in 2008. The worldwide distribution of mosquitoes is misinterpreted only in tropical and subtropical environments. But to a certain extent, it is not true as mosquito can cause annoyance or can also spread pathogens or viruses in temperate latitudes [4–6].

Current studies suggested the progress in the overall global malaria control, and it is estimated that 2 million more cases of malaria have appeared in 2017 as compared with 2016. The number of malaria cases is increasing within the region of the Americas [7]. Similarly, reports of resistance to insecticides increase over time [7, 8]. This fact constitutes a great challenge for malaria vector control programs [9]. The fundamental mechanisms of insecticide resistance in malaria vectors are not clearly identified and recognized. However, the following four basic mechanisms underlying insecticide resistance in mosquitoes were described [10].

1. The modification of the cuticle.

2. Amplified detoxification of the insecticides.

3. Insensitivity of the sites of target of the insecticides.

4. Behavioral avoidance of insecticides.

There are still substantial gaps available to young researchers, particularly in high-dose insecticide resistance in the mosquito population. The increased use of genomic methods has encouraged the study of many facets of mosquito biology, such as the microbiota of mosquito populations, which is related to insecticide resistance [10]. Just like other organisms, mosquito is also hosting various types of microbes, and these microbes are basically acquired during their immature developmental stages, such as from the habitat in which mosquitoes are breeding and also from the food source of mosquitoes from where these mosquitoes take their food [11]. Different ways of obtaining microorganisms have been reported, such as microbes obtained from the environment and/or the food supply, the transmission of the bacteria from the female at the time of egg laying through the transovarian mechanism [12], and transmission from the young stage to the adult stage [13]. These microbes have multiple roles in the mosquito, among which some are also known to the metabolizing nature against the insecticides [14–16] and vigorously change as per the physiology of the host [11, 17]. Hence, the microbiota of the mosquitoes has the capabilities to contribute toward the detoxification of the insecticides and increase the resistance in the host. It is the same phenomenon that has been reported previously in agricultural pests [18–23].

2. Habitat of mosquitoes

Mosquitoes breed almost in every water place such as rivers, swamps, lakes, clean water, large or small water bodies even in permanent and temporary water bodies; this is due to their adaptation mechanism. This leads to the conclusion that there is hardly any water body that didn't lend itself a breeding site for mosquito. In temporary flooded areas, the areas near rivers and lake with the water flow fluctuations, flood waters, mosquitoes such as *Aedes vexans* or *Ochlerotatus sticticus* have developed such adaptation that allows them to breed and their ability to fly in places even far from their breeding sites [24].

Some species of *Ochlerotatus* have also adapted to breed in the harsh environments such as snow-melt, swampy woodlands; these mosquitoes include *Ochlerotatus communis*, *Ochlerotatus cataphylla*, *Ochlerotatus cantans*, *Ochlerotatus hexodontus*, and *Ochlerotatus punctor*. There are some species of mosquitoes that encounter conditions and make them ideal for growth. In the flood plains along coastal areas, the environment contains large amount of salt, thus in these areas, the *Halophilous* species, which prefer salt water or brackish habitats, for example *Ochlerotatus taeniorhynchus, Ochlerotatus sollicitans, Ochlerotatus vigilax, Ochlerotatus caspius, Ochlerotatus detritus*, are in focus in large numbers [24].

The Anopheles larvae developed an associative link with mosquito species in every habitat such as freshwater, salt water, edges of streams, rice fields, mangrove swamps, and grassy ditches or in temporary or permanent water bodies. Some species are known that prefer tree hollows as habitat; these are known as tree species, among which are *Aedes cretinus, Ochlerotatus geniculatus, Orthopodomyia pulcripalpis*, and *Anopheles plumbeus*. Some species of mosquitoes can also breed in small water bodies such as containers, rain water, water drums, tires, cemetery pots, or small clay pots; these species include *Culex pipiens, Aedes aegypti* (*Stegomyia aegypti*), *Aedes albopictus* (*Stegomyia albopicta*), or *Ochlerotatus japonicas* [4, 24]. These adaptations helped mosquitoes to change their habitat, such as Asian Tiger Mosquitoes *Aedes albopictus* that originally found in the tropical regions, but during this climate change, they brought evolution in them as they became photoperiodic sensitive. When the days are shorter, the photoperiodic sensitive female lays different eggs as it lays eggs in longer days. The eggs laid in shorter days are inactive and hatch themselves in suitable seasons, which ensures the species survival in the winter [4].

Medically important mosquitoes are responsible for transporting different valuable pathogens such as viruses, bacteria, and parasites that mostly produce lethal diseases such as Malaria, Dengue, Yellow Fever, Chikungunya fever and Encephalitis. The process of pathogen transmission can be in two ways: (i) mechanical vector (e.g., Myxomatosis in rabbits is caused by Myxoma virus); (ii) biological vector. The latest one is more complicated due to following reasons: (a) It associates in necessary rather obligatory period of replication by the parasite in host. (b) Pathogen's development. (c) Parasitic containment by vector insect. The pathogens that are vectored by insects are one of the most leading causes of the pandemics and epidemics; it is also one of the leading causes of declining and fall of empires, for example, Roman Empire and Greece Empire. The malarial case study in the Roman Empire is best example of fall of Empire. The malaria was a big issue in latter days, and the Roman marshy places were notorious for the "Malaria" (bad air). The blood-sucking mosquitoes make them capable of attaining pathogens from one host, and this behavior makes them capable of passing it to other vertebrate hosts. The physiology of mosquitoes is applicable for the mechanism of transmitting the parasite from one host to other. When certain forms of blood stage parasites (gametocytes) are ingested by a female *Anopheles* mosquito during blood feeding, the gametes mate inside the gut of the female mosquito and beginning of a new life cycle occurs followed by growth and multiplication of parasite in the mosquito. After 10–18 days, a sporozoite form of the parasite is migrated to the salivary glands of the mosquito. When this Anopheles mosquito bites another human, sporozoites are injected into the blood of the human together with the saliva of mosquito. This sporozoite migrates to the liver and begins a new life cycle.

Thus, the infected mosquitoes carry the disease from one human to another human (acting as a "vector"), and infected humans transmit the falciparum parasite to the mosquitoes. Contrary to the human host, the mosquito vectors do not suffer despite the presence of the parasites.

The efficient vectors have a close association with their hosts, and they should have enough long-life span that it should be sufficient for them to make pathogen/parasite enable for the proliferation or to develop the infective stages in the vector. The successful parasite transmission is dependent on the multiple blood meals. If we investigate the stats of mortality and morbidity of vector-borne diseases, the mosquitoes are the most fatal vector to the humanity. The mosquitoes only threaten 3 billion people worldwide alone in subtropical or tropical areas and not only affect the human health but also the socioeconomic factors and political factors [25–28].

3. Microbiota of mosquitoes

A mosquito's gut microbiota contains prokaryotes and eukaryotic community. Mosquito gut microbiota is primarily acquired from the environment, its composition is highly dynamic, varying greatly with species, diet, stage of development of mosquitoes, and geography [29]. Sequencing of the 16S rRNA or18S rRNA hypervariable regions is used as a culture-independent tool for the study of mosquito microbiota composition [30]. Many of the mosquitoes are marine and terrestrial during their developmental periods as adults. Larvae primarily consume organic detritus, single-cell organisms, and small invertebrates, while adults of both sexes usually feed on extra floral nectarines. Results outlined in several recent studies suggest that adult mosquito gut microbiota may have both a positive and a negative effect on vector competency, referring to the capacity of females to obtain, retain, and transmit pathogen to vertebrates. Studies show that the microbes form colonies in mosquitoes, which influences their physiological and metabolic functions control. The mosquitoes have a community of microbes, which includes bacteria, algae, fungi, and viruses. These microbes live in close proximity causing the combined effect on the mosquito's physiology and metabolic functions [31].

3.1 Composition of gut microbiota of mosquitoes

Most of the microbiota in the gut of the mosquitoes is demonstrated as being predominantly Gram-negative of facultative nature, which actually belongs to four different phyla (*Proteobacteria, Firmicutes, Bacteroidetes*, and *Actinobacteria*). These phyla are the most prominent members of the growing insect community, obtaining them primarily from the microenvironments in which they develop. With this, insects can easily proliferate on a regular basis. In addition, multiple members of the bacterial community are known to be part of the gut community and have also been successfully extracted and cultured in mosquitoes. Mosquito's viruses have also been categorized in studies as a part of microbiome. Multiple genera belonging to *Flaviviridae* family are part of mosquitoes' community, which sometimes have the activity of a pathogen in vertebrates. By comparison, the absence of bacteriophages in published research indicates that either viruses infecting bacteria in the intestine are underrepresented, or that few bacteriophages infect bacteria in the intestine of the mosquito [30].

3.2 Gut microbiota acquisition by larvae mosquito

Some species obtain intestine microbiota directly from their parents while others obtain their intestinal microbiota primarily from the environment. Three lines of evidence indicate that growing generation of mosquitoes reacquires the gut microbiota mainly from the environment. Second, laboratory experiments indicate that the mosquito larvae hatch and in their intestine left without bacteria. Second, gut-community composition studies suggest that the majority of microbes found in larvae correlate with those found in their aquatic environment. Third, mosquitoes host highly variable gut communities that it is not expected that the congeners acquired those communities directly. Studies indicate that adult mosquito reproductive tracts contain multiple species of bacteria and some of these bacteria are on the surface of laid female eggs; the majority of these bacteria are acquired of the mosquitoes environment. This can lead to the larvae to develop such microbes that can be ingest directly as eggshell fragments at hatching or inoculation of the aquatic environment in which larvae live. Many species of mosquitoes harbor intracellular bacteria that spread vertically such as bacteria of the genus *Wolbachia*. Additionally, these species are not part of the extracellular microbial population, which is the gut microbiota. Cultural studies initially indicated that mosquito larvae remove their gut microbiota at metamorphosis in a meconium having adults with little gut microbes. Such results have indicated that adults develop a gut microbiota by immersing water from the larval environment and/or feeding on resources such as extrafloral nectarines. However, studies of the composition of the gut bacteria community provide clear evidence that larvae of mosquitoes of genus *Aedes* and *Anopheles* transfer a proportion of their gut microbiota to adults. However, subsequently, the adult gut microbiota may change by consuming microbe containing water, nectar, or other food sources. Vertebrate blood generally contains a few bacteria, but some experiments indicate that the intake of a blood meal changes the composition of the gut microbiota persistently to transiently through alterations in redox status or metabolism. Infection by various vector-borne pathogens can also affect gut microbiota composition through unknown mechanisms [30].

3.3 Microbial variation in gut

As a holobiont, mosquito undergoes a metamorphic transformation from larval stage to adult stage. Microbial mosquito residents (*P. falciparum*) and their larvae refer to the microbial communities that colonize within the target organism (humans). In the adult mosquito, the larvae-associated microflora is replaced by a new set of microbes. This microbiota variation is due to significant changes in the host mosquito that are associated with the environment and feeding habits. This microbial cleaning and acquisition process is termed gut sterilization. Mosquitoes mainly consume bacteria and planktons as nutritious resources during their larval stage. This paves the initial stage of invasion of bacteria that contributes to the inhabitants. Among the microbes, the bacteria colonize more in the midgut than in the reproductive organs and salivary glands [32–34]. Later during adult stages, mosquitoes begin to feed on nectar and blood, which triggers the proliferation of some types of microbes and the decline of the other bacteria. Thus, the host diet and its developmental stage play a crucial role in shaping the gut microbiome [35]. Mosquitoes then begin feeding on nectar and blood during adult stages, it then regulates some types of the proliferation of different microbes and decline of some other bacteria. Therefore, the host diet and its level of growth play a key vital role in the structure of gut microbiome [36]. In the gut of mosquitoes, resident communities can vary from microscopic dominant bacteria to even Protista members. This resident consortium can be changed by the influx of new microbes from their natural habitat. Mosquitoes such as *Anopheles*, *Aedes*, and *Culex* normally lay eggs in water that contains bacteria [35]. Aquatic plants affect the microbial populations of mosquitoes providing microbes to larvae, and many of them are often transferred trans-steadily to adult gut [37–39]. These microbes have a significant impact on the characteristics of mosquito life such as fecundity, reproduction vector competency, and immunity. As per previous earlier studies, the general bacterial flora in mosquitoes includes Gram-negative phylum Proteobacteria (Gammaproteobacteria, Alphaproteobacteria, Betaproteobacteria) phylum Bacteroidetes, Gram-positive phylum Firmicutes including *Clostridia*, *Actinomycetes*, *Spirochetes*, and other species. Naturally, a bacterial community in mosquito gut can reduce the development of *Plasmodium*, a human parasite due to the presence of Gram-negative bacteria. The outer membrane of the cell wall in these Gram-negative bacteria contains lipopolysaccharides, which acts as a physical barrier for harmful agents such as hydrogen peroxide, etc. [40], while Gram-positive bacteria have no such barrier. Furthermore, different Gram-negative bacteria have varying effects against *Plasmodium*. These bacteria produce some metabolites that protect the mosquito. *Plasmodium*, for example, is found to be effective against prodigiosin of red pigment produced by Gram-negative bacteria. The mechanism for this is the upregulation of antimicrobial peptide encoding immune genes (AMP) and a protein containing thioester, which has an antiparasitic effect.

The symbiotic microbes are beneficial for the host in several ways. These require nutritional supplementation, strengthening of the digestive system, and tolerance to environmental perturbation and prevention against parasites. The *Anopheline* gut microbiome is strongly influenced by microbes suspended in its natural habitat. This has been proved by gut analysis of mosquito larvae by Howland [41], who dissected over 1000 larvae of eight species, in where they identified algae in the gut community and associated them to abundance in the food. She concluded that the abundance of algae in the larval food is correlated with algal abundance in the habitats. Also, this has been shown in another study on *Anopheles quadrimaculatus* larvae, a common vector of malaria in the Eastern United States [42] wherein the elimination of algae from a small pond with copper sulfate demonstrated its absence in their food. However, after recolonization the same pond, algal cells were again observed in the larval gut.

Researchers have been identified 98 genera of bacteria in the *Anopheles* mosquitoes, the most common being *Pseudomonas, Aeromonas, Asaia, Comamonas, Elizabethkingia, Enterobacter, Klebsiella, Pantoea*, and *Serratia*. Likewise, Gram-negative bacteria also predominate in *Aedes spp*. The *Anopheline* gut is dominated by resident bacteria of genus *Pantoea* and *Asaia*. These bacteria have shown stable association with *Anopheline* mosquitoes during different life stages. *Pantoea*, natural mosquito symbiont, can cross-colonize several mosquito species and is readily transformed and cultured. This property of *Pantoea* has been proposed for paratransgenic applications [43, 44]. *Asaia* acts as an immunomodulator by producing antimicrobial peptides that interfere with the course of infection particularly its invasion to epithelial tissues and salivary gland [36]. Recent research on two *Anopheles* species *An. gambiae* and *An. coluzzii* from Ghana [45] compared the midgut microbiota of mosquitoes during rainy and dry seasons from urban and rural breeding sites using 454 pyrosequencing. The data suggested that *An. gambia*e and *An. coluzzi* do not differ significantly in their gut microenvironment. *Shewanellaceae* family was observed in both the species. Bacterial families *Enterobacteriaceae* and *Aeromonadaceae* were also associated with *Anopheles* mosquitoes. The only difference observed was among *An. gambiae* collected from the different breeding site during summer. *Aeromonas*, *Shewanella*, and *Thorsellia* were other bacterial genera with variation in abundance according to the breeding sites. This indicates that larval breeding site has a significant impact on the adult mosquito midgut composition. The presence of *Enterobacter* and *Serratia* strain in *Anopheles* mosquito gut has an antiparasitic effect on mosquito. *Enterobacteriaceae* that survived during the rainy season is found to be more in number than that of during the dry season. Two members of this family include *Enterobacter* species and *Thorsellia anopheles*. This Gram-negative *Enterobacter* can directly act on *Plasmodium falciparum* and hinders the development of the parasite. *T. anophelis* was the dominant species in the midgut of *An. gambiae*. This symbiotic association with host mosquito vector attributes to its high tolerance for mosquito midgut alkalinity. *Serratia marcescens* HB3, isolated from laboratory-reared *An. stephensi* mosquitoes, inhibits *Plasmodium* development within the mosquito midgut by interrupting ookinete invasion through the midgut epithelial cells. Phenotypic variation at the cellular and structural levels was observed and directly correlated with the ability to induce resistance against *Plasmodium* invasion [46]. The prevailing environmental conditions have a great influence on the gut microbiome and host-vector competence. One parameter is the influence of chemicals in regulating the bacterial community in mosquito gut. For example, *Pseudomonas aeruginosa* boost the larval development of *Culex quinquefasciatus* in phosphate-rich medium [47].

A part of the mosquito gut microbiota is eukaryotic microorganism such as fungi. Its position as commensal, mutualist, or pathogenic in preserving the ecological balance of mosquitoes is inevitable. During the metamorphic transition, mosquitoes are exposed to fungi in the form of mosquito larvae in water, or by ingestion of fungi in sugar meals, or physical contact with conidia (adult mosquitoes) [48]. Filamentous fungi and yeast are the common fungal isolates present in the midgut and other tissues of mosquitoes. A filamentous fungus comprises some species of *Aspergillus* and *Penicillium* as pathogenic forms and some genera of fungi such as *Beauveria* and *Metarhizium* as entomopathogenic forms [49]. Different genera of yeast such as *Candida*, *Pichia*, and *Wickerhamomyces* have been identified in *Aedes* and *Anopheles* mosquitoes through culture-dependent and culture-independent methods. Earlier explorations in mosquito fungi diversity were based on these types of the culture-dependent method. For example, a yeast strain *Wickerhamomyces anomalus* has been reported in the midgut and reproductive organ of *An. stephensi*, a primary vector of malaria [50]. Recently, with the advent of high-throughput sequencing (HTS) technique, the knowledge about mosquito mycobiome has widened [51]. This HTS approach has been used to analyze the mycobiome formation in *Ae. triseriatus*, from the Japanese E. The series documented the presence of 21 distinct taxonomic fungal operating units (OTUs), of which 15 were identified by both parties. Ascomycota phylum is the major fungal taxa among these two *Aedes* species. Although the existence of mycobiome in mosquito is evident, the tripartite connection between vector, pathogen, and fungus is less known. Hence, there are enough evidences of the fungi present in mosquitoes. These eukaryotic organisms are responsible for the masking of many signals in the organisms.

Mosquito acts as an exclusive host for a large group of viruses, which are insect-specific. A metagenomic approach was used to evaluate viral load in two genera of mosquitoes *Aedes* and Culex. The comparison presented a striking difference in the virome of mosquitoes, where in genus *Aedes* showed a low viral diversity and less abundance than *Culex*. This metagenomic approach led to the identification/discovery of different viral families in mosquitoes such as *Bunyaviridae, Rhabdoviridae, Orthomyxoviridae, Flaviviridae, Mesoviridae, Reoviridae*, unclassified *Chuvirus*, and *Negevirus* groups. Most resident virome acts as commensal microbe due to its inability to infect vertebrate cell lines, prolonged host infection, and vertical transmission [52–54].

3.4 Microbes influence on host vector property

Vectorial capacity is a quantitative measure of several factors such as cellular, biochemical, behavioral, immunological, genetic, and environmental parameters, which can influence vector density, longevity, and vector competence. All these factors are interrelated and can determine the pathogenicity and nonpathogenicity in mosquitoes. *Acetobacteria*, a dominant member of gut microflora, may interact directly or indirectly with invading pathogens. The indirect interaction is by activating innate immune response. Usually pattern recognition receptors (PRRSs) on the host cell recognize preserved surface determinants known as pathogen-associated molecular patterns (PAMPs) that are present/found in microbes exclusively. Such linking activates immune signaling mechanisms such as the road toll or the route to immune deficiency (IMD). A cascade of events leads to the degradation of IF ranging from transcription factor (Cactus), nuclear translocation of NF—ranging from transcription factors (Dif and Dorsal) to antimicrobial peptide (AMP) genes being expressed, in the toll cell signaling pathway. This AMP, produced in the fat body, is secreted into hemolymph where it directly kills the invading microorganism. Genetic research showed that the AMP gene expressions are mainly regulated through the toll pathway and the IMD pathway. The toll pathway is mainly activated by Gram-positive bacteria, human *P. falciparum*, and DENV. The development of Gram-negative bacteria stimulates the IMD pathway, which regulates the antibacterial peptide gene [55–57].

3.5 Applications of microbiome of insects

Microbiome study in the last few decades has led to an understanding of the potential microbial functions. The few examples of which are as follows:

3.5.1 Cellulose and xylan hydrolysis

Termites belong to an extremely successful class of organisms that degrade wood, and they are considered as the potential catalytic sources for efforts aimed to convert wood into biofuels. Researchers have reported the presence of a huge, diverse set of cellulose and xylan-hydrolyzing bacterial genes through the metagenomic and genomic analysis of the communities of bacteria residing in the hindgut of higher wood-feeding *Nasutitermes* species. They have identified a number of previously uncharacterized protein families. Thus, degradation of lignocellulose does not occur by a single enzyme but due to the interaction of many macromolecular complexes that lead to its degradation. These macromolecular complexes have been termed as cellulosomes and are partially known in several microbes. The cellulose degradation of termite was long thought to rely only on microbial gut symbionts. More recently, cellulase gene transcripts have been identified from the termite itself. Similarly, three xylanases genes have been discovered from lepidopteran intestinal tract samples, and one from termite sample. The digestome of the insect gut comprising microbial as well as termite coded enzymes acts together to bring out the complete digestion of lignocelluloses. Many microbes have been identified and play important roles in the conversion of wood into a biofuel, such as ethanol, because of its potential for at least partially replacing fossil fuels in transportation and thereby lowering greenhouse gas emissions.

3.5.2 Vitamin production

The sequencing of genome of *Wigglesworthia* sp., the mycetocyte symbiont of *Glossina brevipalpis*, has been done and the annotation has shown the presence of encoded genes for the formation of thiamin (Vitamin B1), pantothenate (Vitamin B5), riboflavin FAD (Vitamin B2), nicotinamide (Vitamin B3), pyridoxine (Vitamin B6), biotin (Vitamin B7), and folate (Vitamin B9).

3.5.3 Phenolics metabolism and nitrogen fixation

Insects can absorb the atmospheric nitrogen only through the symbiotic association with gut-associated bacteria because the ability to fix nitrogen is widely available among bacteria but apparently absent from all eukaryotes. Nitrogen-fixing *Enterobacter* species have been isolated from the southern pine beetle, which together with some fungal associates may concentrate nitrogen on developing larvae. *Rahnella aquatilis*, *Klebsiella* species, and *Pantoea* species were commonly found in southern pine beetle, and the pine beetle (*Dendroctonus frontalis*) larvae are known to fix nitrogen in other environments. Another important role might be detoxification of conifer defensive compounds, which consists primarily of monoterpenes, diterpenes, and phenolics groups known to be metabolized by bacteria.

3.5.4 Antibiotic resistance

It has been reported in a study that microbial community of gypsy moth midgut shelters genes of hitherto unknown antibiotic resistance. For example, a new group of enzymes beta lactamase was identified from midgut metagenome of gypsy moth. The genes encoding these enzymes were found to be responsible for creating antibiotic resistance in *E. coli*, showing that insects may play some role in propagating resistance genes against important antibiotics.

3.5.5 Signal mimics

Microbes produce metabolites with diverse chemical feature and biological activities. Signal molecules have been reported from the uncultured microbial world through insect gut metagenomics. A study applied the matrix screen to a metagenomic library constructed from the microorganism associated with midgut of gypsy moth. They have reported the identification of a metagenomic clone of gypsy moth midgut microbiomes that produce inducers of quorum sensing and that are chemically different from the earlier quorum sensing inducers. The clone harbored the gene coding for monooxygenase homologue that mediates a pathway of indole oxidation, which resulted in the production of a quorum-sensing compound.

Impact of microbiota on mosquitoes plays critical roles in many mosquito biology processes including feeding, digestion, matting and sexual reproduction, development, immune response, and refractory pathogeny [58].

3.6 Impact of microbiota on mosquito physiology

Scientists have compared transcriptome between septic and aseptic adult female mosquitoes fed various diets and observed that microbiota stimulates some genes involved in digestion and metabolic processes such as glycolysis, gluconeogenesis, and sugar transport. Midgut microbiota, most especially *Enterobacter sp*. in *Ae. aegypti* and *Serratia* sp., have hemolytic activity that can contribute to lysis of the red blood cells (RBCs) and hemoglobin release. Antibiotic treatment of female mosquitoes reduced RBC lysis and egg production within *Ae. aegypti*. Yet not every bacterium supports the growth of the eggs. Various bacterial genera have been used to construct adult mosquitoes that have evolved from gnotobiotic larvae. Tests were carried out on five bacteria (*Aquitalea, Sphingobacterium, Chryseobacterium, Paenibacillus*, and *Comamonas*) that helped with egg development in *Ae. aegypti*. It was observed that *Ae. atropalpus* only was helped by *Comamonas* in the development of eggs [58].

3.7 Metabolic detoxification of insecticides

Three major metabolic gene families are being involved in the mechanism of the detoxification of insecticides in mosquitoes: esterases, cytochrome P450s (P450s), and the S-transferases (GSTs) glutathione. Cytochrome P450s are among those genes families that have the most significant role in both biochemical and the physiological functions of the living organisms. Cytochrome P450s are the most critical and significant to detoxify and also to activate the endogenous compounds as well as the xenobiotics [59]. The largest quantity of the exogenous as well as the endogenous compounds in the metabolic detoxification and the excretion are GSTs, which are dimeric proteins having the property of the solubilization [60–62]. An important property of the GSTs and the P450s is the upregulation at the transcriptional level, which in turn results in the formation of excessive production of proteins; hence, excessive enzymatic activity is being done. Moreover, it also increases the detoxification of the insecticides and toxins of plants with oxidation of compounds, in the insects, and this further leads to the tolerance of these chemical compounds. It was also stated that the production of the resistance against the insecticides required that genes encoding P450s be amplified/duplicated. A large number of organisms have a variety of esterase enzymes being a heterogeneous community of enzymes. The overproduction of these enzymes has been studied extensively as the amplification, and non-frequent overexpression of the genes of esterase enzymes has been proven to have increased detoxifying protein production [63–73].

Researchers have done the comparison of the toxicity level with or without the synergists and conclude that these enzymes are related to detoxification mechanisms in resistance development. In same way, research on resistance to pyrethroids in various species of mosquitoes strongly supports the importance of mitochondrial detoxification in insecticide resistance. Nonetheless, the findings of synergistic studies must be interpreted with caution: while in many cases the use of synergists can correctly indicate the role of detoxification proteins in insecticide resistance, in some cases synergists may be imperfect inhibitors for some of the detoxification enzymes induced by the resistance. Further work is required to support the synergistic study's findings. Metabolic enzyme activity assays are alternative and separate diagnostic tool for detecting the possible involvement of a metabolic enzyme in resistance is to assess elevated levels of enzyme activity and/or an increase in insecticidal metabolism. For permithrin-resistant Cx, the metabolism of permithrin to 4-hydroxypermethrin by microsomal P450 monooxygenases was stated to be significantly greater. *Quinquefasciatus* mosquitoes than vulnerable counterparts thereof [74–80]. Elevated levels of cytochrome P450 monooxygenase, esterase, or GST activities in insecticide-resistant mosquitoes of several species have also been reported; these include *An. albimanus*, *An. gambiae*, *An. stephensi*, *An. funestus*, *Ae. aegypti*, *An. culicifacies*, *Anopheles annularis* [81–85]. Although these types of measurements suggest the critical function of metabolic enzymes in the production of resistance. No specific evidence is available to determine the performance of the metabolic enzymes. Initiation of individual metabolic gene/protein characterization cloning, sequencing of partial or full-length individual metabolic genes, purification of individual metabolic proteins, and screening of resistant mosquito-resistant cDNA libraries have helped to understand the molecular basis of metabolic-detoxification-mediated resistance. This area has been extensively studied in the 20 years since the publication of the first report on 17 partial CYP4 gene sequences from *An. albimanus*. After this, it was followed by the first full-length CYP6E1 sequence from *Cx. quinquefasciatus*, which was calculated using techniques for reaction of the polymerase chain. The availability of individual partial or complete sequences has allowed researchers to identify gene expression and amplification and protein expression. These findings reveal significant details about the metabolic enzyme characteristics associated with increased metabolic detoxification of insecticides in resistant mosquitoes via transcriptional up regulation/DNA amplification. Several P450 genes, including P450 genes from deltamethrin-resistant *Anopheles minimus*, pyrethroid-resistant, have been individually reported to be overexpressed in resistant mosquito species/strains. *Funestus*, Cx-resistant to permithrin *Quinquefasciatus* and Cx-resistant to deltamethrin *Pippiens pallens*. Along with same methodologies, the overregulation of the GST genes especially GSTE-2 was being identified in the mosquito resistant to the DDT, which is *An. gambiae*. And, the findings suggest that the overproduction of the esterase genes can help the amplification of GST genes in the mosquito *Cx. quinquefasciatus*. Certainly, there are a lot of studies that suggest the duplication and amplification of the detoxifying genes. It is very critical in the insecticide resistance phenomenon related to bacteria, since not a single gene analysis shows the complete complexity of this process. It is not clear that how so many of these genes are responsible for the detoxification directly or indirectly in mosquitoes species and what are the methods with which these genes are upregulated. There is no pathway that is completely showing the role in insecticide resistance [86–92].

3.8 Methods to study microbiota of insects

Insect's gut descends from the mouth to anus and is one of the largest organs in insect body. The major microbiome community is present in the insects' gut. Thus, it is very important to carefully isolate the insects' gut microbiota. For this purpose, no specific technique has been standardized up till now. Firstly, we have to carefully disinfect the insects' body by a disinfecting buffer and make dissection to obtain the complete gut. The insects' gut can be separated into three parts, i.e., fore gut, mid gut, and hind gut. After the collection of each part, it is treated with extraction buffer, and metagenomics DNA extraction is made. Cell lysis is a critical step in metagenomics

DNA extraction; thus it is carried out with the help of gentle means such as lysis enzymes. The gut cells are lysed and the remaining gut microbial cellular community is washed. For this purpose, mechanical lysis can also be made like homogenization, bead beating, and shocks to attain complete lysis [93].

3.9 Cultivation of obtained microbiome on the culture

The obtained gut sample is then suspended in saline, phosphate buffers, and then serially diluted to get cultured on the suitable growth medium. The culturing plates are then kept in incubator for 48 h. After this the morphological characteristics are carried for the characterization of bacterial colonies with at least three dilutions. Subsequently, enzyme activities are studied by gene coding for enzymes are cloned and DNA is sequenced for genomic libraries. The cultivated bacteria are then obtained and then used for the DNA extraction. Subsequently, enzyme activities are studied by gene coding for enzymes are cloned and DNA is sequenced for genomic libraries [94].

3.10 Accessing total genome of microbiota

It is not yet universally accepted literature published for the extraction of metagenomics DNA from insects. The major goal is to access unbiased microbial genome of whole communities along with the contamination and degradation of the genome should be taken under consideration. In the DNA isolation the sheering or DNA damage should be taken with care so that the DNA with high molecular weight can be obtained, which can then be used to create DNA libraries through BAC vectors. The DNA should be free from downstream of the applications such as cloning and PCR so, for this purpose no macromolecules should be attached to DNA [95].

3.11 Specified gene enrichment in DNA

Genes are the functional units, they control the phenotypes of a particular organism. For the quest of specific function, gene enrichment technique is used, which in return increases the efficiency of cloning prospective and also leads to the discovery of uncharacterized genes from a microbial community. The typical methods for the enrichment are to control the environment of the community by exposing them to pressure, temperature, pH, light, or electric shock. This in return controls the phenotype of the genes. The enrichment techniques include suppressive subtractive hybridization phage display and affinity capture [96, 97].

3.12 Whole-genome sequence analysis

With the emergence of the field of genomics techniques in the last decade, the studies about the insecticide resistance have been revolutionized. With the help of the WGS analysis of the mosquitoes, mainly *Ae. aegypti*, *An. gambiae*, *Cx. quinquefasciatus*, and the *An. darlingi*, is one of the major achievements, which have boosted the development of the high-throughput analysis through the genomic studies. Also have enhanced the knowledge of the basic and most critical biological processes, which are responsible for this resistance of the insecticides in the mosquitoes. Furthermore, these high-throughput techniques guarantee the most novel and innovative approaches for the control of the mosquitoes as the vector and hence reducing the mosquito borne-disease on the global scale. The collective data on the EST known as expressed sequence tags and some of the most very known and easily accessible techniques such as NGS (Next-Generation Sequencing), oligonucleotide microarray, applied quantitative trait loci analysis, and suppression subtractive hybridization have the most significant impact on the studies related to the expression. These expression analysis has a very significant role in making a new perspective of the role of the genes in insecticide resistance on the genomic level. These high-throughput techniques allow the researchers to study the mechanism of the insecticide resistance on the whole-genome level. Also very highly complex biological pathways have been developed with the help of the whole-genome investigation of the mosquitoes. With the help of the analysis of the genome, we have found enough knowledge on the complexities of the presence of the genes inside the genome of mosquitoes, which in turn detoxifies the insecticides in the mosquito populations. Some examples are 31 GSTs, 51 esterases, and 111 P450s sequences of genes in the mosquito belonging to *An. gambiae*. Also, 26 GSTs, 49 esterases, and 160 P450 sequences of genes in the mosquito belonging to *Ae. aegypti* [89]. And 35 GSTs, 71 esterases, and 204 P450 genes sequences in the *Cx. quinquefasciatus*. Lastly, 30 GSTs, 20 esterases, and 89 of P450s sequences of genes in *An. Darlingi* [98–105].

For itself, the cover interaction/expression relationship among the detoxification at the metabolic level and the multiple of the genes involved in detoxification have been shown in multiple genera of mosquitoes. There is evidence in which the DDT and pyrethroids resistance include genes such as GSTs genes, P450 genes which were overexpressing in the species of *Anopheles gambiae*, *Ae. Aegypti*, and *Anopheles funestus*. This has been explored in species resistant to DDT and pyrethroids, including multiple P450 and GST genes that are overexpressed or that interact in DDT/pyrethroid-resistant in *An. gambiae*, pyrethroid-resistant *An. funestus*, pyrethroid-resistant, *Ae. aegypti*. Also, multiple P450 genes that are overexpressed in DDT and pyrethroid-resistant *Ae. aegypti* and pyrethroid-resistant *An. gambiae*. Collectively, with the help of these explorations, it is widely accepted that there are various genes that are regulating and interacting in the mechanism of the resistance in the mosquitoes. With high-throughput technologies, the researchers understand the expressing genes involved in insecticide resistance. With the help of novel technique of SSH/cDNA, Liu et al. discovered 22 new genes, which were overexpressing in the *Cx. quinquefasciatus* for the pyrethroid resistance. The genes for P450 were 2 in number, for EST genes, 20 new genes were described and all of these genes were responsible for the transduction of the signal in insecticides resistance. Likewise, another high-throughput technique known as EST/cDNA microarray analysis has been revealing the overexpression of the genes responsible for the DDT resistance. Some of these genes belong to those species not already studied and they were directly involved in the mechanism of the resistance. Some of these genes encoding calcium/sodium, peptidases and lipid/carbohydrates metabolism. The genes involved in the detoxification with the help of metabolism and some other genes, which are identified newly, have been proven to have a very significant role in the resistance against insecticides, and the relationship among the phenotype of resistance and the overexpression of the genes, thought to have the most significant role, is yet not clear [106–117].

Numerous strategies have been used for the validation of the overexpression of the genes and the resistance phenotype, to analyze the exact phenomenon of the resistance in the mosquitoes. These strategies include the in vitro protein metabolism assay, in vivo silencing of genes with the help of the RNAi techniques and also the modeling, these techniques are opted as they can fill up the gap between the conventional proteomics and genomics and the novel area of the field named as functional genomics. The in vitro functional studies and the in silico presentation functional validation are being done for the confirmation of the theory that overexpressed genes are involved in the metabolization of the insecticides in the mosquitoes or not, this is very important to determine as it will narrow down the number and names of genes, which are actually involved in the insecticide resistance. Mitchell et al. have performed a functional study on the DDTs metabolism with the help of the *An. gambiae* P450 reductase and recombinant CYP6M2. Same studies have also been done for the assessment of the abilities of the recombinant CYP6M2 from the mosquitoes *An. gambiae* is used for the metabolism of pyrethroids and the *An. funestus* have the recombinant CYP6P9a and CYP6P9b. In an insect-baculovirus expression system, CYP6Z1 of *An. gambiae* and CYP6P7 and CYP6AA3 in *An. minimus* are capable of metabolizing DDT and pyrethroids, respectively. In silico 3-D homology modeling and molecular docking of metabolic enzyme substrate interactions are new and effective tools for understanding the relationship between protein structures and substrates, which can provide reasonable explanations for substrate specificities and differences in metabolism. Six regions of P450 proteins, designated substrate-recognition sites (SRS1 6; 46), contribute to the function of P450s, with SRS1, SRS4, SRS5, and SRS6 involved in the formation of catalytic sites and SRS2 and SRS3 participating in substrate access channel configuration. With this new computer modeling system to complement highly complex functional metabolism studies, researchers can now confidently state that several mosquito P450s, including CYP6Z1, CYP6AA3, CYP6P7, and CYP6M2, are important in insecticide resistance. This approach explains both how the molecular structures (proteins and chemicals) interact and how changes in the insect's metabolism are caused by allelic variation [118–121].

3.13 Metagenomics expression libraries

On the basis of functional genes, metagenomics libraries are made by the help cloning vectors and the gene expressions are observed by functional assays. These gene expressions are then stored in metagenomics databases to help the researcher to access the previously unknown/uncharacterized genes. Furthermore, the characteristics of functional gene such as enzyme activities are expressed with a proficient vector. Heterologous expression of a gene in the host cells is impeded by various steps such as transcription, translation, and posttranslational process or maturation. Few metagenomics expression data of genes, which are isolated from the functional expression library technique, are listed in **Table 1**.

3.14 Metagenomic analysis of microbiomes

16S rRNA sequencing became the standard and normal method of determining the structure of a human microbiome population. The V1V3 and V3V5 regions of the hypervariable 16S rRNA gene help to distinguish the taxonomic structure of different bacterial species. To study the composition of microbiota, researchers categorize this gene into Operational Taxonomic Unit (OTU). Sanger sequencing was the primary instrument for sampling the entire amplicon range (16S rDNA). However, people discovered that species diversity can be classified utilizing shorter DNA stretches with higher sequence coverage and thus the developments of NGS, i.e., Roche 454 pyrosequencing, Illumina, and Ion Torrent sequencing are also used

Sr. no.	Insect source	Enzyme/gene	Potential application	Reference
1.	*Reticulitermes flavipes*	RfBGluc-1 beta-glucosidase	Digestion of lignocellulose	[122]
2.	*Rotschildia lebaeu* (Lepidoptera)	Xylanase	Degradation of xylane	[123]
3.	Termites (Nasutitermitidae)	Endo-1, 4-xylanase	Degradation of xylane	[124]
4.	*Nasutitermes ephratae*	Glycosyl hydrolase	Digestion of lignocellulose	[125]

Table 1.
Examples of insect's source with their enzymes and genes isolated by the metagenomics functional expression analysis.

for the meta-genomic sequencing. Numerous analytical methods for studying the 16S rRNA sequences of microbes were also developed later to better understand their biology in the microbials. Nonetheless, even though we have strong coverage and longer sequencing reads using 16S rRNA sequencing, it would still be challenging to access the genomic details of low-abundance species. Therefore, recent work has moved to the use of high-throughput data techniques to develop both the qualitative and quantitative microbiome DNA information, mRNA transcripts, metabolites, and microbial community proteins. Metagenomic methods will help give a more detailed functional view of microorganisms and their functions within the microbiome. Shotgun metagenomic sequencing was the first step in this direction in which the whole genomic DNA of human/environmental bacteria samples were analyzed with a view to identifying all species and recognizing the microbe's gene function potential. Another example is the HMP Unified Metabolic Analysis Network (HUMAnN), which performs metabolic and functional metagenomic data reconstructions [126]. This technique was performed on 102 individuals at seven key locations in the human body, namely diarrhea, dorsal tongue, and anterior nares. For various sites, they established the main metabolic pathways, genes, and functional modules that were distinct across individuals. Glycosaminoglycan degradation, phosphate and amino acid transport within this microbiota have been shown to be more involved in the vaginal microbiome; these methods have also been applied for insect's microbiome. Computational modeling strategies such as metabolic genome scale models (GEMs) have been developed to integrate and interpret data for research purpose based on the increased experimental data produced by the high-throughput strategies. Throughout recent years, meta-omics results are used on a genome scale throughout tandem with metabolic models (GEMs). The genome size of metabolic models and metagenomic data were taken as feedback by using MAMBO (Metabolomic Analysis of Metagenomes using fBa and Optimization). The use of in vitro, ex vivo, and in situ laboratory evidence with in silico models serves as an outstanding testing tool for the discovery in human microbiomes of the elusive microbial microbe–microbe and microbe–host relationships that suggest major therapeutic progresses. Each of the respective omic data types provides useful knowledge in characterizing the organism's working, and certain data types are incorporated more directly into the modeling formalism than others. For example, Vanee et al. used a proteomics-derived model to describe the *Thermobifida fusca* microbe's metabolism functionalities where the growth rates seen in experimental and silico results were almost similar [127].

3.15 Homology-based analysis of metagenome sequenced DNA

Compared with functional/expression analysis, homology-based metagenomics are more precise as they target the gene on the basis of the data present and existing conserved genomics databases. Sequence-based screening methods depend on the existing conserved sequences and hence, may not help to identify brand new nonhomologous enzymes [128]. The sequence-based search combined with powerful bioinformatics tools has led to a higher rate of identification of novel genes than function-based methods do. Bioinformatics tools for sequence mining have been developed, based not only on homology of the primary sequence but also on the predicted protein structures. Gene function can be predicted with the improvement of the protein sorting and modeling tools, the putative active sites. Some tools of gene finding such as MetaGene has been used in order to predict 90% of shotgun sequences [129]. Many recent publications identify metagenome sequence databases that look for genes and enzymes that would be useful for commercial development in prospecting. For example, 71 million base pairs of sequence data were created by sequencing a metagenome library of hindgut microbiota from the largest family of wood-feeding termites. By detecting complete domains using global alignment, over 700 homologous domains of the glycoside hydrolase catalytic site corresponding to 45 different carbohydrate active enzyme families were identified, including a rich diversity of putative cellulases and hemicellulases [130].

3.16 Insecticide resistance

Numerous studies have shown that the individual mosquito species are involved in multiple mechanisms of resistance. In particular, two mechanisms increased metabolic detoxification of insecticides and reduced target protein sensitivity, which is the most critical target of insecticide. The insensitivity of the target site has been studied very extensively and has been accepted due to its extreme importance. The relationship between the genes related to the resistance on the regulation level of genes has provided with a very excellent example showing that how precisely these resistances develop in the insects. In the coding region, the overexpression and the amplification of mutant result in the structural differences inside the proteins and are linked with the resistance of the insecticides in the populations of mosquitoes. The overexpression at the transcriptional level of these genes shows resistance to the insecticides in mosquitoes. Collectively it is very easy for the researchers to conclude that these resistances are not only being transmitted from one generation to the other, but also it is being regulated at gene level. It is not yet clear which genes are directly or indirectly involved in the resistance and also how many are involved in the phenomenon [131–137].

Author details

Sahar Fazal[1], Rabbiah Manzoor Malik[1,2*], Ahmad Zafar Baig[1], Narjis Khatoon[1], Huma Aslam[1], Aiza Zafar[1] and Muneeba Ishtiaq[1]

1 Capital University of Science and Technology, Islamabad, Pakistan

2 Wah Medical College, Wah Cantt, Pakistan

*Address all correspondence to: rabbiahmanzoor@gmail.com

References

[1] Tolle MA. Mosquito-borne diseases. Current Problems in Pediatric and Adolescent Health Care. 2009;**39**:97-140

[2] Zhao Y, Zhang X, Shu S, Sun Y, Feng X, Zhang S. Yellow Fever: A Re-Emerging Threat. Health, 2018;**10**:1431-1448. DOI: 10.4236/health.2018.1010110

[3] Harbach RE, Howard TM. Index of currently recognized mosquito species (diptera: Culicidae). European Mosquito Bulletin. 2007;**23**:1-66

[4] Becker N, Petric D, Zgomba M, Boase C, Madon M, Dahl C, et al. Mosquitoes and Their Control. Switzerland, AG: Springer Science & Business Media; 2010

[5] Depoortere E, Salmaso S, Pompa M, Guglielmetti P, Coulombier D. Chikungunya in Europe. Lancet. 2008;**371**:723

[6] Ashfaq M, Hebert PD, Mirza JH, Khan AM, Zafar Y, Mirza MS. Analyzing mosquito (diptera: Culicidae) diversity in Pakistan by dna barcoding. PLoS One. 2014;**9**:e97268

[7] Alonso P, Noor AM. The global fight against malaria is at cross roads. The Lancet. 2017;**390**:2532-2534

[8] W. H. Organization. Global report on insecticide resistance in malaria vectors: 2010-2016. World Health Organization; 2018

[9] Quiñones ML, Norris DE, Conn JE, Moreno M, Burkot TR, Bugoro H, et al. Insecticide resistance in areas under investigation by the international centers of excellence for malaria research: A challenge for malaria control and elimination. The American Journal of Tropical Medicine and Hygiene. 2015;**93**:69-78

[10] Riveron JM, Tchouakui M, Mugenzi L, Menze BD, Chiang M-C, Wondji CS. Insecticide resistance in malaria vectors: An update at a global scale. In: Towards Malaria Elimination—A Leap Forward. London, United Kingdom: IntechOpen; 2018

[11] Guégan M, Zouache K, Démichel C, Minard G, Potier P, Mavingui P, et al. The mosquito holobiont: Fresh insight into mosquito–microbiota interactions. Microbiome. 2018;**6**:1-17

[12] Coon KL, Vogel KJ, Brown MR, Strand MR. Mosquitoes rely on their gut microbiota for development. Molecular Ecology. 2014;**23**:2727-2739

[13] Lindh J, Borg-Karlson A-K, Faye I. Transstadial and horizontal transfer of bacteria within a colony of *Anopheles gambiae* (diptera: Culicidae) and oviposition response to bacteria-containing water. Acta Tropica. 2008;**107**:242-250

[14] Barr AR, Al-Azawi A. Notes on Oviposition and the Hatching of Eggs of *Aedes* and *Psorophora* mosquitoes (Diptera: Culicidae). University of Kansas; 1953

[15] Clements AN et al. The Biology of Mosquitoes: Development, Nutrition and Reproduction. Vol. 1. London: Chapman & Hall; 1992

[16] Becker N, Zgomba M, Petric D, Ludwig M. Comparison of carbon dioxide, octenol and a host-odour as mosquito attractants in the upper rhine valley, Germany. Medical and Veterinary Entomology. 1995;**9**:377-380

[17] Minard G, Mavingui P, Moro CV. Diversity and function of bacterial microbiota in the mosquito holobiont. Parasites & Vectors. 2013;**6**:1-12

[18] Kikuchi Y, Hayatsu M, Hosokawa T, Nagayama A, Tago K, Fukatsu T. Symbiont-mediated insecticide resistance. Proceedings of the National Academy of Sciences. 2012;**109**:8618-8622

[19] Xia X, Sun B, Gurr GM, Vasseur L, Xue M, You M. Gut microbiota mediate insecticide resistance in the diamondback moth, *Plutella xylostella* (l.). Frontiers in Microbiology. 2018;**9**:25

[20] Xia X, Zheng D, Zhong H, Qin B, Gurr GM, Vasseur L, et al. Dna sequencing reveals the midgut microbiota of diamondback moth, *Plutella xylostella* (l.) and a possible relationship with insecticide resistance. PLoS ONE. 2013;**8**:e68852

[21] Itoh H, Tago K, Hayatsu M, Kikuchi Y. Detoxifying symbiosis: Microbe-mediated detoxification of phytotoxins and pesticides in insects. Natural Product Reports. 2018;**35**:434-454

[22] Dada N, Sheth M, Liebman K, Pinto J, Lenhart A. Whole metagenome sequencing reveals links between mosquito microbiota and insecticide resistance in malaria vectors. Scientific Reports. 2018;**8**:1-13

[23] Soltani A, Vatandoost H, Oshaghi MA, Enayati AA, Chavshin AR. The role of midgut symbiotic bacteria in resistance of *Anopheles stephensi* (diptera: Culicidae) to organophosphate insecticides. Pathogens and Global Health. 2017;**111**:289-296

[24] Mohrig W. Die culiciden deutschlands. Anzeiger für Schådlingskunde. 1969;**42**:126-127

[25] Kettle D. Medical and Veterinary Entomology. Wallingford, UK: Cab International; 1995

[26] Woodring J, Davidson E. Biological control of mosquitoes. In: The Biology of Disease Vectors. Colorado: University Press of Colorado; 1996. pp. 530-548

[27] Lehane M. Managing the blood meal. In: Biology of Blood-Sucking Insects. New York: Published in the United States of America by Cambridge University Press; 2005. pp. 84-96

[28] Bruce-Chwatt LJ, De Zulueta J, et al. The Rise and Fall of Malaria in Europe: A Historico-Epidemiological Study. Newyork: Published for the Regional Office for Europe of the World Health Organization; 1980

[29] Wang S, Dos-Santos AL, Huang W, Liu KC, Oshaghi MA, Wei G, et al. Driving mosquito refractoriness to *Plasmodium falciparum* with engineered symbiotic bacteria. Science. 2017;**357**:1399-1402

[30] Strand MR. Composition and functional roles of the gut microbiota in mosquitoes. Current Opinion in Insect Science. 2018;**28**:59-65

[31] Pidiyar VJ, Jangid K, Patole MS, Shouche YS. Studies on cultured and uncultured microbiota of wild *Culex quinquefasciatus* mosquito midgut based on 16S ribosomal rna gene analysis. The American Journal of Tropical Medicine and Hygiene. 2004;**70**:597-603

[32] Zouache K, Raharimalala FN, Raquin V, Tran-Van V, Raveloson LHR, Ravelonandro P, et al. Bacterial diversity of field-caught mosquitoes, *Aedes albopictus* and *Aedes aegypti*, from different geographic regions of Madagascar. FEMS Microbiology Ecology. 2011;**75**:377-389

[33] Noden BH, Vaughan JA, Pumpuni CB, Beier JC. Mosquito ingestion of antibodies against mosquito midgut microbiota

improves conversion of ookinetes to oocysts for *Plasmodium falciparum*, but not *P. yoelii*. Parasitology International. 2011;**60**:440-446

[34] Molloy JC, Sinkins SP. Wolbachia do not induce reactive oxygen species-dependent immune pathway activation in *Aedes albopictus*. Viruses. 2015;**7**:4624-4639

[35] Gusmão DS, Santos AV, Marini DC, Bacci M Jr, Molina MAB, Lemos FJA. Culture-dependent and culture-independent characterization of microorganisms associated with *Aedes aegypti* (diptera: Culicidae) (l.) and dynamics of bacterial colonization in the midgut. Acta Tropica. 2010;**115**:275-281

[36] Chavshin AR, Oshaghi MA, Vatandoost H, Pourmand MR, Raeisi A, Enayati AA, et al. Malpighian tubules are important determinants of *Pseudomonas* transstadial transmission and longtime persistence in *Anopheles stephensi*. Parasites & Vectors. 2015;**8**:1-7

[37] Pumpuni CB, Demaio J, Kent M, Davis JR, Beier JC. Bacterial population dynamics in three anopheline species: The impact on *Plasmodium* sporogonic development. The American Journal of Tropical Medicine and Hygiene. 1996;**54**:214-218

[38] Briones AM, Shililu J, Githure J, Novak R, Raskin L. *Thorsellia anophelis* is the dominant bacterium in a Kenyan population of adult *Anopheles gambiae* mosquitoes. The ISME Journal. 2008;**2**:74-82

[39] Chavshin AR, Oshaghi MA, Vatandoost H, Pourmand MR, Raeisi A, Enayati AA, et al. Identification of bacterial microflora in the midgut of the larvae and adult of wild caught *Anopheles stephensi*: A step toward finding suitable paratransgenesis candidates. Acta Tropica. 2012;**121**:129-134

[40] Kumar S, Molina-Cruz A, Gupta L, Rodrigues J, Barillas-Mury C. A peroxidase/dual oxidase system modulates midgut epithelial immunity in *Anopheles gambiae*. Science. 2010;**327**:1644-1648

[41] Howland LJ. Bionomical investigation of English mosquito larvae with special reference to their algal food. The Journal of Ecology. 1930:81-125

[42] Coggeshall LT et al. Relationship of plankton to anopheline larvae. American Journal of Hygiene. 1926;**6**(4):556-559

[43] Bisi DC, Lampe DJ. Secretion of anti-*Plasmodium* effector proteins from a natural *Pantoea agglomerans* isolate by using PelB and HlyA secretion signals. Applied and Environmental Microbiology. 2011;**77**:4669-4675

[44] Djadid ND, Jazayeri H, Raz A, Favia G, Ricci I, Zakeri S. Identification of the midgut microbiota of *An. stephensi* and *An. maculipennis* for their application as a paratransgenic tool against malaria. PLoS ONE. 2011;**6**:e28484

[45] Akorli J, Gendrin M, Pels NAP, Yeboah-Manu D, Christophides GK, Wilson MD. Seasonality and locality affect the diversity of *Anopheles gambiae* and *Anopheles coluzzii* midgut microbiota from Ghana. PLoS ONE. 2016;**11**:e0157529

[46] Bando H, Okado K, Guelbeogo WM, Badolo A, Aonuma H, Nelson B, et al. Intra-specific diversity of *Serratia marcescens* in *Anopheles* mosquito midgut defines *Plasmodium* transmission capacity. Scientific Reports. 2013;**3**:1641

[47] Peck GW, Walton WE. Effect of bacterial quality and density on growth and whole body stoichiometry of *Culex quinquefasciatus* and *Culex tarsalis* (diptera: Culicidae). Journal of Medical Entomology. 2006;**43**:25-33

[48] Lynch PA, Grimm U, Thomas MB, Read AF. Prospective malaria control using entomopathogenic fungi: Comparative evaluation of impact on transmission and selection for resistance. Malaria Journal. 2012;**11**:383

[49] Scholte E-J, Knols BG, Samson RA, Takken W. Entomopathogenic fungi for mosquito control: A review. Journal of Insect Science. 2004;**4**:19

[50] Ricci I, Damiani C, Scuppa P, Mosca M, Crotti E, Rossi P, et al. The yeast *Wickerhamomyces anomalus* (*Pichia anomala*) inhabits the midgut and reproductive system of the Asian malaria vector *Anopheles stephensi*. Environmental Microbiology. 2011;**13**:911-921

[51] Muturi EJ, Bara JJ, Rooney AP, Hansen AK. Midgut fungal and bacterial microbiota of *Aedes triseriatus* and *Aedes japonicus* shift in response to La Crosse virus infection. Molecular Ecology. 2016;**25**:4075-4090

[52] Bolling BG, Weaver SC, Tesh RB, Vasilakis N. Insect-specific virus discovery: Significance for the arbovirus community. Viruses. 2015;7:4911-4928

[53] Vasilakis N, Tesh RB. Insect-specific viruses and their potential impact on arbovirus transmission. Current Opinion in Virology. 2015;**15**:69-74

[54] Shi M, Neville P, Nicholson J, Eden J-S, Imrie A, Holmes EC. High-resolution metatranscriptomics reveals the ecological dynamics of mosquito-associated rna viruses in Western Australia. Journal of Virology. 2017;**91**

[55] Beerntsen BT, James AA, Christensen BM. Genetics of mosquito vector competence. Microbiology and Molecular Biology Reviews. 2000;**64**:115-137

[56] Kingsolver MB, Huang Z, Hardy RW. Insect antiviral innate immunity: Pathways, effectors, and connections. Journal of Molecular Biology. 2013;**425**:4921-4936

[57] Christophides GK, Vlachou D, Kafatos FC. Comparative and functional genomics of the innate immune system in the malaria vector *Anopheles gambiae*. Immunological Reviews. 2004;**198**:127-148

[58] Coon KL, Brown MR, Strand MR. Gut bacteria differentially affect egg production in the anautogenous mosquito *Aedes aegypti* and facultatively autogenous mosquito *Aedes atropalpus* (diptera: Culicidae). Parasites & Vectors. 2016;**9**:1-12

[59] Liu N. Insecticide resistance in mosquitoes: Impact, mechanisms, and research directions. Annual Review of Entomology. 2015;**60**:537-559

[60] Ketterman AJ, Saisawang C, Wongsantichon J. Insect glutathione transferases. Drug Metabolism Reviews. 2011;**43**:253-265

[61] Ranson H, Hemingway J. Mosquito glutathione transferases. Methods in Enzymology. 2005;**401**:226-241

[62] Ranson H, Rossiter L, Ortelli F, Jensen B, Wang X, Roth CW, et al. Identification of a novel class of insect glutathione s-transferases involved in resistance to DDT in the malaria vector *Anopheles gambiae*. Biochemical Journal. 2001;**359**:295-304

[63] Scott JG. Cytochromes p450 and insecticide resistance. Insect Biochemistry and Molecular Biology. 1999;**29**:757-777

[64] Rosenthal GA, Berenbaum MR. Herbivores: Their Interactions with Secondary Plant Metabolites: Ecological

and Evolutionary Processes. Vol. 2. San Diego, California: Academic Press; 2012

[65] Li X, Schuler MA, Berenbaum MR. Molecular mechanisms of metabolic resistance to synthetic and natural xenobiotics. Annual Review of Entomology. 2007;**52**:231-253

[66] Schuler MA. The role of cytochrome p450 monooxygenases in plant–insect interactions. Plant Physiology. 1996;**112**:1411

[67] Schuler MA. P450s in plant–insect interactions. Biochimica et Biophysica Acta (BBA)-Proteins and Proteomics. 2011;**1814**:36-45

[68] Kasai S, Weerashinghe IS, Shono T. P450 monooxygenases are an important mechanism of permethrin resistance in *Culex quinquefasciatus* say larvae. Archives of Insect Biochemistry and Physiology: Published in Collaboration with the Entomological Society of America. 1998;**37**:47-56

[69] Riveron JM, Irving H, Ndula M, Barnes KG, Ibrahim SS, Paine MJ, et al. Directionally selected cytochrome P450 alleles are driving the spread of pyrethroid resistance in the major malaria vector *Anopheles funestus*. Proceedings of the National Academy of Sciences. 2013;**110**:252-257

[70] Wondji CS, Irving H, Morgan J, Lobo NF, Collins FH, Hunt RH, et al. Two duplicated P450 genes are associated with pyrethroid resistance in *Anopheles funestus*, a major malaria vector. Genome Research. 2009;**19**:452-459

[71] Pasteur N, Raymond M. Insecticide resistance genes in mosquitoes: Their mutations, migration, and selection in field populations. Journal of Heredity. 1996;**87**:444-449

[72] Raymond M, Chevillon C, Guillemaud T, Lenormand T, Pasteur N. An overview of the evolution of overproduced esterases in the mosquito *Culex pipiens*. Philosophical Transactions of the Royal Society of London. Series B: Biological Sciences. 1998;**353**:1707-1711

[73] Vaughan A, Hemingway J. Mosquito carboxylesterase estα 21 (a2). Cloning and sequence of the full-length cdna for a major insecticide resistance gene worldwide in the mosquito *Culex quinquefasciatus*. Journal of Biological Chemistry. 1995;**270**:17044-17049

[74] Brogdon WG, McAllister JC, CorwinAM,Cordon-RosalesC.Independent selection of multiple mechanisms for pyrethroid resistance in guatemalan *Anopheles albimanus* (diptera: Culicidae). Journal of Economic Entomology. 1999;**92**:298-302

[75] Cuamba N, Morgan JC, Irving H, Steven A, Wondji CS. High level of pyrethroid resistance in an *Anopheles funestus* population of the Chokwe district in Mozambique. PLoS ONE. 2010;**5**:e11010

[76] Enayati AA, Vatandoost H, Ladonni H, Townson H, Hemingway J. Molecular evidence for a kdr-like pyrethroid resistance mechanism in the malaria vector mosquito *Anopheles stephensi*. Medical and Veterinary Entomology. 2003;**17**:138-144

[77] Kasai S, Shono T, Yamakawa M. Molecular cloning and nucleotide sequence of a cytochrome p450 cdna from a pyrethroid-resistant mosquito, *Culex quinquefasciatus* Say. Insect Molecular Biology. 1998;**7**:185-191

[78] Liu H, Cupp EW, Micher KM, Guo A, Liu N. Insecticide resistance and cross-resistance in Alabama and Florida strains of *Culex quinquefaciatus*. Journal of Medical Entomology. 2004;**41**:408-413

[79] McAbee RD, Kang K-D, Stanich MA, Christiansen JA, Wheelock CE, Inman AD, et al. Pyrethroid tolerance in *Culex pipiens pipiens* var *molestus* from Marin county, California. Pest Management Science: formerly Pesticide Science. 2004;**60**:359-368

[80] Xu Q, Liu H, Zhang L, Liu N. Resistance in the mosquito, *Culex quinquefasciatus*, and possible mechanisms for resistance. Pest Management Science: formerly Pesticide Science. 2005;**61**:1096-1102

[81] Vulule J, Beach R, Atieli F, McAllister J, Brogdon W, Roberts J, et al. Elevated oxidase and esterase levels associated with permethrin tolerance in *Anopheles gambiae* from Kenyan villages using permethrin-impregnated nets. Medical and Veterinary Entomology. 1999;**13**:239-244

[82] Casimiro S, Coleman M, Mohloai P, Hemingway J, Sharp B. Insecticide resistance in *Anopheles funestus* (diptera: culicidae) from Mozambique. Journal of Medical Entomology. 2014;**43**:267-275

[83] Marcombe S, Mathieu RB, Pocquet N, Riaz M-A, Poupardin R, Sélior S, et al. Insecticide resistance in the dengue vector *Aedes aegypti* from martinique: Distribution, mechanisms and relations with environmental factors. PLoS ONE. 2012;**7**:e30989

[84] Morou E, Dowd AJ, Rajatileka S, Steven A, Hemingway J, Ranson H, et al. A simple colorimetric assay for specific detection of glutathione-S transferase activity associated with DDT resistance in mosquitoes. PLoS Neglected Tropical Diseases. 2010;**4**:e808

[85] Gunasekaran K, Muthukumaravel S, Sahu S, Vijayakumar T, Jambulingam P. Glutathione S transferase activity in Indian vectors of malaria: A defense mechanism against DDT. Journal of Medical Entomology. 2011;**48**:561-569

[86] Scott JA, Collins FH, Feyereisen R. Diversty of cytochrome P450 genes in the mosquito, *Anopheles albimanus*. Biochemical and Biophysical Research Communications. 1994;**205**:1452-1459

[87] Rongnoparut P, Boonsuepsakul S, Chareonviriyaphap T, Thanomsing N. Cloning of cytochrome P450, CYP6P5, and CYP6AA2 from *Anopheles minimus* resistant to deltamethrin. Journal of Vector Ecology: Journal of the Society for Vector Ecology. 2003;**28**:150-158

[88] Amenya D, Naguran R, Lo T-C, Ranson H, Spillings B, Wood O, et al. Over expression of a cytochrome P450 (CYP6P9) in a major African malaria vector, *Anopheles funestus*, resistant to pyrethroids. Insect Molecular Biology. 2008;**17**:19-25

[89] Liu N, Li T, Reid WR, Yang T, Zhang L. Multiple cytochrome P450 genes: Their constitutive overexpression and permethrin induction in insecticide resistant mosquitoes, *Culex quinquefasciatus*. PLoS ONE. 2011;**6**:e23403

[90] Gong M-Q, Gu Y, Hu X-B, Sun Y, Ma L, Li X-L, et al. Cloning and overexpression of cyp6f1, a cytochrome P450 gene, from deltamethrin-resistant *Culex pipiens pallens*. Acta Biochimica et Biophysica Sinica. 2005;**37**:317-326

[91] Ortelli F, Rossiter LC, Vontas J, Ranson H, Hemingway J. Heterologous expression of four glutathione transferase genes genetically linked to a major insecticide-resistance locus from the malaria vector *Anopheles gambiae*. Biochemical Journal. 2003;**373**:957-963

[92] Mouches C, Pasteur N, Berge JB, Hyrien O, Raymond M, de Saint

Vincent BR, et al. Amplification of an esterase gene is responsible for insecticide resistance in a California Culex mosquito. Science. 1986;**233**:778-780

[93] Rajendhran J, Gunasekaran P. Strategies for accessing soil metagenome for desired applications. Biotechnology Advances. 2008;**26**:576-590

[94] Streit W, Bjourson A, Cooper J, Werner D. Application of subtraction hybridization for the development of a rhizobium *Leguminosarum* biovar *phaseoli* and *Rhizobium tropici* group-specific dna probe. FEMS Microbiology Ecology. 1999;**13**:59-67

[95] Shi W, Syrenne R, Sun J-Z, Yuan JS. Molecular approaches to study the insect gut symbiotic microbiota at the omics age. Insect Science. 2010;**17**:199-219

[96] Galbraith EA, Antonopoulos DA, White BA. Suppressive subtractive hybridization as a tool for identifying genetic diversity in an environmental metagenome: The rumen as a model. Environmental Microbiology. 2004;**6**:928-937

[97] Goldman E, Rosenberg AH, Zubay G, Studier WF. Consecutive low-usage leucine codons block translation only when near the 5 end of a message in *Escherichia coli*. Journal of Molecular Biology. 1995;**245**:467-473

[98] Nene V, Wortman JR, Lawson D, Haas B, Kodira C, Tu ZJ, et al. Genome sequence of *Aedes aegypti*, a major arbovirus vector. Science. 2007;**316**:1718-1723

[99] Holt RA, Subramanian GM, Halpern A, Sutton GG, Charlab R, Nusskern DR, et al. The genome sequence of the malaria mosquito *Anopheles gambiae*. Science. 2002;**298**:129-149

[100] Arensburger P, Megy K, Waterhouse RM, Abrudan J, Amedeo P, Antelo B, et al. Sequencing of *Culex quinquefasciatus* establishes a platform for mosquito comparative genomics. Science. 2010;**330**:86-88

[101] Marinotti O, Cerqueira GC, De Almeida LGP, Ferro MIT, Loreto ELdS, Zaha A, et al. The genome of *Anopheles darlingi*, the main neotropical malaria vector. Nucleic Acids Research. 2013;**41**:7387-7400

[102] Severson DW, Behura SK. Mosquito genomics: Progress and challenges. Annual Review of Entomology. 2012;**57**:143-166

[103] Ranson H, Claudianos C, Ortelli F, Abgrall C, Hemingway J, Sharakhova MV, et al. Evolution of supergene families associated with insecticide resistance. Science. 2002;**298**:179-181

[104] Strode C, Wondji CS, David J-P, Hawkes NJ, Lumjuan N, Nelson DR, et al. Genomic analysis of detoxification genes in the mosquito *Aedes aegypti*. Insect Biochemistry and Molecular Biology. 2008;**38**:113-123

[105] Yang T, Liu N. Genome analysis of cytochrome P450s and their expression profiles in insecticide resistant mosquitoes, *Culex quinquefasciatus*. PLoS ONE. 2011;**6**:e29418

[106] David J-P, Strode C, Vontas J, Nikou D, Vaughan A, Pignatelli PM, et al. The *Anopheles gambiae* detoxification chip: a highly specific microarray to study metabolic-based insecticide resistance in malaria vectors. Proceedings of the National Academy of Sciences. 2005;**102**:4080-4084

[107] Djouaka RF, Bakare AA, Coulibaly ON, Akogbeto MC, Ranson H, Hemingway J, et al. Expression of the

cytochrome P450S, CYP6P3 AND CYP6M2 are significantly elevated in multiple pyrethroid resistant populations of *Anopheles gambiae* ss. from Southern Benin and Nigeria. BMC Genomics. 2008;**9**:1-10

[108] Müller P, Donnelly MJ, Ranson H. Transcription profiling of a recently colonised pyrethroid resistant *Anopheles gambiae* strain from Ghana. BMC Genomics. 2007;**8**:36

[109] Müller P, Warr E, Stevenson BJ, Pignatelli PM, Morgan JC, Steven A, et al. Field-caught permethrin-resistant *Anopheles gambiae* overexpress CYP6P3, A P450 that metabolises pyrethroids. PLoS Genetics. 2008;**4**:e1000286

[110] Bariami V, Jones CM, Poupardin R, Vontas J, Ranson H. Gene amplification, ABC transporters and cytochrome P450s: Unraveling the molecular basis of pyrethroid resistance in the dengue vector, *Aedes aegypti*. PLoS Neglected Tropical Diseases. 2012;**6**:e1692

[111] Irving H, Riveron J, Ibrahim S, Lobo N, Wondji C. Positional cloning of rp2 QTL associates the P450 genes CYP6Z1, CYP6Z3 and CYP6M7 with pyrethroid resistance in the malaria vector *Anopheles funestus*. Heredity. 2012;**109**:383-392

[112] Nikou D, Ranson H, Hemingway J. An adult-specific CYP6 P450 gene is overexpressed in a pyrethroid-resistant strain of the malaria vector, *Anopheles gambiae*. Gene. 2003;**318**:91-102

[113] Lumjuan N, Rajatileka S, Changsom D, Wicheer J, Leelapat P, Prapanthadara L-A, et al. The role of the *Aedes aegypti* epsilon glutathione transferases in conferring resistance to DDT and pyrethroid insecticides. Insect Biochemistry and Molecular Biology. 2011;**41**:203-209

[114] Ding Y, Ortelli F, Rossiter LC, Hemingway J, Ranson H. The *Anopheles gambiae* glutathione transferase supergene family: Annotation, phylogeny and expression profiles. BMC Genomics. 2003;**4**:35

[115] Itokawa K, Komagata O, Kasai S, Okamura Y, Masada M, Tomita T. Genomic structures of Cyp9m10 in pyrethroid resistant and susceptible strains of *Culex quinquefasciatus*. Insect Biochemistry and Molecular Biology. 2010;**40**:631-640

[116] Liu N, Liu H, Zhu F, Zhang L. Differential expression of genes in pyrethroid resistant and susceptible mosquitoes, *Culex quinquefasciatus* (s.). Gene. 2007;**394**:61-68

[117] Vontas J, Blass C, Koutsos A, David J-P, Kafatos F, Louis C, et al. Gene expression in insecticide resistant and susceptible *Anopheles gambiae* strains constitutively or after insecticide exposure. Insect Molecular Biology. 2005;**14**:509-521

[118] Mitchell SN, Stevenson BJ, Müller P, Wilding CS, Egyir-Yawson A, Field SG, et al. Identification and validation of a gene causing cross-resistance between insecticide classes in *Anopheles gambiae* from Ghana. Proceedings of the National Academy of Sciences. 2012;**109**:6147-6152

[119] Stevenson BJ, Bibby J, Pignatelli P, Muangnoicharoen S, ONeill PM, Lian L-Y, et al. Cytochrome P450 6M2 from the malaria vector *Anopheles gambiae* metabolizes pyrethroids: Sequential metabolism of deltamethrin revealed. Insect Biochemistry and Molecular Biology. 2011;**41**:492-502

[120] Chiu T-L, Wen Z, Rupasinghe SG, Schuler MA. Comparative molecular modeling of *Anopheles gambiae*

CYP6Z1, a mosquito P450 capable of metabolizing DDT. Proceedings of the National Academy of Sciences. 2008;**105**:8855-8860

[121] Duangkaew P, Pethuan S, Kaewpa D, Boonsuepsakul S, Sarapusit S, Rongnoparut P. Characterization of mosquito CYP6P7 and CYP6AA3: Differences in substrate preference and kinetic properties. Archives of Insect Biochemistry and Physiology. 2011;**76**:236-248

[122] Mattiacci L, Dicke M, Posthumus MA. Beta-glucosidase: An elicitor of herbivore-induced plant odor that attracts host-searching parasitic wasps. Proceedings of the National Academy of Sciences. 1995;**92**:2036-2040

[123] Brennan CA, Anderson KV. Drosophila: The genetics of innate immune recognition and response. Annual Review of Immunology. 2004;**22**:457-483

[124] Beaugrand J, Chambat G, Wong VW, Goubet F, Rémond C, Paës G, et al. Impact and efficiency of GH10 and GH11 thermostable endoxylanases on wheat bran and alkali-extractable arabinoxylans. Carbohydrate Research. 2004;**339**:2529-2540

[125] Warnecke F, Luginbühl P, Ivanova N, Ghassemian M, Richardson TH, Stege JT, et al. Metagenomic and functional analysis of hindgut microbiota of a wood-feeding higher termite. Nature. 2007;**450**:560-565

[126] Sen P, Orešič M. Metabolic modeling of human gut microbiota on a genome scale: An overview. Metabolites. 2019;**9**:22

[127] Abubucker S, Segata N, Goll J, Schubert AM, Izard J, Cantarel BL, et al. Metabolic reconstruction for metagenomic data and its application to the human microbiome. PLoS Computational Biology. 2012;**8**:e1002358

[128] Himmel ME et al. Biomass Recalcitrance: Deconstructing the Plant Cell Wall for Bioenergy. United States of America: Wiley-Blackwell; 2009

[129] Selengut JD, Haft DH, Davidsen T, Ganapathy A, Gwinn-Giglio M, Nelson WC, et al. TIGRFAMS and genome properties: Tools for the assignment of molecular function and biological process in prokaryotic genomes. Nucleic Acids Research. 2007;**35**:D260-D264

[130] Noguchi H, Park J, Takagi T. Metagene: Prokaryotic gene finding from environmental genome shotgun sequences. Nucleic Acids Research. 2006;**34**:5623-5630

[131] Hemingway J, Field L, Vontas J. An overview of insecticide resistance. Science. 2002;**298**:96-97

[132] Li T, Liu N. Inheritance of permethrin resistance in *Culex quinquefasciatus*. Journal of Medical Entomology. 2014;**47**:1127-1134

[133] Ranson H, Nguessan R, Lines J, Moiroux N, Nkuni Z, Corbel V. Pyrethroid resistance in African anopheline mosquitoes: What are the implications for malaria control? Trends in Parasitology. 2011;**27**:91-98

[134] Xu Q, Wang H, Zhang L, Liu N. Kdr allelic variation in pyrethroid resistant mosquitoes, *Culex quinquefasciatus* (s.). Biochemical and Biophysical Research Communications. 2006;**345**:774-780

[135] Li T, Zhang L, Reid W, et al. Sodium channel gene expression associated with pyrethroid resistant house flies and German cockroaches. Gene. 2006;**379**:62-67

[136] Yang T, Liu N. Permethrin resistance variation and susceptible reference line isolation in a field population of the mosquito, *Culex quinquefasciatus* (diptera: Culicidae). Insect Science. 2014;**21**:659-666

[137] Nabeshima T, Mori A, Kozaki T, Iwata Y, Hidoh O, Harada S, et al. An amino acid substitution attributable to insecticide-insensitivity of acetylcholinesterase in a Japanese encephalitis vector mosquito, *Culex tritaeniorhynchus*. Biochemical and Biophysical Research Communications. 2004;**313**:794-801

Chapter 5

Influence of Climatic Factors on the Abundance and Profusion of Mosquitoes in Eastern Province, Saudi Arabia

Assad Al-Thukair, Yasin Jemal and Alexis Nzila

Abstract

This study was performed to evaluate the change in seasonal abundance and distribution of individual mosquito vectors (Culex, Anopheles, and Aedes) in relation to the climatic factors in Eastern Province, Saudi Arabia, for the study period of 2014. The association between mosquito abundance and environmental parameters was investigated using bivariate and multivariate analysis. The study showed the range of temperature and relative humidity required for individual mosquito larvae abundance varies for Culex, Anopheles, and Aedes. However, no variation was observed in the range of temperature and relative humidity required for the abundance of adult Culex and Anopheles. The results revealed a negative relationship between mosquito larval/adult abundance and temperature (Total number of larva/adult is 671/11 in July, While it is 2462/221 in January). There is a link between relative humidity and rainfall, as the three climatic factors together were responsible for 33.1% (R^2 = 0.331), 54.6% (R^2 = 0.546), and 86.6% (R^2 = 0.866) of the variance on Culex, Anopheles, and Aedes larvae, respectively. The effects of the three climatic parameters of temperature, relative humidity, and rainfall on mosquito larval and adult abundance were discussed. In addition, influences of other environmental factors on larval/adult mosquito distribution and abundance were also explained.

Keywords: mosquitoes, climate factors, Saudi Arabia

1. Introduction

Mosquitoes have a higher impact than any other bug because of the diseases they spread. Mosquito-borne infections are a substantial hazard to human health and are one of the leading causes of morbidity and mortality worldwide [1–5]. The mosquito vector, the human host, and the environment are all involved in the development of these diseases [6].

Over one billion people are affected and over one million people die each year because of vector-borne diseases, the majority of which are caused by mosquitos [5].

Zika virus, Malaria, Dengue Fever, Japanese Encephalitis, Yellow Fever, West Nile Virus, Filariasis, and Rift Valley Fever are the communal mosquito-borne diseases MBDs [5, 7–9]. In Saudi Arabia, dengue fever, malaria, and rift valley fever are among the MBDs reported by many researchers in many parts of the kingdom [10–20].

Complex factors influence mosquito dispersal and abundance, including MBDs [21, 22]. Climate parameters such as temperature, relative humidity, and rainfall, on the other hand, are critical determinants of mosquito vector survival, production, growth, abundance, and dispersal [23–26]. The temperature has been proven to have an impact on mosquito abundance, activity, and presence in both temporary and permanent habitats. It has an impact on the parasite's development and the time it takes from egg to adult mosquito [27–31]. Rainfall has a similar effect on mosquito dispersion by giving or sustaining more breeding grounds. On the other hand, clearing out small breeding sites and lowering the temperature, has a detrimental impact [6, 31]. The number of females laying eggs, the number of eggs laid, the frequency of feeding, and the metabolic rate of adult mosquitos are all affected by changes in relative humidity. Aside from climatic considerations, mosquito distribution and abundance were substantially impacted by the spatial distribution of breeding regions, habitat, land use patterns, preferred hosts, and flight distance [32, 33]. The association between climatic parameters such as temperature, relative humidity, and rainfall has been studied in several research [34–37]. However, no research has been done on the impact of climatic parameters (temperature, relative humidity, and rainfall) on mosquito abundance in Saudi Arabia's Eastern Province.

The objective of this research is to determine how seasonal abundance and distribution of individual mosquito vectors (Culex, Anopheles, and Aedes) alter in connection to climatic parameters such as temperature, relative humidity, and rainfall in Saudi Arabia's Eastern Province.

2. Material and methods

2.1 Study area

The Eastern Province of Saudi Arabia is bordered to the north by the Northern Province, Kuwait to the northeast, and the Sultanate of Oman to the south by the Arabian Gulf. It has a variety of geographical characteristics, including sandy soil, coastal lowlands, industrialized areas, and agricultural areas. It is characterized by an arid climate with a temperature rising from 15°C in January to a maximum of about 42°C in the August-September period. The average annual rainfall ranges from around 100 mm in the north and northeast during winter to less than 10 mm in Rub al-Khali [38].

Several environmental factors influence the abundance and distribution of mosquitoes in the area. These factors include temperature, relative humidity, and precipitation, the presence of palm gardens/vegetables that hold a large volume of rainwater, widespread salt marshes, and irrigation ditches. Poor sanitary sewerage system in the areas also causes the accumulation of large volume of sewage water which serves as good breeding habitat for mosquitoes in the study area [18]. 322 larvae breeding sites were assessed for the presence of mosquito larvae in eight locations. However, only 206 sites (64.0%) found positive with mosquito larvae. Those locations include;

Abu Main (5 sites), Umm As Sahik (19 sites), Safwa (10 sites), Al-Awjam (22 sites), Dammam (12 sites), Al-Qatif and its surrounding area (81 sites), Buqayq (32 sites) and Al-Sarar (25 sites). Those sites showed their diverse ecological characteristic and abundance of mosquito species **Figure 1**.

2.2 Data collection

The larval and adult mosquito data was collected in collaboration with the Ministry of Health branch in Dammam. Data collection was carried out from January to December 2014. The monthly data collected were compiled for each study site for 2014. A sampling of mosquito larvae was carried out in various

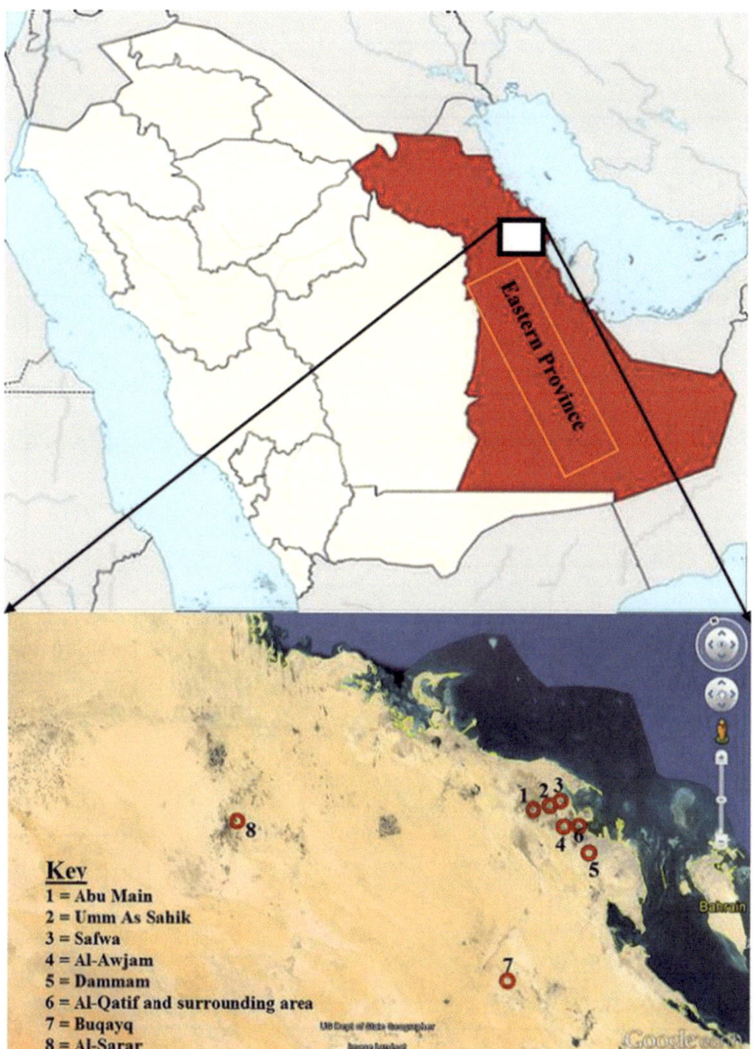

Figure 1.
Map showing study sites in Eastern Province, Saudi Arabia [39].

breeding habitats (ditches, sewages, stagnant and surface waters) by taking 3-5 scoops of water for each sampling location to check for the presence of larvae [18]. Mosquito larvae were identified using a dissecting microscope. Electric flycatchers and cow sheets with spray are applied to catch adult mosquitoes mainly from cattle barns.

The meteorological data of temperature, relative humidity, and precipitation were obtained from the Presidency of Meteorology and Environment (PME) Dammam for the period noted above. Temperature is defined as a mean average of minimum and maximum temperature, measured in degree Celsius (°C). Relative humidity (RH), expressed in percentage (%), is the average monthly humidity based on the daily records. Precipitation/rainfall is the amount of rainfall in the month, measured in millimeters.

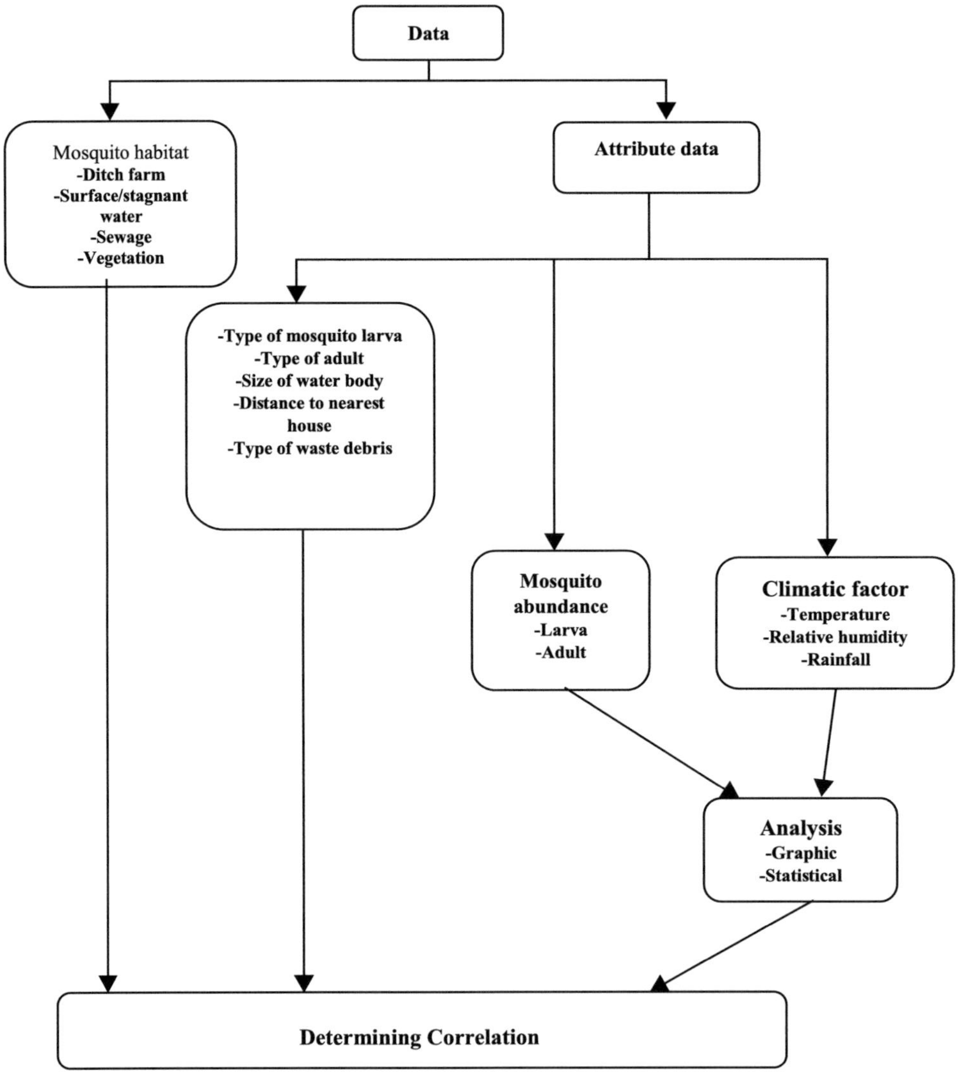

Figure 2.
Diagram showing steps processes of the study.

2.3 Data analysis

Data was analyzed to determine the relationship between mosquito abundance and climatic factors. Bivariate analysis was carried out to determine the relationship between mosquito abundance and each climatic factor (temperature, relative humidity, and rainfall). Multivariate regression analysis was performed to identify the overall effect of temperature, relative humidity, and rainfall in mosquito abundance. A descriptive analysis was carried out to determine the trends of mosquito abundance and climatic factors. The results of the bivariate analysis are expressed in Pearson correlation coefficient using sigma plot software (Systat Software Inc).

A systematic procedure was carried out to study mosquito distribution and abundance in Eastern Province, Saudi Arabia **Figure 2**.

3. Results

Table 1 shows the number of mosquito larvae and adult mosquitos collected in the Eastern Province of Saudi Arabia during the study year (2014). From January to December 2014, 31041 mosquito larvae and 2036 adult mosquitos were collected across all sites. Qatif and the surrounding area had the most adults and larvae, followed by Awjam and Umm As Sahik.

Culex mosquito larvae accounted for 20345 (65.54%) of the total 31041 mosquito larvae collected, whereas Aedes and Anopheles mosquito larvae accounted for 5641 (18.17%) and 5055 (16.28%) respectively. In contrast, 1528 (75.05%) of the 2036 adult mosquitos collected were Culex, while 508 (24.95%) were Anopheles. Throughout the year, however, no adult Aedes mosquitos were collected at any of the sites. In each study site, **Table 2** showed the relative distribution and number of larval and adult mosquitos. The larval and adult Culex were found in many habitats throughout the research area, according to the findings.

Some mosquito species were captured as larvae but not as adults in this investigation. In the study region, Aedes mosquitos were gathered as larvae but not as adults throughout the year. Adult Culex and Anopheles were also not collected throughout the year in Buqayq and Al-Sarar. During the study period, neither larval nor adult Anopheles were obtained from the Dammam area **Table 2**. The relationship between mosquito larvae (Culex, Anopheles and Aedes) abundance and climatic factors of temperature, relative humidity, and rainfall demonstrated in **Figure 3**. A high number of Culex larvae were observed throughout December, February, March, and April, whereas many Anopheles larvae were gathered during November, December, March, April, and June. The high number of Aedes larvae were observed during November, December, and February, as shown. **Figure 3** also revealed that a significant number of total mosquito larvae were collected in the months of November, December, February, March, and April.

Figure 4 depicts the link between adult mosquito abundance (Culex and Anopheles) and climatic parameters (temperature, relative humidity, and rainfall). Specifically, throughout the months of December, February, and March, many adult Culex and Anopheles were gathered. This figure also shows that in November, December, January, February, March, and April, 2014 a large number of total adult mosquitos were seen. The statistical analyses performed between larval and adult mosquito abundance and climatic factors are given in **Table 3**. These statistical analyses were executed for Abu Main, Umm As-Sahik, Safwa, Al-Awjam, Dammam,

Stage type	Month												Total
	Jan	Feb	Mar	Apr	May	Jun	Jul	Aug	Sep	Oct	Nov	Dec	
Larval													
Culex	1525	1987	2718	2303	1493	1550	410	1505	1483	1680	1547	2144	20345
Anopheles	387	462	643	582	368	561	203	257	298	285	504	505	5055
Aedes	550	896	630	250	278	247	58	210	100	398	1005	1019	5641
Total	2462	3345	3991	3135	2139	2358	671	1972	1881	2363	3056	3668	31041
Adult													
Culex	169	274	273	163	38	44	11	55	36	40	165	260	1528
Anopheles	52	115	107	29	11	0	0	4	2	3	28	157	508
Aedes	0	0	0	0	0	0	0	0	0	0	0	0	0
Total	221	389	380	192	49	44	11	59	38	43	193	417	2036

Table 1.
Time-based dispersal and abundance of larvae and adult type in Eastern Province, Saudi Arabia 2014.

Stage	Area	Culex	Aedes	Anopheles	Total
Larval	Abu-Main	690	235	242	1167
	Umm As Sahik	1275	355	668	2298
	Safwa	770	250	557	1577
	Al-Awjam	1132	343	670	2145
	Dammam	915	248	0	1163
	Al-Qatif and surrounding area	13123	3215	2788	19126
	Buqayq	885	190	48	1123
	Al-Sarar	1555	805	82	2442
	Total	20345	5641	5055	31041
Adult	Abu-Main	59	0	69	128
	Umm As-Sahik	291	0	81	372
	Safwa	25	0	3	28
	Al-Awjam	255	0	86	341
	Dammam	6	0	0	6
	Al-Qatif and surrounding area	892	0	269	1161
	Buqayq	0	0	0	0
	Al-Sarar	0	0	0	0
	Total	1528	0	508	2036

Table 2.
Spatial distribution and abundance of larvae and adult by mosquito type.

and Al-Qatif, including Buqayq and Al Sarar for larvae, with the exception of Buqayq and Al Sarar for the adult since no adult mosquitoes were collected from these sites during field visits. **Table 3** illustrated the negative correlation between temperature and Culex (except in Umm-As Sahik), Anopheles, and Aedes larvae. However, positive relationship between relative humidity and rainfall except in some sites. The multivariate regression analysis, on the other hand, explained that the three climatic factors together were responsible for 33.1% (R^2 = 0.331), 54.6% (R^2 = 0.546), and 86.6% (R^2 = 0.866) of the variance on Culex, Anopheles and Aedes larvae, respectively, in Eastern Province of Saudi Arabia.

Table 3 also clearly shows that adult Culex mosquito abundance had a negative correlation with temperature except in Safwa. Specifically, in Umm As Sahik, Awjam, and Qatif and the surrounding area, a strong negative correlation between adult Culex and the temperature was observed with correlation values of −0.726, −0.717, and −0.850, respectively. However, positive correlation with relative humidity, with highest correlation values of 0.716, 0.773, and 0.592 in Umm As Sahik, Awjam, and Qatif and surrounding area, respectively, but a negative correlation with relative humidity in Safwa site. It is also evident from **Table 3** that adult Culex mosquito abundance had a moderate to low positive correlation with rainfall except (negative) in Safwa and Dammam.

Similarly, **Table 3** clearly shows that adult Anopheles mosquito abundance had a strong negative correlation with temperature. The table also demonstrated a negative correlation between Adult Anopheles abundance and rainfall (except

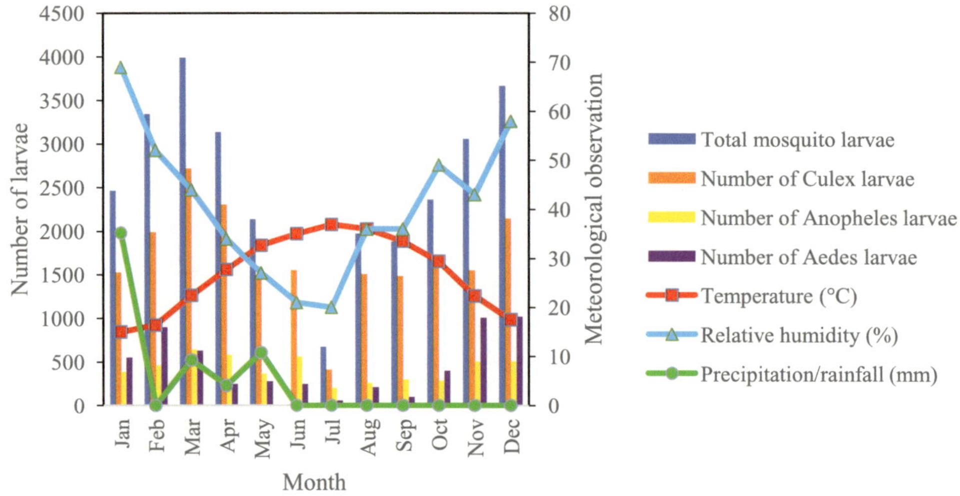

Figure 3.
The temporal relationship between climatic factors and mosquito larvae.

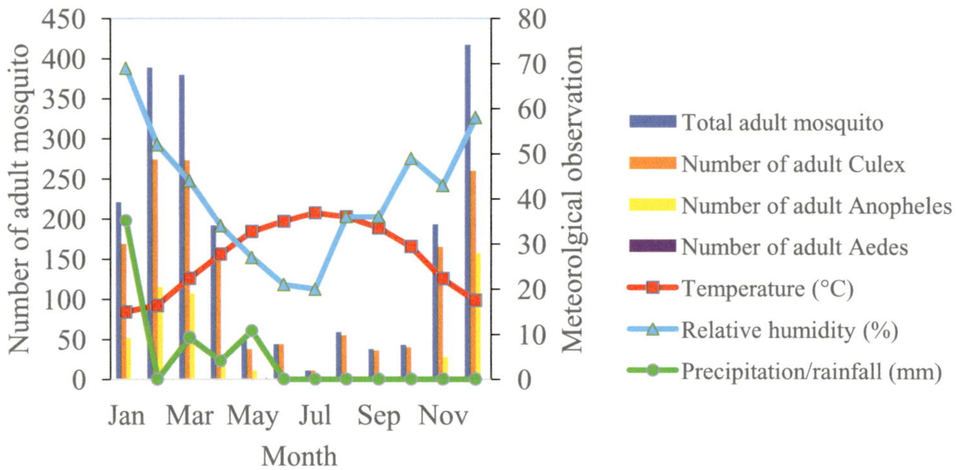

Figure 4.
The temporal relationship between climatic factors and adult mosquitoes.

in Umm-As Sahik and Al-Awjam) while a strong positive correlation with relative humidity in all sites.

The current study also demonstrated the combined effect of the three climatic factors on the abundance of adult Culex and Anopheles mosquitoes. The multivariate regression model for three climatic factors (temperature, RH, and rainfall) explained 86% (R^2 = 0.860) and 73.9% (R^2 = 0.739) of the variance in adult Culex and Anopheles mosquito abundance, respectively. It showed also that the three climatic factors together were responsible for 33.1% (R^2 = 0.331), 54.6% (R^2 = 0.546) and 86.6% (R^2 = 0.866) of the variance on Culex, Anopheles and Aedes larvae, respectively. This means that 86% and 73.9% of the variance are accounted for the three parameters and the remaining 14% and 26.1% are attributed to other factors such as the presence of the vegetation, waste materials, water reservoirs, ditches, and others. Comparing the two adults, the adult Anopheles mosquito was more influenced

Type	Correlation and significance association	AM	US	SA	AW	DA	QS	BU	AS	EP
					Larvae					
Culex	Culex abundance and temperature	−0.817**	0.268	−0.532	−0.161	−0.304	−0.456	−0.724**	−0.350	−0.538
	Culex abundance and RH	0.703*	−0.025	0.522	0.117	0.204	0.351	0.684*	0.159	0.424
	Culex abundance and rainfall	0.351	0.075	0.629*	0.431	0.244	−0.160	0.719**	0.537	0.059
Anopheles	Anopheles abundance and temperature	−0.749**	−0.576	−0.793**	−0.698*	a	−0.242	−0.655*	−0.446	−0.481
	Anopheles abundance and RH	0.600*	0.396	0.583*	0.463	a	−0.094	0.498	0.320	0.151
	Anopheles abundance and rainfall	0.165	0.200	0.399	0.407	a	−0.138	0.487	0.388	0.058
Aedes	Aedes abundance and temperature	−0.881**	−0.523	−0.898**	−0.370	−0.452	−0.718**	−0.498	−0.202	−0.848**
	Aedes abundance and RH	0.753**	0.389	0.720**	0.232	0.453	0.575	0.324	0.129	0.670*
	Aedes abundance and rainfall	0.753**	0.323	0.384	0.041	0.039	−0.102	0.610*	0.190	0.034
					Adult					
Culex	Culex abundance and temperature	−0.489	−0.726**	0.073	−0.717**	−0.186	−0.850**	a	a	−0.876**
	Culex abundance and RH	0.212	0.716**	−0.192	0.773**	0.048	0.592*	a	a	0.650*
	Culex abundance and rainfall	0.068	0.057	−0.112	0.344	−0.152	0.174	a	a	0.174
Anopheles	Anopheles abundance and temperature	−0.548	−0.875**	−0.472	−0.848**	a	−0.633*	a	a	−0.802**
	Anopheles abundance and RH	0.509	0.688*	0.602*	0.772**	a	0.426	a	a	0.627*
	Anopheles abundance and rainfall	−0.031	0.238	−0.926	0.551	a	−0.078	a	a	0.090

***Correlation is significant at 0.01 level.*
**Correlation is significant at 0.05 level.*
[a]Cannot be computed.
Note: AM = Abu Main, US = Umm As Sahik, SA = Safwa, AW = Awjam, DM= Dammam, QS = Qatif and its surrounding area, BU = Buqayq, AS = Al-Sarar, EP = Eastern Province.

Table 3.
The correlation coefficient between climatic factors, and abundance of adult and larval.

by other environmental factors than by climatic factors compared to the adult Culex mosquito which is more influenced by climatic factors than by other environmental factors in the Eastern Province, Saudi Arabia.

Overall, both Culex and Anopheles larvae had a moderate negative association with temperature in Saudi Arabia's Eastern Province, but Aedes larvae had a substantial negative correlation with temperature. On the other hand, low, moderate, and a strong positive correlation were observed between Anopheles, Culex, and Aedes larvae, and relative humidity, respectively. Rainfall and the three mosquito larvae types in the study area had a low positive link, according to the current study. Adult Culex and Anopheles both displayed a strong negative connection with temperature, with the highest values of −0.876 and −0.802, respectively, and a substantial positive correlation with relative humidity, with correlation values of 0.650 and 0.627, respectively. In Eastern Province, Saudi Arabia, both adult mosquitoes had a favorable link with rainfall in general.

4. Discussion

Understanding the impact of climatic conditions on mosquito distribution and abundance is critical for mosquito control efforts. The range and abundance of individual mosquito types are influenced by climatic conditions such as temperature, relative humidity, and rainfall [32, 34].

In the Eastern Province of Saudi Arabia, this study gave a clear explanation of the relationship between mosquito abundance and meteorological conditions. The response of larvae and adult mosquitoes to each climatic factors varied depending on season and site as shown in graphical **Figures 3** and **4**, and statistical analyses in **Table 3**. Other environmental factors, such as the presence of vegetation, irrigation activities, and poor environmental sanitation, were also shown to have an impact on the distribution and abundance of individual mosquito vectors in the study. In several ecosystems in the research region, the Culex mosquito was found to be the most abundant and widely spread. The reasons for the larval and adult Culex's widespread range and abundance in Saudi Arabia's Eastern Province are similar to prior investigations [10–20]. Agricultural expansion, the presence of irrigation ditches/canals, ponds, and extensive farming, according to Alahmed [18], contribute to the wide dispersion and incidence of mosquitos in Saudi Arabia's Eastern Province. Muturi et al. [40] observed that the presence of floating vegetation in the aquatic habitat, turbid/polluted water, and the presence of water reservoirs such as irrigation canals/dits in the area all influence the distribution of Culex larvae and have been linked to the presence of Culex larvae.

Calhoun et al. [41] reported a higher number of Culex larvae in oily/rusty water when compared to clean water. Similarly, Ohta and Kaga [42] found that substantial irrigation activities enhance mosquito growth, lengthen mosquito annual growing periods, and raise mosquito maximum generation numbers by altering natural water in their environment. It was also shown that irrigation systems not only aid mosquito growth during dry seasons but also help to stabilize growth during rainy seasons. Temperatures ranging from 16.4 to 27.7°C are ideal for Culex larvae's growth and survival, while temperatures ranging from 17.5 to 35°C and 16.4 to 22.3°C are ideal for Anopheles and Aedes larvae development and survival, respectively. Temperatures of 16.4 to 22.4°C, on the other hand, support substantial growth and survival of adult Culex and Anopheles. On the other hand, the overall data of larvae/adult clearly indicate that temperatures ranging from 16.4 to 27.7°C are ideal for larvae development and survival, whereas temperatures ranging from 15 to 27.7°C promote a high abundance and spread of adult mosquito in Eastern province.

High environmental temperatures greater than 30°C decreases the survival of the Culex mosquito [43]. However, Hopp and Foley [44] and Tun *et al.* [27] reported that high temperatures speed up the growth and survival of larval and adult stages of the Culex mosquito. Similarly, the increase in environmental temperatures decreases the survival and development of larval and adult stages of Anopheles mosquito [45]. Bayoh and Lindsay [29] also found a decrease in Anopheles larvae survival as environmental temperature increases. However, Minakawa *et al.* [34] reported that the influence of temperature on Anopheles mosquito was significant. The influence of temperature on mosquito development, survival, and productivity is difficult to predict at a precise range, as evidenced by these and other studies [23]. During the summer, the average temperature in the research region exceeded 35°C, which is unfavorable for mosquito larval and adult growth. In July, when the temperature was 36.9°C, just a few larval and adult mosquitos were found, as shown in **Figures 3** and **4**. Overall, high larval and adult mosquitos were collected at temperatures ranging from 16.4 to 27.7°C and 15 to 27.7°C, respectively. Temperatures between 20 and 29°C have been found to be advantageous for mosquito growth in several studies [23, 36–37, 46]. The study also demonstrated that moderate relative humidity influences the increase of the larval and adult stages of the mosquito. Abundant Culex and Anopheles larvae were observed at average relative humidity that ranges from 34 to 58%. Unlike to this, a high number of Aedes larvae was collected at mean relative humidity that ranges from 43 to 58%. On the other hand, a high number of both adult Culex and Anopheles mosquitoes were observed at a relative humidity that ranges between 44 and 58% (**Figures 3** and **4**).

The survival and developmental phases of mosquitoes are influenced by relative humidity, according to various research. The lifespan of mosquitos is shown to increase as humidity rises, while high humidity increases mosquito density and abundance [18, 23, 25, 35–37]. Costa *et al.* [30] observed that when the temperature and relative humidity are both lower, the number of female Aedes mosquitos depositing eggs and their egg production (oviposition) increases. In contrast, Hopp and Foley [44] reported that as temperature and humidity rise, the Aedes mosquito produces more eggs and larvae counts. Low humidity, on the other hand, was associated with a lower number of Culex, Anopheles, and Aedes larvae, as well as a lower abundance of adult Culex and Anopheles mosquitos, according to this study. As the relative humidity drops throughout the summer, only a small number of larval and adult mosquitos are gathered. In all study sites, the number of larval and adult mosquitos increased throughout the months of October, November, December, January, February, and March, 2014 when relative humidity was high (**Figures 3** and **4**).

The effect of rainfall on mosquito larvae was not seen in the current investigation **Figure 3**. Even though the fact that the average annual rainfall in Eastern Province is 5 mm, the influence of rainfall on adult mosquitos was visible in the number of adult mosquitos during the wet months. In comparison to the dry seasons, higher adult mosquito activity was recorded during the rainy months of January, February, March, and April **Figure 4**. Rainfall has a beneficial or negative impact on mosquito numbers, either by supplying more/maintaining breeding places or by flushing mosquito larvae from small breeding sites [25, 31, 35–37, 47, 48].

The bivariate analysis indicated that the response of the larval and adult mosquito vectors of Culex and Anopheles as well as Aedes larvae to each climatic factors such as temperature, relative humidity, and rainfall varied by site. As shown in **Table 3**, both stages of the larval and adult forms of an individual mosquito of Culex and Anopheles including Aedes larvae were found negatively correlated with temperature while positively correlated to relative humidity and rainfall.

Similarly, from the multivariate regression analysis, the response of the individual mosquito vectors of both stages that are the larval and adult Culex and Anopheles as well as Aedes larvae, to the combined effect of the three climatic factors varied, depending on the site. From the regression model, it is understood that Aedes larvae were more influenced by climatic factors than Culex and Anopheles larvae, which were more affected by other environmental factors. It seems that Culex and Anopheles larvae are more influenced by the presence of vegetation, waste material, water reservoirs, and ditches. The presence of floating and terrestrial vegetation, poor environmental sanitation, and extensive irrigation activities that create water reservoirs such as ditches are among the major environmental factors for mosquito abundance and their wide distribution in many habitats [39, 41, 42, 49].

The vast spread of Culex larvae could be attributable to favorable climatic conditions in the research area, as well as their capacity to develop and survive in a variety of aquatic breeding sites. They can also thrive in polluted and saline aquatic habitats. Aside from water quality, the presence of floating vegetation and waste materials (such as plastics, papers, old tires, and rags) in the aquatic habitat also contributed to the wide distribution and abundance of Culex larvae, as these environmental factors provide appropriate access for adult Culex mosquitos to lay their eggs and for their larvae to develop and survive. Irrigation activities in the study area also contribute to the larvae's distribution and abundance by creating water reservoirs such as ditches where mosquito larvae can breed.

The presence of some mosquito types as larvae but not as an adult in some sites may be due to the differences in adult behavior such as feeding and resting behavior (as some mosquito species are indoor feeders and indoor resting while others are outdoor feeders and indoor resting) attributed to unavailability of adult mosquitoes and they did not come close to the trapping or sampling location placed outside houses during the data collection period [18]. The other reason for the unavailability of adult mosquitoes was limited access to the human residence since adult mosquitoes were collected from rooms of cattle during the morning time (day).

5. Conclusion

Mosquito control programs benefit greatly from an awareness of the effects of climatic conditions on mosquito vectors. Mosquito abundance can be predicted by anticipating temperature, relative humidity, and rainfall, and then present and future mosquito control measures can be planned and implemented. As a result, this research provides comprehensive information on the impact of climatic conditions on the abundance of specific mosquito vectors in Saudi Arabia's Eastern Province. However, further research is needed to determine the impact of global warming, irrigation activities, land use, and the biological characteristics of mosquito breeding sites on mosquito distribution and abundance before large-scale control methods can be implemented.

Acknowledgements

The authors would like to thank King Fahd University of Petroleum and Minerals (KFUPM) for the support to conduct the study. The authors are grateful to the Ministry of Health, Dammam Branch, and Presidency of Meteorological and Environment, Dammam, for providing required logistic support and meteorological data, for the study.

Author details

Assad Al-Thukair[1]*, Yasin Jemal[2] and Alexis Nzila[1]

1 Life Science Department, King Fahd University of Petroleum and Minerals (KFUPM), Dhahran, Saudi Arabia

2 Earth Science Department, King Fahd University of Petroleum and Minerals (KFUPM), Dhahran, Saudi Arabia

*Address all correspondence to: thukair@kfupm.edu.sa

References

[1] Pratt HD, Barnes RC, Littig KS. Mosquitoes of Public Health Importance and their Control: Training Guide. Atlanta, Georgia, USA: Insect Control Series; 1963

[2] World Health Organization. Vector Control: Methods for use by individuals and communities. Geneva, Switzerland: World Health Organization; 1997

[3] Gratz NG. Emerging and resurging vector-borne diseases. Annual Review Entomology. 1999;**44**:51-75

[4] Gandhi G, Srinivasulu N, Naik KG, Naik BR. Original research article remote sensing and geographical information system application for mosquito intervention: A Case Study of Grater Hyderabad. International Journal of Current Microbiology and Applied Sciences. 2013;**2**:560-568

[5] World Health Organization. A Global Brief on Vector-borne Diseases. Geneva, Switzerland: World Health Organization; 2014

[6] Ceccato P, Connor SJ, Jeanne I, Thomson MC. Application of geographical information systems and remote sensing technologies for assessing and monitoring malaria risk. Parassitologia. 2005;**47**:81-96

[7] Lehane M. The Biology of Blood-sucking Insects. 2nd ed. Cambridge, UK: Cambridge University Press; 2005

[8] Matthews G. Integrated Vector Management: Controlling Vectors of Malaria and Other Insect Vector Borne Diseases. London, UK: Imperial College; 2011

[9] World Health Organization. Current Zika Product Pipeline. Geneva, Switzerland: World Health Organization; 2016

[10] Bashwari LA, Mandil AM, Bahnassy AA, Al-Shamsi MA, Bukhari HA. Epidemiological profile of malaria in a university hospital in the eastern region of Saudi Arabia. Saudi Medical Journal. 2001;**22**:133-138

[11] Fakeeh M, Zaki AM. Dengue in Jeddah, Saudi Arabia, 1994-2002. Dengue Bulletin. 2003;**27**:13-18

[12] Madani TA, Al-Mazzou YY, Al-Jeffri MH, Mishkhas AA, Al-Rabeah AM, Turkistani AM, et al. Rift Valley Fever Epidemic in Saudi Arabia: Epidemiological, clinical and laboratory characteristics. Oxford Journals. 2003;**37**:1084-1092

[13] Flick R, Bouloy M. Rift Valley fever virus. Current Molecular Medicine. 2005;**5**:827-834

[14] Al-Tawfiq JA. Epidemiology of travel-related malaria in a non-malarious area in Saudi Arabia. Saudi Medical Journal. 2006;**27**:86-89

[15] Al-Qabati AG, Al-Afaleq AI. Cross-sectional, longitudinal and prospective epidemiological studies of Rift Valley Fever in Al-Hasa Oasis, Saudi Arabia. Journal of Animal and Veterinary Advances. 2010;**9**:258-265

[16] El-Gilany AH, Eldeib A, Hammad S. Clinico-epidemiological features of dengue fever in Saudi Arabia. Asian Pacific Journal of Tropical Medicine. 2010;**3**:220-223. DOI: 10.1016/S1995-7645(10)60013-2

[17] Ahmed AM, Shaalan EA, Aboul-Soud MAM, Tripet F,

Al-Khedhairy AA. Mosquito vectors survey in the AL-Ahsaa District of Eastern Saudi Arabia. Journal of Insect Science. 2011;**11**:1-11. DOI: 10.1673/031.011.17601

[18] Alahmed AM. Mosquito fauna (Diptera: Culicidae) of the Eastern Region of Saudi Arabia and their seasonal abundance. Journal of King Saud University Science. 2012;**24**:55-62. DOI: 10.1016/j.jksus.2010.12.001

[19] Khormi HM, Kumar L. Using geographic information system and remote sensing to study common mosquito- borne diseases in Saudi Arabia. Journal of Food, Agriculture and Environment. 2013;**11**:14-17

[20] Aziz AT, Al-Shami SA, Mahyoub JA, Hatabbi M, Ahmad AH, Rawi CSM. An update on the incidence of dengue gaining strength in Saudi Arabia and current control approaches for its vector mosquito. Parasites & Vectors. 2014;7:258. DOI: 10.1186/1756-3305-7-258

[21] Craig M, Le Sueur D, Snow B. A climate-based distribution model of malaria transmission in sub-Saharan Africa. Parasitology Today. 1999;**15**:105-111. DOI: 10.1016/S0169-4758(99)01396-4

[22] Reisen WK, Cayan D, Tyree M, Baker MC, Eldridge B, and Dettinger M. Impact of climate variation on Mosquito abundance in California. Journal of Geographical Sciences. 2006;**16**:430-438. DOI: 10.1007/s11442-006-0406-6

[23] Reiter P. Climate change and mosquito-borne disease. Environmental Health Perspectives. 2001;**109**:141-161. DOI: 10.2307/3434853

[24] Zhou G, Munga S, Minakawa N. Spatial relationship between adult malaria vector abundance and environmental factors in western Kenya highlands. American Journal of Tropical Medicine and Hygiene. 2007;77:29-35

[25] Bashar K, Tuno N. Seasonal abundance of Anopheles mosquitoes and their association with meteorological factors and malaria incidence in Bangladesh. Parasites & Vectors. 2014;7:442. DOI: 10.1186/1756-3305-7-442

[26] Palaniyandi M, Anand P, Maniyosai R. Spatial cognition: A geospatial analysis of vector-borne disease transmission and the environment, using remote sensing and GIS. International Journal of Mosquito Research. 2014;**1**:39-54

[27] Tun-Lin W, Burkot TR, Kay BH. Effects of temperature and larval diet on development rates and survival of the dengue vector Aedes aegypti in north Queensland, Australia. Medical and Veterinary Entomology. 2000;**14**:31-37. DOI: 10.1046/j.1365-2915.2000.00207.x

[28] Bayoh MN, Lindsay SW. Effect of temperature on the development of the aquatic stages of Anopheles gambiae sensu stricto (Diptera: Culicidae). Bulletin of Entomological Research. 2003;**93**:375-381. DOI: 10.1079/BER2003259

[29] Bayoh MN, Lindsay SW. Temperature-related duration of aquatic stages of the Afrotropical malaria vector mosquito Anopheles gambiae in the laboratory. Medical and Veterinary Entomology. 2004;**18**:174-179. DOI: 10.1111/j.0269-283X.2004.00495.x

[30] Costa EAPDA, Santos EMDM, Correia JC, Albuquerque CMRD. Impact of small variations in temperature and humidity on the reproductive activity and survival of Aedes aegypti (Diptera, Culicidae). Revista Brasileira

de Entomologia. 2010;**54**:488-493. DOI: 10.1590/S0085-56262010000300021

[31] Byun R, Webb CE. Guidelines for Mosquito Risk Assessment and Management in Constructed Wetlands. Sydney, Australia: Sydney Western Region; 2012

[32] Lindsay SW, Martens WJM. Malaria in the African highlands: Past, present and future. Bulletin of the World Health Organization. 1998;**76**:33-45

[33] Gimnig J, Hightower A, Hawley W. Application of geographic information systems to the study of the ecology of mosquitoes and mosquito-borne diseases. In: Willem T, Pim M, Robert B, editors. Environmental Change and Malaria Risk: Global and Local Implications. Atlanta, USA: Frontis; 2005. pp. 27-39

[34] Minakawa N, Sonye G, Mogi M, Githeko A, Yan G. The effects of climatic factors on the distribution and abundance of malaria vectors in Kenya. Journal of Medical Entomology. 2002;**39**:833-841. DOI: 10.1603/0022-2585-39.6.833

[35] Murty US, Rao MS, Arunachalam N. The effects of climatic factors on the distribution and abundance of Japanese encephalitis vectors in Kurnool district of Andhra Pradesh, India. Journal of Vector Borne Diseases. 2010;**47**:26-32

[36] Alshehri MSA. Dengue fever outburst and its relationship with climatic factors. World Applied Sciences Journal. 2013;**22**:506-515. DOI: 10.5829/idosi.wasj.2013.22.04.443

[37] Tian H-Y, Bi P, Cazelles B, Zhou S, Huang S-Q, Yang J, et al. How environmental conditions impact mosquito ecology and Japanese encephalitis: An eco-epidemiological approach. Environment International. 2015;**79**:17-24. DOI: 10.1016/j.envint.2015.03.002

[38] Thomas J. Eastern Saudi Arabia: Topography, Geography and Vegetation. 2012. Available from: http://www.onislam.net/content/english/hajj/services/01.shtml

[39] Jemal Y, Al-Thukair AA. Combining GIS application and climatic factors for mosquito control in Eastern Province, Saudi Arabia. Saudi Journal of Biological Sciences. 2018;**8**:1593-1602. DOI: 10.1016/j.sjbs.2016.04.001

[40] Muturi EJ, Shililu JI, Gu W, Jacob BG, Githure JI, Novak RJ. Larval habitat dynamics and diversity of Culex mosquitoes in rice agro-ecosystem in Mwea, Kenya. American Journal of Tropical Medicine and Hygiene. 2007;**76**:95-102

[41] Calhoun LM, Avery M, Jones L, Gunarto K, King R, Roberts J, et al. Combined sewage overflows (CSO) are major urban breeding sites for Culex quinquefasciatus in Atlanta, Georgia. American Journal of Tropical Medicine and Hygiene. 2007;**77**:478-484

[42] Ohta S, Kaga T. Effect of irrigation systems on temporal distribution of malaria vectors in semi-arid regions. International Journal of Biometeorology. 2014;**58**:349-359. DOI: 10.1007/s00484-012-0630-y

[43] Westbrook CJ, Reiskind MH, Pesko KN, Greene KE, Lounibos LP. Larval environmental temperature and the susceptibility of Aedes albopictus Skuse (Diptera: Culicidae) to Chikungunya virus. Vector Borne and Zoonotic Diseases. 2010;**10**:241-247. DOI: 10.1089/vbz.2009.0035

[44] Hopp MJ, Foley JA. Worldwide fluctuations in dengue fever case related

to climate variability. Climate Research. 2003;**25**:85-94. DOI: 10.3354/cr025085

[45] Christiansen-Jucht C, Parham PE, Saddler A, Koella JC, Basáñez M-G. Temperature during larval development and adult maintenance influences the survival of Anopheles gambiae s.s. Parasites and Vectors. 2014;7:489. DOI: 10.1186/s13071-014-0489-3

[46] World Health Organization. Climate Change and Human Health. Geneva, Switzerland: World Health Organization; 1996

[47] Koenraadt CJM, Githeko AK, Takken W. The effects of rainfall and evapotranspiration on the temporal dynamics of Anopheles gambiae s.s. and Anopheles arabiensis in a Kenyan village. Acta Tropica. 2004;**90**:141-153. DOI: 10.1016/j.actatropica.2003.11.007

[48] Hu W, Tong S, Mengersen K, Oldenburg B. Rainfall, mosquito density and the transmission of Ross River virus: A time-series forecasting model. Ecological Modelling. 2006;**196**:505-514. DOI: 10.1016/j.ecolmodel.2006.02.028

[49] Chaikoolvatana A, Singhasivanon P, Haddawy P. Utilization of a geographical information system for surveillance of Aedes aegypti and dengue hemorrhagic fever in north-eastern Thailand. Dengue Bulletin. 2007;**31**:75-82

Section 2

Mosquito Control and New Technologies

Chapter 6

Vector Control Strategies

Wilber Gómez-Vargas and Giovani Esteban Zapata-Úsuga

Abstract

Vector-borne diseases, mainly dengue and malaria, are serious public health problems in the world; for the control of Aedes and Anopheles mosquitoes, there are several strategies such as biological, genetic, chemical, physical, and cultural. For the application of these control strategies, it is important to take into account the integrated vector management promoted by the World Health Organisation, taking into account the local context. This chapter shows the most important recent advances in vector control methods. The efforts of researchers in the development and evaluation of these and new control methods, the political will of governments, funding from the business sector, and community participation are essential to the success of these strategies.

Keywords: Aedes, Anopheles, new technologies, vector-borne diseases, vector control

1. Introduction

Globally, dengue remains a serious public health problem due to increasingly severe epidemics [1] and the emergence of new arboviruses, such as chikungunya and Zika, and the re-emergence of other arboviruses that were already under control, such as yellow fever, which has recorded cases in urban settings for the first time in more than 50 years [2]. As for malaria, although in recent years there has been progressing in its reduction, it still continues to affect many communities, especially children in Africa [3]. World Health Organisation (WHO) warns of the growing threat of resistance from malaria vectors and parasites, and the challenges of the COVID-19 pandemic [3].

Mosquito control of vectors *Aedes* and *Anopheles* measures include biological control, genetic control, chemical control, physical control, and cultural control.

Related to biological control, several studies have been reported recently that species of some fungal genera, for example, *Streptomyces*, *Pycnoporus, Pestalotiopsis*, *Culicinomyces*, *Leptoneglia*, *Beauveria Metarhizium, Cochliobolus and Aspergillus* and bacterial genera, for example, *Wolbachia*, *Bacillus,* and *Pseudomonas* display a potent ability to kill many species of mosquitoes, including those of the genera *Aedes* and *Anopheles*, mainly. Kairomones and pheromones are being developed. Nematode control for *Aedes* has been little studied, while for *Anopheles,* it has seen more development and interest in recent years.

As for genetic control, advances in the sterile insect technical (SIT), the insect incompatibility insect (IIT), and control by genetic manipulation are highlighted, mainly in *Aedes* control. SIT has been implemented mainly in *Anopheles arabiensis*.

IntechOpen

In terms of chemical vector control, advances are directed towards the development of new insecticides extracted from plants and the use of the method Autodissemination Augmented by Males (ADAM) that can be useful for small and cryptic containers of *Aedes aegypti* and useful in the control of *Anopheles arabiensis*.

Physical control has been progressing in ovitraps and acoustic larvicides that are promising for control of *A. aegypti*. In Anopheles control, the use of mosquito nets is highlighted.

Concerning cultural control, communication for mobilisation and behavioural impact (COMBI), approaches to social participation and eco-health are of vital importance in control programmes.

The WHO in its global vector control response 2017–2030 [4], noted the urgent need for the development and integration of innovative mosquito control methods, mainly *Aedes* and *Anopheles* vectors. New control strategies targeting these species are being developed, but their impact on arboviral diseases and malaria transmitted by these vectors has not yet been demonstrated. To this end, the WHO has adopted Integrated Vector Management [IVM], defined as "a rational decision-making process for the optimal use of vector control resources" [5], which provides countries with long-term sustainable and ecologically sound control methods that can reduce dependence on insecticides and protect populations where vector-borne diseases are prevalent, improving the effectiveness and efficiency of national vector control programmes [6].

The objective of this chapter is to review the progress made over the last 10 years in the control of the *Aedes* and *Anopheles* vectors.

2. Control *Aedes* mosquitoes

2.1 Biological control

2.1.1 Traditional strategies

Species *A. aegypti* and *Aedes albopictus* are the most prominent vectors in the transmission of arboviruses, such as dengue, chikungunya, yellow fever, and Zika [7]. Worldwide, biological control of these species, mainly *Ae. aegypti* has been specifically geared towards larvae, and the most commonly used control method has been biolarvicide *Bacillus thuringiensis* var. *israelensis* (*Bti*) and larvivores fish [8].

2.1.2 Bacterial control

An important and promising development dwells in the use of endosymbiont gram-negative bacteria *Wolbachia*. The strain being used in field trials is the wMel strain of *Wolbachia pipientis*. It consists of the artificial infection of *Ae. aegypti* (wAlbB) or *Ae. albopictus* (wPip) with the bacteria, mainly transmitted vertically, which intervenes in the manipulation of the host's reproduction to optimise its maternal transmission through eggs, favouring females, and inducing different distortion phenotypes among sexes of the progeny through mechanisms of parthenogenesis, feminization, and cytoplasmatic incompatibility (CI) [9–12]. *Wolbachia* is also present in somatic tissues, it can, therefore, be acquired from infected embryonic lineages or pass from cell to cell [13]. Furthermore, these bacteria can also block the replication of arboviruses (pathogenic interference) in populations of field mosquitoes [14, 15].

After *Wolbachia* is established in the local mosquito population, there is no need for further releases. It could also be genetically modified to prevent the vector from becoming infected, a phenomenon known as paratransgenesis [16]. Nevertheless, the use of *Wolbachia* as a control strategy is under scrutiny due to uncertainties related to the longevity of the viral suppression and the possibility of concomitant adaptative changes in the vector mosquito, the bacteria, or the virus [17]. Consequently, the use of mosquitoes infected with *Wolbachia* has not been approved in most countries due to insufficient knowledge of the potential dangers of this control method [18]. Pilot tests are currently being conducted by the World Mosquito Program in 12 countries in Asia, Central and South America, and the Pacific region [19].

Recently with the advances in nanotechnology, the bacterial products are produced from the synthesis of nanoparticles method that has been used with *B. thuringiensis* in third instar larvae of *Ae. aegypti* resulting in a 65% mortality [LC50: 0.10 ppm and LC90: 0.39 ppm] [20]. In another study, the ovicidal, pupicidal, and larvicidal efficacy of silver nanoparticles synthesised by *Bacillus marisflavi* strain isolated from marine habitat in species of *Ae. aegypti, Culex quinquefasciatus* and *Anopheles stephensi* have been demonstrated. The use of nanoparticles and their rapid synthesis of AgNPs against vectors, especially *Ae. aegypti*, would be a good biological control tool. However, the current research has some limitations, such as the cost-effective analysis and possible contamination of nanoparticles in the ambient or their effects on other useful microbes [21].

On the other hand, bacteria-derived metabolites may be a potential substitute for insecticides that have developed resistance. A study showed that secondary metabolites from extremophilic bacteria *Bacillus* and *Pseudomonas* sp., which caused larvae mortality of *Ae. aegypti* and *Cu. quinquefasciatus* of 100% at a concentration of 100 ppm [22].

2.1.3 Fungal control

Nowadays, there is an ample selection of fungal products with larvicide properties against vector *Ae. aegypti*. One of such products is chitinase enzymes from *Streptomyces cacaoi* subsp. *cacaoi*-M20 directed at the chitin required by the larvae, in which at the concentrations of 75 μl, 125 μl, 250 μl, and 500 μl no pupa formation and adult emergence were observed in experiments conducted [23]. Other promising products are ethyl acetate extracts from fungi, such as fungus *Pycnoporus sanguineus* which had a larvicidal activity of LC_{50} = 156.8 ppm and relative potency (0.612) and *Pestalotiopsis virgulate* with a larvicidal activity of LC_{50} = 101.8 ppm and relative potency (1.634), against *Ae. aegypti* larvae [24].

Studies with entomopathogenic fungi have proven promising in vector control such as *Culicinomyces clavisporus* that showed LC50 (≤ 3.6 × 105 conidia/ml) after a 3-day exposure and LT50 (≤ 1.3 days) at 106 conidia/ml against *Ae. aegypti* larvae [25] and *Leptoneglia chapmanii* where the persistence and pathogenicity decreased over time regardless of location, the assays showed that the mortality of *Ae. aegypti* larvae was significantly lower ($p < 0.05$) in containers located outside without sun protection (89% at first week and 9% at sixth week) compared with the containers located indoors (97% at first week and 42% at sixth week) and outside with shade (89% at first week and 29% at sixth week) [26, 27]. Another new fungus is *Isaria tenuipes* (formerly *Paecilomyces tenuipes*) a common fungal species that frequently affects major agricultural pests usually belonging to the group lepidopteran but this study showed that the fungus heavily damaged the internal gut cells and external physiology of *Ae. aegypti* larvae and its non-toxic activity against aquatic predators, such as *Toxorhynchites splendens*, this fungus will add on to its biologically safe insecticides [28].

As for adult control, particularly of *Ae. aegypti*, new methods of control have been developed in recent years, such as autodissemination of entomopathogenic fungi, mainly using isolates *Metarhizium anisoplae* and *Beaveria bassiana* in the laboratory [29, 30]. This process "uses a sexual or other attractants to concentrate individuals of one sex and spread the fungi in natural populations" [31]. *M. anisoplae* transmitted by males killed 85% of females in sexual encounters and reduced female fecundity by 99% [29]. *B. bassiana* killed 90% of the females confined with a fungus-contaminated male in 15 days and reduced female fecundity by 96% [30].

Recently with the advances in nanotechnology, products produced from the synthesis of nanoparticles aided by fungal are being studied. For example, the larvicide activity of silver nanoparticles (AgNPs) synthesised by fungus *Cochliobolus lunatus*, where a 100% mortality was observed at concentrations of 10 and 5 ppm against all instars treated [2nd, 3rd y 4th] [32]. In another study, cerium oxide nanoparticles were synthesised through *Aspergillus niger*, which resulted in 100% mortality of first instar larvae of *Ae. aegypti* at a dosage of 0.250 mg/L [33].

2.1.4 Entomopathogenic nematodes

Few studies are interested in the effect of nematodes on *Ae. aegypti* control, a study published in Argentina in 2014, was tested the infectivity of *Heterorhabditis bacteriophora* on *Ae. aegypti* larvae, and larval mortality rates ranges of 0–84% [34]. In another study conducted in Mexico, strains of *Heterorhabditis bacteriophora* and *Steinernema carpocapsae* were tested for their pathogenicity as infective juveniles (IJs) against larvae of *Ae. aegypti* (L.) of third- and fourth-instar mosquito larvae. Strain M5 of *S. carpocapsae* caused 100% mortality at the 200 IJ/larva concentration, with a median lethal concentration (LC_{50}) of 42 IJ/larva (LC_{90} = 91 IJ/larva). Strain M18 of *Heterohabditis bacteriophora* caused 73% mortality at 200 IJ/larva, with an LC_{50} = 72 and LC_{90} = 319 IJ/larva [35]. In a study, the larvicidal potential against some mosquito species of several nematodes isolated from soil was evaluated under laboratory conditions. The nematode *Steinernema abassi* showed 97.33% of mortality against *Ae. aegypti* [36]. These researches would lead to the development of an eco-friendly mosquito control agent.

2.2 Genetic control

2.2.1 Sterile insect technical (SIT)

Over the last decades, the Sterile Insect Technique (SIT), one of the most important methods of genetic control, has greatly developed [37]. This technique, specific to each species, consists of mass-rearing of male insects, genetically modified or not [through chemicals or radiation], to be released in target areas in quantities sufficient for them to compete with wild males for wild females and mate with them. They will, therefore, sterilise the females or transfer to their progeny lethal modifications or modifications that prevent pathogenic transmission, contributing to the reduction of target populations. Sustained liberation of sterile males will reduce the target population or potentially eradicate isolated populations [16, 18, 38]. Since the 1960s and 1970s, SIT has been successfully used against *Cu. quinquefasciatus* in the USA [39], *An. albimanus* in El Salvador [40] and the control of tsetse fly in Africa [41]. Pilot trials in the USA in which gamma-irradiated sterile male *Ae. aegypti* and *Anopheles quadrimaculatus* were released, showed no apparent suppression of populations after 43–48 weeks in the treated areas [42].

The application of SIT against mosquitoes must take into account mass-rearing procedures, sterilisation methods, transport and release methods, and trapping systems [43]. The application of SIT in vectors requires the release of males only because it maximises the effectiveness of releases, the efficiency of breeding efforts, and manages the public perception and stringent regulations that exist even for the release of small numbers of potentially disease-transmitting females. One of the advantages of releasing sterile males is the control of cryptic breeding sites, as these males locate their mates who then lay non-viable eggs, allowing for more effective control of these sites which are difficult to control with insecticides [43].

Nowadays, the viability of SIT for mosquitos *Aedes* is being evaluated with pilot trials by institutions and governments from different countries, such as Brazil, China, Cuba, French Polynesia, Italy, Mauritius, Mexico, Reunion, Singapore, Spain, Sudan, Thailand, and the United States [43].

2.2.2 Incompatible insect technique (IIT)

This technique of incompatible insects is related to SIT, as instead of releasing sterile males, Wolbachia-infected males are released which, after mating with a wild female, do not produce viable offspring [44]. This technique exploits the biological mechanism of cytoplasmic incompatibility present in *Wolbachia* to produce infected but not sterilised males as is the case with radiation and genetic modification which impose a large fitness burden or suffer from complicated regulatory pathways [44]. Recently, studies combining the SIT and Incompatible Insect Technique (IIT) have been carried out for *Ae. aegypti* and *Ae. albopictus* [45, 46]. This technique involves triple-infecting laboratory mosquitoes with *Wolbachia* strains (*Ae. albopictus* is naturally infected with wAlbA and wAlbB; the triple infection incorporates wPip) and irradiating the pupae to sterilise females. However, for this combination to be deemed the safest solution for the suppression of vector populations, perfect sexual identification mechanisms must be developed [46].

2.2.3 Control by genetic manipulation

Among the genetic control techniques, the most advanced strategy is the release of insects carrying a self-limiting gene (RISL) [10]. According to Zheng et al. [46], this method consists of inserting a self-limiting gene into the genome of the vector that interrupts its development, thus preventing it from reaching the adult stage, and then mass-producing them and releasing them into the wild to compete with wild populations. The purpose of this technique is to suppress the local populations and reduce the likelihood of disease transmission. It should be noted that sustained release of transgenic males is necessary to maintain suppression of wild *Ae. aegypti* populations. However, one of the disadvantages of this technique is that males carrying the lethal gene may be less competitive in mating than wild males, leading to low population suppression [10].

At the present time, mosquito control techniques, such as genetic handling strategies to produce "female killers", consisting of releasing males with a gene that is lethal to the females and will cause conditioned sterilisation or selective lethality, continue to evolve [47]. Another technique is Homing Endonuclease Genes (HEG), which grant resistance to infection and determine fertility and sex differentiation in mosquitoes are also being used [48]. Finally, a genetic technique based on CRISPR, to propagate target genes through traditional Mendelian inheritance, is being developed under laboratory conditions. Its most recent advancement has a binary focus to simultaneously interrupt the genes that are essential for female viability and male fertility of *Ae. aegypti*, that can suppress and eliminate populations at any life stage resulting in the survival of sterile males. It requires two breeding strains, one expressing Cas9 and the other expressing guide RNAs (gRNAs) known as precision-guided sterile insect technique (pgSIT), which compared with SIT and IIT not require the use of radiation, *Wolbachia*, or antibiotics, and will not persist in the environment longterm [49].

2.3 Chemical control

2.3.1 Traditional control

Insecticides have played a predominant role in vector control programmes. Accordingly, controlled release larvicide temephos has been commonly used in *Ae. aegypti* larvae control. In regards to adult mosquito control, it has been carried out through ultra-low volume (ULV) spatial spraying with organophosphate insecticides, such as malathion and pyrimiphos-methil, and with pyrethroids, such as deltamethrin, cypermethrin, and cyfluthrin, in addition to personal protection with repellents [50]. Recently, PAHO has recommended indoor residual spraying (IRS) of insecticides in urban areas to control *Ae. aegypti*, a measure in place to control malaria vectors [51]. However, intensive use of insecticides has led to the development of resistance in vector populations [52], environmental pollution, destruction of beneficial fauna, and the subsequent loss of balance in different ecosystems [53].

2.3.2 Control by autodissemination augmented by males (ADAM)

At present, innovative strategies using biorational insecticides, which present minimal impacts on human beings and the environment, are evolving. The most interesting and promising strategy implemented has been the Autodissemination Augmented by Males (ADAM), which consists of the use of males *Ae. aegypti* or *Ae. albopictus* that have been mass-reared, dusted with pyriproxyfen (PPF) or methoprene (insect growth regulators) and then released and thus transfer lethal concentrations directly contaminate larval habitats or indirectly contaminate them via mating with females that then visit such sites [54]. This substance acts analogously to the juvenile hormone and interferes in the metamorphoses of *Aedes* larvae in breeding grounds or resting grounds during oviposition, thus, reducing mosquito populations [55]. These compounds have advantages that include their "high toxicity to immature mosquitoes, low toxicity to adult mosquitoes, a substantial amount of prior research and environmental assessment, and its classification as a low risk insecticide" [53]. This strategy has been successfully implemented under field conditions in *Ae. aegypti* control in Brazil, Peru, and the USA [54, 56–58]. Likewise, it has been tested for *Ae. albopictus* under laboratory and field conditions in the USA [53, 59]. Brelsfoard et al.; [58] clarify that this technique should be integrated into existing control programmes and can be overlaid onto existing autocidal methods (e.g., SIT and IIE) and can offer effective control to the small and cryptic containers.

2.3.3 Development of the new insecticides

New insecticides have been developed to control mosquito resistance. Fludora Co-Max®, for example, combines two active ingredients with different modes of action (flupyradifurone, a butenolide, and transfluthrin, a pyrethroid), and has shown 100% mortality of resistant *Aedes* in the USA and Brazil through vehicle-mounted ULV spraying [60]. Another laboratory-tested insecticide that has shown 100% mortality in *Ae. aegypti* control is chlorfenapyr (CFP), a pyrrole insecticide repurposed from agriculture that could potentially be used for indoor residual spraying [60].

Studies have shown mortality of *Ae. aegypti*, *Ae. albopictus* and other vector's larvae with essential oils or plant extracts such as *Pergularia daemia* [61], *Plumeria rubra* [62], *Gmelina asiatica* [63], *Annnona squamosa* [64], *Polianthus tuberosa* [65], *Ambrosia arborescens* [66], *Solanum mammosum* [67], *Annona glabra* [68], *Plumbago auriculata* [69], and *Marsilea quadrifolia* [70]. All these studies show promise for the development of new insecticides for vector control.

2.3.4 Use of nanotechnology in the manufacture of plant-based products

The development of new compounds from plants is motivated by increasing resistance to insecticides. As of late, there have been developments in mosquito larvicides made from silver nanoparticles [AgNPs] synthesised by plants, this method is rapid, cost-effective, environmentally friendly, and safe for humans and it has exceptional properties such as bacterial activity, high resistance to oxidation and high thermal conductivity. The larvicidal effect is still unknown but it is assumed that AgNPs penetrate through the larval membrane causing death [71].

2.4 Physical control

Several strategies for physical control of *Ae. aegypti* have been developed, that is, physically interrupting larvae and pupae respiration through disturbances in air contact above the water surface with oils, surfactants, and polystyrene pearls [72] and mechanical barriers, such as lids, curtains, mosquito nets, and ovitraps [73].

New ovitraps are promising tools for the control, recent studies in laboratory and field, showed that the autocidal gravid ovitraps (AGO) which attract and capture gravid females looking for a place to lay their eggs [74] and attractive toxic sugar bait (ATSB) that use the staple sugar feeding behaviour of males of *Ae. aegypti* in nature for their control [75] have been shown to reduce the *Ae. aegypti* population.

Acoustic larvicidal are innovative technologies designed for the physical control of *Ae. aegypti*. This system uses sound waves that transmit acoustic energy across the water by causing rapid and traumatic vibrations, thus breaking the walls of the dorsal tracheal trunk and resulting in instant death. Furthermore, the lowest resonating energies affect other structures, inhibiting the emergence of larvae. In conclusion, mortality is the result of both effects [76, 77]. The lowest frequencies (20–50 kHz) are known to be more effective as larvicidal than higher frequencies (>100 kHz) [77]. However, when other aquatic insects, such as Diptera, Hemiptera, and Coleoptera that have open tracheal systems, are exposed to the acoustic beam for a prolonged period they may be adversely affected [78]. But other studies in which this acoustic control system has been used have shown high larval mortality of *Ae. aegypti* and *Cu. quinquefasciatus* (100%), both laboratory and field conditions and did not affect larvae predators, such as *Methanofollis formosanus*, *Poecilia reticulata* (Guppy fish), *Xiphophorus helleri* (Swordtail fish), *Micronecta grisea* (small water-boatmen) and *Indoplanorbis exustus* (freshwater snails) [76, 77, 79]. The promising nature of this system resides in the low risk of resistance development in target mosquito populations and this equipment can be used as a complement to the chemical or biological larvicides that have been used in control programmes under specific operational conditions [78].

2.5 Cultural control

2.5.1 Communication for mobilisation and behavioural impact (COMBI)

Since 2003, WHO has promoted the integrated management strategy for dengue prevention and control. Within this strategy is Communication for Behavioural Impact (COMBI) methodology. According to Parks and Lloyd [80], COMBI plans communication and social mobilisation that promotes the acquisition of recommended healthy practices and encourages the adoption and maintenance of those behaviours by involving individuals and families through the promotion of objectives with integrated strategies that contribute to the achievement of such objectives. Behavioural change has been shown to be essential for the prevention of arboviruses, such as dengue, so it is important to have a better understanding of the perception of the risk of becoming ill. This approach has been implemented in Asia and the Americas for several years, leaving lasting lessons in which goals, achievements, and difficulties were identified [81–83]. Lessons learned in the Americas show that it has been evidenced that meeting behavioural objectives, integration of multidisciplinary teams, formative research, community mobilisation, and advocacy have favoured the implementation of COMBI, however, the constant change of personnel, lack of political will due to the fact that these programmes are difficult to implement because they take longer to reflect impact compared to a low-cost approach Information, Education and Communication (IEC), which is limited to communication through home visits, leaflets and different vertical actions [83].

2.5.2 Approaches to social participation

Community involvement is a key element for the successful control of Ae. aegypti, studies conducted mainly in the 2000s in several countries suggest that integrated community-based control of *Ae. aegypti* under different approaches reduced vector density and had an impact on dengue transmission [84–88]. These approaches, such as Socialisation of Evidence for Participatory Action [SEPA], have been used in mobilising communities for vector control in Nicaragua and Mexico, known as The Green Way, which is based on cluster randomised controlled trial added community engagement in dengue prevention. These studies aimed to prove the hypothesis that informed mobilisation adds to the effectiveness of programmes managed by local governments [89–93]. In Cuba, other approaches have been implemented, such as Rifkin's approaches to community participation in health programmes, Shediac-Rizkallah and Bone's approaches to sustainability [86, 94, 95], and the evaluation of community participation in health programmes and the theory of education [96–98]. In China, Bishop's five-step learning process approach for community empowerment in vector control was applied [99].

2.5.3 Ecosystem approaches to health

In recent years, three approaches to community participation in *Ae. aegypti* control have gained relevance: eco-health, the socio-ecological system, and the political theory of health.

Eco-health integrates factors from the micro and macro contexts, that is, ecological [latitude, altitude, temperature, humidity, and precipitation], biological [natural and artificial surroundings related to vector and virus], and social factors [demographic, economic, political, and cultural, including programmes for the prevention and control of dengue] [100]. Studies have been carried out in the Americas and Asia [101, 102] to determine the weight of ecological and social factors in dengue vector infestation, and to analyse their implementation [103].

Based on systemic thinking, the socio-ecological system approach makes human beings a part of nature [104]. This model focuses on the interactions between human and natural systems along with a series of spatial, temporal, and organisational scales; for instance, the individual, the community, and the society [105]. It has been implemented, for the most part, in the city of Machala, Ecuador [106–109].

The political ecology of health analyses how health is positioned within socio-environmental networks that lead to illness and examines the contextual realities in decision making for resource use in health matters. Constructs about health authored by individual participants and institutions through the relations between social and environmental systems emerge within these networks [110]. In Ecuador, researchers tried to establish the social and environmental interactions of illnesses transmitted by *Ae. aegypti*, and concluded that the vulnerability of the population to these arboviral diseases stems from the socio-political limitations of community action and poverty, combined with a fragile public health system that undertakes incomplete, sporadic efforts to control such diseases [111]. Another recent study that has used this approach in the city of Maputo, Mozambique [112], took into consideration the patterns of distribution and storage of water, as well as the biophysical characteristics that make stored water more attractive to vector *Ae. aegypti*. In Maputo, all families store water, but different communities do it in different ways depending on their socio-economic situation. Therefore, it is dependent on an explicit analysis of power relations. Poor people store water both inside and outside of their homes, while wealthier people do it in closed tanks on top of their residences. The latter do not see nor live close to the stored water.

3. *Anopheles* mosquito control

3.1 Biological and genetic control

3.1.1 Biological control with bacteria

An alternative to the use of insecticides is the use of entomopathogenic bacteria, which has been implemented in some countries since the beginning of the century, when, in 1904, Meyer and Neide described the first bacterium, which attacks mosquito larvae, *Bacillus sphaericus* [113]. To date, about 35 strains of this bacterium are known to exist worldwide and are still effective on *Anopheles* [114]. Another bacterium, which has been widely used is *B. thuringiensis var. israelensis*, which is currently considered highly effective [115, 116]. The application of these larvicides although effective in controlling *Anopheles* has financial limitations in addition to the shortage of personnel trained in the ecology and biology of the vectors, the lack of organisational structures, and the predominance of vertical control programmes [117].

Another bacterium, which has recently been evaluated, is *Wolbachia*. It has been tested for the control of *Ae. aegypti*. *Wolbachia* is maternally transmitted intracellular bacteria, which invade insect populations, by manipulating their reproduction and immunity, thus, limiting the spread of numerous human pathogens including *Plasmodium*, but the activity of these bacteria in *Anopheles* control programmes has not been explored. Inhibition of *Plasmodium falciparum* in *Anopheles gambiae* under laboratory conditions has been reported [118] and the same author demonstrated that the native microbiome of *A. gambiae* and *An. stephensi* prevents vertical transmission of *Wolbachia* [119]. On the other hand, there are records of natural infection of this bacterium in wild *Anopheles*, as reported in West Africa where *Wolbachia* was found in *An. gambiae* from the field [120] and in larvae of *An. stephensi* [121]. On the same continent, but in sub-Saharan Africa, *Wolbachia* was found in low densities in species of the gambiae complex (*An. moucheti* and *An. demeilloni*) [122]. Similar reports were recorded in Central Africa by the World Mosquito Program [123]. Reports have also been made in Malaysia where they recorded 17 *Anopheles* species, of which eight species were positive for the natural occurrence of *Wolbachia* [124].

3.1.2 Entomopathogenic fungus

Metarhizium anisopliae and *Beauveria bassiana*, are the two entomopathogenic fungi well recognised in the literature, these can infect mosquitoes early in life and kill them, depending on the exposure dose and fungus isolate, after 3–14 days. In addition, these fungi have shown that interfere with *Plasmodium* parasite development in the *Anopheles* mosquito [125].

The discovery of new mosquitocides from fungal extracts for *Anopheles* species is promising, that is, the extract from *Penicillium toxicarium* has exhibited high toxicity to mosquito larvae and adults on *A. gambiae* [126]. Other studies showed that the fungal extracts of *Trichoderma asperellum* had a larvicidal effect *in vitro* on *Anopheline* larvae [127, 128].

3.1.3 Biological control with nematodes

The use of Mermithid worms (Nematoda, Mermithidae) for the control of *Anopheles* larvae has been used for several years. The nematode with which the first reported work began was the species *Romanomermis culicivorax*. This is an obligate endoparasite of mosquito larvae and has been recorded in *An. stephensi*, *An. albimanus*, *An. gambiae*, *Culex,* and *Aedes*, the advantage is that it does not affect animals, plants, and humans. In the United States, the nematode has been used to control insects, such as *Anopheles freeborni* and several species of *Culex,* and is classified by the United States Department of Agriculture as a safe and innocuous biological product for mosquito control [129]. In Brazil, in 2000, a bioplant was created in the facilities of the Federal University of the State of Roraima, for rearing *Romanomermis iyengari* as a control strategy in larval breeding sites of *Anopheles* sp. in breeding sites in Boa Vista - Roraima [130]. In Mexico, applications of a dose of 2000–3000 pre-parasitic juvenile *R. iyengari* per square metre produced an infection rate of approximately 85–100% in *An. pseudopunctipennis* larvae, thus reducing the risk of malaria transmission to people living nearby breeding sites [131].

New studies have been carried out in recent years, the nematode *R. culicivorax* was used in the North Atlantic Autonomous Region in Nicaragua and showed efficiency in controlling larval densities of *Anopheles albimanus* [132]. In another study, isolated nematodes were subsequently cultured and evaluated their larvicidal potential against the larvae of several mosquitoes. The nematode *Heterohabditis indica* showed 97.33% of mortality against *An. stephensi* [36]. In a recent study in Africa, the nematode *R. iyengari* was mass-produced, and the pre-parasitic stage (J2) was used for laboratory and field experiments. In field experiments, the monthly applications of 3500–5000 pre-parasitic nematodes per m^2 eliminated larval mosquito development in *Anopheles* and mixed breeding sites [133]. In Benin, West Africa evaluated coconut coir fibres as a replacement for coarse sand to improve yields in largescale production of *R. iyengari* because this method has the potential for facilitating the wider distribution of this nematode for use against malaria vectors in West Africa [134].

3.1.4 Biological control with kairomones

Female mosquito vectors use physical and chemical signals to locate their blood food source in vertebrate hosts, such as transpiration of CO2, octenol, lactic acid, and a variety of sweat compounds released in respiration and excretions, producing characteristic odours of substances called kairomones, which are chemicals produced by other organisms different to the insects but which attract them [135]. This is a new area to integrate vector control systems since they are just starting with the first studies conducted in Africa where it incorporated a system of traps with kairomones as attractants as a means of control *An. gambiae*. Thus, the first Kairomone [Methyl mercaptan] has already been identified, which attracts this species of *Anopheles*, which will open the possibility to conduct similar studies in other countries and thus, expand more on this control method [136]. These studies allow to do new research and the search for new strategies of this type in other malarial countries, which can become an alternative control model.

3.1.5 Biological control with pheromones

The use of pheromones in odour traps for the surveillance and control of mosquito vectors is considered a new and viable component of integrated vector management programmes. Few works have been conducted, by using these substances, due to the difficulty of synthesising them in the laboratory. A study shows pheromone release in the reproductive frenzy of some *Anopheles* species has been reported at the laboratory level in species, such as *An. arabiensis* and *An. gambiae* and five species of importance in the transmission in Africa (*An. gambiae*, *An. coluzzii*, *An. arabiensis*, *An. merus,* and *An. funestus*) in semi-field experiments [137]. It is important to further expand these types of studies, replicate them, and set the foundations for the next generation of attractants and traps to be used in vector-borne disease control programmes.

3.1.6 Sterile insect technique (SIT) in Anopheles

In recent years, the possibility of using the sterile insect technique (SIT) as part of the programmes against mosquitoes has received increased attention, this is due to the resistance developed by parasites to drugs and vectors to insecticides [138]. The most developed model for SIT is with the species *Anopheles arabiensis* but when considering a mosquito release programme, one of the first issues to be addressed is how to eliminate/separate the hematophagous vector females, several studies have investigated this issue, because sex separation increases the efficiency of an SIT programme [139, 140]. So much progress has been made in these researches that in the study of Kaiser et al., [141] three separate releases were performed within a 2-year period. Approximately 5000–15,000 laboratory-reared male *An. arabiensis* (KWAG) were produced and marked for mark–release–recapture experiments, this study showed that marked males were found in swarms with wild males, indicating that laboratory-reared males are able to locate and participate in mating swarms.

3.2 Chemical and physical control

Indoor residual spraying (IRS) and the use of long-lasting insecticidal nets (LLINs) have been effective control strategies for malaria vector control, leading to a reduction in cases between 2002 and 2017 [142, 143]. However, there are two major problems—first, the use of these strategies alone or in combination will not eliminate malaria; and second, insecticide resistance of the main malaria vectors is widespread and increasing [142]. According to the literature, few advances have been made in the development of new insecticides for malaria vector control. In this regard, a combination of the neonicotinoid clothianidin and the pyrethroid deltamethrin (Fludora Fusion) was recently developed as a new vector control tool, which has been effective in managing resistance [144].

One study demonstrated in large-cage SFS experiments the autodissemination of PPF by the malaria vector *Anopheles arabiensis*, which provides proof of principle for the autodissemination of PPF to breeding habitats by malaria vectors. Bioassay of water samples from artificial habitats in these experiments resulted in significantly lower emergence rates in treated chambers (0.16 ± 0.23) compared to controls (0.97 ± 0.05) ($p < 0.0001$) [145]. To this end, Kiware et al., [146] conducted deterministic mathematical models to describe that use only field-measurable input parameters and capture the biological processes that mediate PPF autodissemination.

3.3 Cultural control

3.3.1 Combi

The COMBI methodology is a very local and targeted methodology that integrates health education in a language of its own, community mobilisation, and social, anthropological, and biological research, directed in a sharp and intelligent way towards specific and precise health behavioural outcomes [80]. This methodology differs from traditional approaches, achieving generational changes in vector-borne disease control and prevention programmes, but which are subject to political will for their continuity and execution. For example, in Colombia, the COMBI strategy was implemented in several departments (Antioquia, Cauca, Chocó, Córdoba, and Valle del Cauca) articulated with vector-borne disease control programmes, where the behavioural objective was the use of nets [83]. In rural areas of Sudan, a study was conducted where it was assessed the effectiveness of COMBI strategy in enhancing the utilisation of long-lasting insecticidal nets (LLINs) among mothers of underfive

Control	Vectors	Strategies	Advantages	Disadvantages
Biological	*Aedes*	*Bacillus thuringiensis var. israelensis*	No resistance Selective and safe Acceptable for treating drinking water sources and containers. Long-lasting, moderately costly, and eco-friendly	Low residual action in polluted habitats.
	Anopheles	*Bacillus sphaericus*	No resistance Selective and safe Acceptable for treating drinking water sources and containers Long-lasting, moderately costly, and eco-friendly	Low residual action in polluted habitats.
	Anopheles	Kairomones and pheromones*	Selective and safe	Understudy
	Aedes, Anopheles	Larvivorous fish Nematodes	Well accepted in several countries, needs a delivery mechanism and maintenance. Adequate for treating large and/or permanent mosquito habitats. Eco-friendly	The intense work to maintain the organisms in the containers depend on the above environmental factors, in addition to the emptying of reservoirs, and escape or death of the organisms. For fish its resistance to temperature and the physicochemical characteristics of the water, especially to chlorine.
		Fungi*	The specific pathogenic capacity to mosquito larvae and the prolonged period of persistence. Laboratory maintenance. Eco-friendly	Require maintenance or large-scale infrastructure. Require demanding long-term maintenance. Delay in generating mortality. Their viability is affected by environmental factors such as temperature, pH, salinity and organic matter content in the water, as well as by external factors such as ultraviolet A radiation from the sun.
		Wolbachia*	Wolbachia can invade and persist in wild mosquito populations. Low-cost, self-sustaining form control. Persistence and varying invasiveness of the modifications induced, with the need to consider the evolution and long-term effects of the factors responsible for these modifications, including their potential for transfer to other species. Helps to reduce the use of insecticide and can be combined with the conventional techniques.	*Wolbachia* has not been approved in most countries due to insufficient knowledge of the potential dangers of this control method. Complicated regulatory pathways.

Control	Vectors	Strategies	Advantages	Disadvantages
Genetic	*Aedes, Anopheles*	Sterile Insect Technical (SIT)*	The major benefit of minimising the direct impact of vector control on health and the environment; the potential for unintended replacement of the target population by the population of another vector species; no large-scale maintenance or infrastructure required; helping to reduce the use of insecticide and can be combined with the conventional techniques.	Require demanding long-term maintenance, the disadvantage of being rather inflexible, or even uncontrollable (e.g., of the expected spread affecting an entire species). SIT and genetic manipulation impose a large fitness burden and suffer from complicated regulatory pathways
		Incompatible Insect Technique (IIT)*		
		Genetic manipulation (Female Killers, HEG, pgSIT)*		
Chemical	*Aedes, Anopheles*	Insecticides and bioinsecticides*	Effective for all stages of mosquitoes. It has demonstrated entomological and epidemiological efficacy.	Insecticide resistance, Low acceptability, and limited sense of security in the community Costly and time-consuming Requires high coverage Poor persistence Regulatory and environmental constraints Needs skilled, experienced staff Constraints for the treatment of cryptic breeding sites
		Autodissemination Augmented by Males (ADAM)*	High toxicity to immature mosquitoes, low toxicity to adult mosquitoes, a substantial amount of prior research and environmental assessment, and its classification as a low-risk insecticide. Effective control to the small and cryptic containers.	Insecticide resistance Degradation of insecticide
Physical	*Aedes*	Oils, surfactants, and polystyrene pearls	Effective control of the small containers.	Environmentally unfriendly
		Ovitraps*	Low cost Possible to combine with community participation Sustainable, able to be reused for several seasons.	Insecticide resistance Degradation of insecticide Costly and time-consuming Requires high coverage
		Acoustical larvicides*	Effective control of the small containers. This method can be used as a complement to the chemical or biological larvicides Reduce the use of insecticide	Costly and time-consuming Requires high coverage Poor persistence Regulatory and environmental constraints
	Aedes, Anopheles	Mosquito nets, curtains, lids	Individual-and community-based action Residual activity with long-lasting technology.	Insecticide resistance Low protection against UV Degradation of insecticide

Control	Vectors	Strategies	Advantages	Disadvantages
Cultural	*Aedes, Anopheles*	COMBI	There is evidence that community participation contributes to the reduction of the vector population.	The constant change of personnel and lack of political will due to the fact that these programmes are difficult to implement because they take longer to reflect impact compared to a low-cost approach IEC.
		Approaches to social participation		
		Ecosystem approaches to health*		

New strategies.

Table 1.
Advantages and disadvantages of vector control strategies.

children, the study demonstrated the usefulness of COMBI strategy for increasing awareness about malaria, developing a positive perception towards malaria prevention and, increasing the utilisation of LLINs [147].

3.3.2 Approaches to social participation and eco-health

Community motivation to participate in entomological projects is an important premise. A qualitative approach was used to survey the factors motivating members of the local community to assist in the implementation of Target Malaria's entomological research activities in Bana, Western Burkina Faso. The results showed a degree of consistency around five categories of motivation: (a) enhance domestic protection from mosquitoes and malaria, (b) contribute to a future world free of the disease, (c) acquire knowledge and skills, (d) earn financial compensation, and (e) gain social prestige for the village [148]. A cluster-randomised controlled trial conducted in Malawi combined the interventions to the current national malaria control strategies of Malawi with community-based larval source management and structural house improvements for 2 years in rural, southern Malawi and demonstrated to reduce malaria transmission below the level reached by current interventions alone [149].

In a recent study, community participation is key to the success of IVM implementation at the local level. The project promoted the adoption and sustainability of IVM and scale-up of IVM-related activities as well as increased community participation and partnership in malaria control through outreach, capacity-building, and collaboration with other stakeholders in the area. Thus, it is that between 2016 and 2018 the project was able to reach 25,322 people in the community advocacy and social mobilisation initiatives [150].

The community-based interventions and research to action based on an ecosystem framework (eco-health) provided information in an integrative way characterising annual dynamics among indigenous communities. The research was conducted with the Bari of Karikachaboquira and the Wayúu of Marbacella and El Horno in Colombia, using qualitative and participatory methods, including seasonal graphics, semi-structured interviews, geo-referencing routes, and participatory observation, an eco-health calendar was obtained for each community, linking the socioecological dynamics to specific diseases, especially malaria. The eco-health calendar allows the integration of eco-bio-social factors in a layout that breaks conceptual and cultural barriers [151].

Table 1 shows the advantages and disadvantages of the *Aedes* and *Anopheles* vector control strategies.

4. Conclusions

Many mosquito vector control strategies have been developed in recent years, but these strategies must take into account the local context and their application must be guided by integrated vector management.

In vector control strategies, various advances are being developed worldwide in all forms of control, for example, regardless of biological and genetic control the extensive development of the use of other species of fungi, *Wolbachia* bacteria, the sterile male technique, and the genetic manipulation of insects, which have already been tested in field conditions, may bring interesting results for inclusion in traditional control programmes in the future. A great development is expected in the use of the CRISP technique in gene editing in mosquitoes for later release.

A great development is expected in the use of autodissemination augmented by males, which is a technique that offers many advantages and can be used in combination with traditional control methods.

It is possible that in the future, the use of insecticides will be limited by the development of the above control strategies; however, it is necessary to develop other alternatives that arise from plants where the use of nanotechnology can play an important role.

These advances are essential, but the communities that ultimately benefit from all this development must be taken into account.

The efforts of researchers in the development and evaluation of these and new control methods, the political will of governments, funding from the business sector, and community participation are essential to the success of these strategies.

Author details

Wilber Gómez-Vargas[1]* and Giovani Esteban Zapata-Úsuga[2]

1 Epidemiology and Biostatistics and Researcher Colombian Institute of Tropical Medicine, CES University, Medellín, Colombia

2 Entomology, National University of Colombia, Medellín, Colombia

*Address all correspondence to: wgomez@ces.edu.co

References

[1] Bhatt S, Gething PW, Brady OJ, Messina JP, Farlow AW, Moyes CL, et al. The global distribution and burden of dengue. Nature. 2013;**496**(7446):504-507

[2] WHO. Technical Report: Recommendations for Scientific Evidence-Based Yellow Fever Risk Assessment in the Americas. Washington, D.C.: WHO; 2013. p. 49

[3] World Health Organization. World Malaria Report 2021 [Internet]. Geneva: WHO; 2021. Available from: https://apps.who.int/iris/handle/10665/350147. [Accessed: 2 January 2022]

[4] WHO. Global vector response 2017-2030 [Internet]. 2017. Available from: https://www.who.int/publications/i/item/9789241512978

[5] Pan American Health Organization. Handbook for Integrated Vector Management. Washington, DC: Organización Panamericana de la Salud, Oficina Sanitaria Panamericana, Oficina Regional de la Organización Mundial de la Salud; 2012. p. 68

[6] Organización Panamericana de la Salud. Documento operativo de aplicación del manejo integrado de vectores adaptado al contexto de las Américas. Washington, D.C.: OPS; 2019. p. 68

[7] Kraemer MU, Sinka ME, Duda KA, Mylne AQ, Shearer FM, Barker CM, et al. The global distribution of the arbovirus vectors Aedes aegypti and ae. Albopictus. eLife. 2015;**4**:e08347

[8] Araújo AP, Araujo Diniz DF, Helvecio E, de Barros RA, de Oliveira CMF, Ayres CFJ, et al. The susceptibility of Aedes aegypti populations displaying temephos resistance to Bacillus thuringiensis israelensis: A basis for management. Parasites & Vectors. 2013;**6**(1):297

[9] McMeniman CJ, Lane RV, Cass BN, Fong AWC, Sidhu M, Wang YF, et al. Stable introduction of a life-shortening Wolbachia infection into the mosquito Aedes aegypti. Science. 2009;**323**(5910):141-144

[10] Calvitti M, Marini F, Desiderio A, Puggioli A, Moretti R. Wolbachia density and cytoplasmic incompatibility in Aedes albopictus: Concerns with using artificial Wolbachia infection as a vector suppression tool. Bourtzis K, editor. PLoS One. 2015;**10**(3):e0121813

[11] Bonneau M, Landmann F, Labbé P, Justy F, Weill M, Sicard M. The cellular phenotype of cytoplasmic incompatibility in Culex pipiens in the light of cidB diversity. PLoS Pathogens. 2018;**14**(10):e1007364

[12] PAHO. Evaluation of Innovative Strategies for Aedes aegypti Control: Challenges for their Introduction and Impact Assessment. Washington, D.C: PAHO; 2019

[13] Pietri JE, DeBruhl H, Sullivan W. The rich somatic life of Wolbachia. MicrobiologyOpen. 2016;**5**(6):923-936

[14] Bourtzis K, Dobson SL, Xi Z, Rasgon JL, Calvitti M, Moreira LA, et al. Harnessing mosquito–Wolbachia symbiosis for vector and disease control. Acta Tropica. 2014;**132**:S150-S163

[15] Dutra HLC, Rocha MN, Dias FBS, Mansur SB, Caragata EP, Moreira LA. Wolbachia blocks currently circulating Zika virus isolates in Brazilian Aedes aegypti mosquitoes. Cell Host & Microbe. 2016;**19**(6):771-774

[16] Bouyer J, Marois E. Genetic control of vectors. In: Pests and Vector-Borne Diseases in the Livestock Industry. Wageningen, The Netherlands: Wageningen Academic Publishers; 2018. pp. 435-451

[17] Yen PS, Failloux AB. A review: Wolbachia-based population replacement for mosquito control shares common points with genetically modified control approaches. Pathogens. 2020;**9**(5):404

[18] World Health Organization, The International Atomic Energy Agency. Guidance Framework for Testing the Sterile Insect Technique as a Vector Control Tool against aedes-Borne Diseases [Internet]. Geneva: World Health Organization; 2020. p. 189. Available from: https://apps.who.int/iris/handle/10665/331679. [Accessed: 4 January 2022]

[19] Ross PA, Turelli M, Hoffmann AA. Evolutionary ecology of Wolbachia releases for disease control. Annual Review of Genetics. 2019;**53**(1):93-116

[20] Najitha Banu A, Balasubramanian C, Moorthi PV. Biosynthesis of silver nanoparticles using Bacillus thuringiensis against dengue vector, Aedes aegypti (Diptera: Culicidae). Parasitology Research. 2014;**113**(1):311-316

[21] Thelma J, Balasubramanian C. Ovicidal, larvicidal and pupicidal efficacy of silver nanoparticles synthesized by Bacillus marisflavi against the chosen mosquito species. PLoS One. 2021;**16**(12):e0260253

[22] Nabar BM, Lokegaonkar S. Larvicidal activity of microbial metabolites extracted from extremophiles against vector mosquitoes. International Journal of Mosquito Research. 2015;**2**(3):161-163

[23] Janaki T. Larvicidal activity of Streptomyces cacaoi subsp. cacaoi-M20 against Aedes aegypti. International Journal of Botany Studies. 2016;**1**(2):47-49

[24] Bucker A, Bucker NCF, de Souza AQL, da Gama AM, Rodrigues-Filho E, da Costa FM, et al. Larvicidal effects of endophytic and basidiomycete fungus extracts on Aedes and Anopheles larvae (Diptera, Culicidae). Revista da Sociedade Brasileira de Medicina Tropical. 2013;**46**(4):411-419

[25] Rodrigues J, Campos VC, Humber RA, Luz C. Efficacy of Culicinomyces spp. against Aedes aegypti eggs, larvae and adults. Journal of Invertebrate Pathology. 2018;**157**:104-111

[26] Rueda ME, Tavares I, López CC, García J. Leptolegnia chapmanii como alternativa biológica para el control de Aedes aegypti. Biomédica. 2019;**39**(4): 798-810

[27] Rueda Páramo ME, López Lastra CC, García JJ. Persistence and pathogenicity of a native isolate of Leptolegnia chapmanii against Aedes aegypti larvae in different anthropic environments. Biocontrol Science and Technology. 2015;**25**(2):238-243

[28] Karthi S, Vasantha-Srinivasan P, Ganesan R, Ramasamy V, Senthil-Nathan S, Khater HF, et al. Target activity of Isaria tenuipes (Hypocreales: Clavicipitaceae) fungal strains against dengue vector Aedes aegypti (Linn.) and its non-target activity against aquatic predators. Journal of Fungi. 2020;**6**(4):196

[29] Reyes-Villanueva F, Garza-Hernandez JA, Garcia-Munguia AM, Tamez-Guerra P, Howard AF, Rodriguez-Perez MA. Dissemination of Metarhizium anisopliae of low and high virulence by mating behavior in Aedes aegypti. Parasites & Vectors. 2011;**4**(1):171

[30] García-Munguía AM, Garza-Hernández JA, Rebollar-Tellez EA, Rodríguez-Pérez MA, Reyes-Villanueva F. Transmission of Beauveria bassiana from male to female Aedes aegypti mosquitoes. Parasites & Vectors. 2011;**4**(1):24

[31] Baverstock J, Roy HE, Pell JK. Entomopathogenic fungi and insect behaviour: From unsuspecting hosts to targeted vectors. BioControl. 2010;**55**(1):89-102

[32] Salunkhe RB, Patil SV, Patil CD, Salunke BK. Larvicidal potential of silver nanoparticles synthesized using fungus Cochliobolus lunatus against Aedes aegypti (Linnaeus, 1762) and Anopheles stephensi Liston (Diptera; Culicidae). Parasitology Research. 2011;**109**(3):823-831

[33] Gopinath K, Karthika V, Sundaravadivelan C, Gowri S, Arumugam A. Mycogenesis of cerium oxide nanoparticles using aspergillus Niger culture filtrate and their applications for antibacterial and larvicidal activities. Journal of Nanostructure in Chemistry. 2015;**5**(3):295-303

[34] Peshiutta ML, Cagnolo SR, Almirón WR. Susceptibilty of larvae of Aedes aegypti (Linnaeus) (Diptera: Culicidae) to entomopathogenic nematode Heterorhabtiditidis bacteriophora (Ponar) (Rhabditida: Heterorhabditidae). Revista de la Sociedad Entomológica Argentina. 2014;**73**(3-4):99-108

[35] Treviño-Cueto D, Subbotin SA, Sanchez-Peña SR. Larvicidal activity of Entomopathogenic nematodes isolated from Mexico against Aedes aegypti (Diptera: Culicidae). Journal of Entomological Science. 2021;**56**(1):12-23

[36] Aiswarya D, Raja Ramalingam K, Chinnaperumal K, Govindasamy B, Paramasivam D, Dhayalan A, et al. Isolation and growth inhibition potential of entomopathogenic nematodes against three public health important mosquito vectors. Experimental Parasitology. 2019;**197**:76-84

[37] Alphey L, McKemey A, Nimmo D, Neira Oviedo M, Lacroix R, Matzen K, et al. Genetic control of Aedes mosquitoes. Pathogens and Global Health. 2013;**107**(4):170-179

[38] Facchinelli L, Valerio L, Ramsey JM, Gould F, Walsh RK, Bond G, et al. Field cage studies and progressive evaluation of genetically-engineered mosquitoes. PLoS Neglected Tropical Diseases. 2013;**7**(1):e2001

[39] Patterson RS, Weidhaas DE, Ford HR, Lofgren CS. Suppression and elimination of an island population of Culex pipiens quinquefasciatus with sterile males. Science. 1970;**168**(3937):1368-1370

[40] Weidhaas DE, Breeland SG, Lofgren CS, Dame DA, Kaiser R. Release of Chemosterilized males for the control of Anopheles albimanus in El Salvador. IV. Dynamics of the test population. The American Journal of Tropical Medicine and Hygiene. 1974;**23**:298-308

[41] Vreysen MJB, Saleh KM, Ali MY, Abdulla AM, Zhu ZR, Juma KG, et al. Glossina austeni (Diptera: Glossinidae) eradicated on the island of Unguja, Zanzibar, using the sterile insect technique. Journal of Economic Entomology. 2000;**93**(1):123-135

[42] Weidhaas DE, Schmidt CH, Seabrook EL. Field studies on the release of sterile males for the control of Anopheles quadrimaculatus. Mosquito News. 1962;**22**:283-290

[43] Lees RS, Carvalho D, Bouyer J. Potential impact of integrating the sterile

insect technique into the fight against disease-transmitting mosquitoes. In: Sterile Insect Technique Principles and Practice in Area-Wide Integrated Pest Management. 2nd ed. IAEA. New York: CRC Press; 2021. pp. 1081-1118

[44] Pagendam DE, Trewin BJ, Snoad N, Ritchie SA, Hoffmann AA, Staunton KM, et al. Modelling the Wolbachia incompatible insect technique: Strategies for effective mosquito population elimination. BMC Biology. 2020;**18**(1):161

[45] Kittayapong P, Kaeothaisong N, Ninphanomchai S, Limohpasmanee W. Combined sterile insect technique and incompatible insect technique: Sex separation and quality of sterile Aedes aegypti male mosquitoes released in a pilot population suppression trial in Thailand. Parasites & Vectors. 2018;**11**(S2):657

[46] Zheng X, Zhang D, Li Y, Yang C, Wu Y, Liang X, et al. Incompatible and sterile insect techniques combined eliminate mosquitoes. Nature. 2019;**572**(7767):56-61

[47] Windbichler N, Papathanos PA, Crisanti A. Targeting the X chromosome during spermatogenesis induces Y chromosome transmission ratio distortion and early dominant embryo lethality in Anopheles gambiae. Stern DL, editor. PLoS Genetics. 2008;**4**(12):e1000291

[48] Deredec A, Burt A, Godfray HCJ. The population genetics of using homing endonuclease genes in vector and Pest management. Genetics. 2008;**179**(4):2013-2026

[49] Li M, Yang T, Bui M, Gamez S, Wise T, Kandul NP, et al. Suppressing mosquito populations with precision guided sterile males. Nature Communications. 2021;**12**(1):5374

[50] Jing Q, Wang M. Dengue epidemiology. Global Health Journal. 2019;**3**(2):37-45

[51] Pan-American Health Organization. Manual for Indoor Residual Spraying in Urban Areas for Aedes aegypti Control. Washington, DC: Pan American Health Organization; 2019. p. 60

[52] Santacoloma L, Chaves B, Brochero HL. Estado de la susceptibilidad de poblaciones naturales del vector del dengue a insecticidas en 13 localidades de Colombia. Biomédica. 2012;**32**:3

[53] Mains JW, Brelsfoard CL, Dobson SL. Male mosquitoes as vehicles for insecticide. PLoS Neglected Tropical Diseases. 2015;**9**(1):e0003406

[54] Devine GJ, Perea EZ, Killeen GF, Stancil JD, Clark SJ, Morrison AC. Using adult mosquitoes to transfer insecticides to Aedes aegypti larval habitats. PNAS. 2009;**106**(28):11530-11534

[55] Hustedt JC, Boyce R, Bradley J, Hii J, Alexander N. Use of pyriproxyfen in control of Aedes mosquitoes: A systematic review. PLoS Neglected Tropical Diseases. 2020;**14**(6):e0008205

[56] Abad-Franch F, Zamora-Perea E, Ferraz G, Padilla-Torres SD, Luz SLB. Mosquito-disseminated Pyriproxyfen yields high breeding-site coverage and boosts juvenile mosquito mortality at the Neighborhood scale. PLoS Neglected Tropical Diseases. 2015;**9**(4):e0003702

[57] Abad-Franch F, Zamora-Perea E, Luz SLB. Mosquito-disseminated insecticide for citywide vector control and its potential to block arbovirus epidemics: Entomological observations and Modeling results from Amazonian Brazil. PLoS Medicine. 2017;**14**(1):e1002213

[58] Brelsfoard CL, Mains JW, Mulligan S, Cornel A, Holeman J, Kluh S, et al. Aedes

aegypti males as vehicles for insecticide delivery. Insects. 2019;**10**(8):230

[59] Suman DS, Wang Y, Faraji A, Williams GM, Williges E, Gaugler R. Seasonal field efficacy of pyriproxyfen autodissemination stations against container-inhabiting mosquito Aedes albopictus under different habitat conditions: Field efficacy of pyriproxyfen autodissemination stations against mosquitoes. Pest Management Science. 2018;**74**(4):885-895

[60] Corbel V, Durot C, Achee NL, Chandre F, Coulibaly MB, David JP, et al. Second WIN international conference on "integrated approaches and innovative tools for combating insecticide resistance in vectors of arboviruses", October 2018. Singapore: Parasites & Vectors. 2019;**12**(1):331

[61] Patil CD, Borase HP, Patil SV, Salunkhe RB, Salunke BK. Larvicidal activity of silver nanoparticles synthesized using Pergularia daemia plant latex against Aedes aegypti and Anopheles stephensi and nontarget fish Poecillia reticulata. Parasitology Research. 2012;**111**(2):555-562

[62] Patil CD, Patil SV, Borase HP, Salunke BK, Salunkhe RB. Larvicidal activity of silver nanoparticles synthesized using Plumeria rubra plant latex against Aedes aegypti and Anopheles stephensi. Parasitology Research. 2012;**110**(5):1815-1822

[63] Muthukumaran U, Govindarajan M, Rajeswary M, Hoti SL. Synthesis and characterization of silver nanoparticles using Gmelina asiatica leaf extract against filariasis, dengue, and malaria vector mosquitoes. Parasitology Research. 2015;**114**(5):1817-1827

[64] Velayutham K, Ramanibai R. Larvicidal activity of synthesized silver nanoparticles using isoamyl acetate identified in Annona squamosa leaves against Aedes aegypti and Culex quinquefasciatus. The Journal of Basic and Applied Zoology. 2016;**74**:16-22

[65] Rawani A. Mosquito larvicidal activity of green silver nanoparticle synthesized from extract of bud of Polianthus tuberosa L. International Journal of Nanotechnology and Application. 2017;**1**:12

[66] Morejón B, Pilaquinga F, Domenech F, Ganchala D, Debut A, Neira M. Larvicidal activity of silver nanoparticles synthesized using extracts of Ambrosia arborescens (Asteraceae) to control Aedes aegypti L. (Diptera: Culicidae). Journal of Nanotechnology. 2018;**20**:1-8

[67] Pilaquinga F, Morejón B, Ganchala D, Morey J, Piña N, Debut A, et al. Green synthesis of silver nanoparticles using Solanum mammosum L. (Solanaceae) fruit extract and their larvicidal activity against Aedes aegypti L. (Diptera: Culicidae). PLoS One. 2019;**14**(10):e0224109

[68] Amarasinghe LD, Wickramarachchi PASR, Aberathna AAAU, Sithara WS, De Silva CR. Comparative study on larvicidal activity of green synthesized silver nanoparticles and Annona glabra (Annonaceae) aqueous extract to control Aedes aegypti and Aedes albopictus (Diptera: Culicidae). Heliyon. 2020;**6**(6):e04322

[69] Govindan L, Anbazhagan S, Altemimi AB, Lakshminarayanan K, Kuppan S, Pratap-Singh A, et al. Efficacy of antimicrobial and Larvicidal activities of green synthesized silver nanoparticles using leaf extract of Plumbago auriculata lam. Plants. 2020;**9**(11):1577

[70] Ishwarya R, Saravanan K, Selvaraj D, Govindarajan M, Alharbi NS,

Kadaikunnan S, et al. Antibacterial greener silver nanoparticles synthesized using Marsilea quadrifolia extract and their eco-friendly evaluation against Zika virus vector, Aedes aegypti. Green Processing and Synthesis. 2021;**10**(1):742-755

[71] Feng X, Ma H, Huang S, Pan W, Zhang X, Tian F, et al. Aqueous–organic phase-transfer of highly stable gold, silver, and platinum nanoparticles and new route for fabrication of gold Nanofilms at the oil/water Interface and on solid supports. The Journal of Physical Chemistry. B. 2006;**110**(25):12311-12317

[72] Lee SJ, Kim JH, Lee SC. Effects of oil-film layer and surfactant on the siphonal respiration and survivorship in the fourth instar larvae of Aedes togoi mosquito in laboratory conditions. Scientific Reports. 2018;**8**(1):5694

[73] Lima EP, Goulart MOF, Rolim Neto ML. Meta-analysis of studies on chemical, physical and biological agents in the control of Aedes aegypti. BMC Public Health. 2015;**15**(1):858

[74] Sharp TM, Lorenzi O, Torres-Velásquez B, Acevedo V, Pérez-Padilla J, Rivera A, et al. Autocidal gravid ovitraps protect humans from chikungunya virus infection by reducing Aedes aegypti mosquito populations. Pimenta P, editor. PLoS Neglected Tropical Diseases. 2019;**13**(7):e0007538

[75] Sissoko F, Junnila A, Traore MM, Traore SF, Doumbia S, Dembele SM, et al. Frequent sugar feeding behavior by Aedes aegypti in Bamako, Mali makes them ideal candidates for control with attractive toxic sugar baits (ATSB). Lanz-Mendoza H, editor. PLoS One. 2019;**14**(6):e0214170

[76] Britch SC, Nyberg H, Aldridge RL, Swan T, Linthicum KJ. Acoustic control of mosquito larvae In artificial drinking water containers. Journal of the American Mosquito Control Association. 2016;**32**(4):341-344

[77] Kalimuthu K, Tseng LC, Murugan K, Panneerselvam C, Aziz AT, Benelli G, et al. Ultrasonic technology applied against mosquito larvae. Applied Sciences. 2020;**10**(10):3546

[78] Fredregill CL, Motl GC, Dennett JA Jr, Bueno R, Debboun M. Efficacy of two larvasonictm units against Culex larvae and effects on common aquatic nontarget organisms in Harris County, Texas. Journal of the American Mosquito Control Association. 2015;**31**(4):5

[79] Tawatsin A, Thavara U, Siriyasatien P, Permpoonburana S. Development of a novel ultrasonic sound-generated device: The physical tool for controlling immature stages of mosquitoes transmitting dengue haemorrhagic fever (Aedes aegypti) and Filariasis (Culex quinquefasciatus). Biomedical Journal of Scientific & Technical Research. 2019;**19**(3):14308-14314

[80] Parks W, Lloyd L. Planning Social Mobilization and Communication for Dengue Fever Prevention and Control: A Step-by-Step Guide. Geneva: World Health Organization; 2004

[81] OPS/OMS. Sistematización de lecciones aprendidas en proyectos COMBI en dengue en la Región de las Américas. Costa Rica: Organización Panamericana de Salud; 2011

[82] Asian Development Bank, World Health Organization. Managing regional public goods for health: Community-based dengue vector control. Mandaluyong City, Philippines: Asian Development Bank; 2013

[83] Rodriguez Reyes AJ, Roncancio Melgarejo CP, Misnaza Castrillón SP.

Estrategias de comunicación para impactar conductas (COMBI) en enfermedades vectoriales en América Latina. Revista Médica de Risaralda. 2020;**26**(1):78-91

[84] Kay B, Nam VS. New strategy against Aedes aegypti in Vietnam. Public Health. 2005;**365**:5

[85] Kittayapong P, Bhumiratana A, Yoksan S, Chansang U, Chansang C. Suppression of dengue transmission by application of integrated vector control strategies at Sero-positive GIS-based foci. American Journal of Tropical Medicine and Hygiene. 2008;**78**(1):70-76

[86] Toledo Romani ME, Vanlerberghe V, Perez D, Lefevre P, Ceballos E, Bandera D, et al. Achieving sustainability of community-based dengue control in Santiago de Cuba. Social Science & Medicine. 2007;**64**(4):976-988

[87] Cáceres-Manrique FDM, Vesga-Gómez C, Angulo-Silva ML. Empoderamiento para la prevención y control del Dengue. Revista de Salud Pública. 2010;**12**(5):798-806

[88] Pérez D, Robert E, Pérez EJ, Vanlerberghe V, Lefèvre P, Ridde V. A realist synthesis of community-based interventions in vector-borne diseases. American Journal of Tropical Medicine and Hygiene. 2021;**104**(4):1202-1210

[89] Andersson N, Nava-Aguilera E, Arosteguí J, Morales-Perez A, Suazo-Laguna H, Legorreta-Soberanis J, et al. Evidence based community mobilization for dengue prevention in Nicaragua and Mexico (Camino Verde, the green way): Cluster randomized controlled trial. BMJ. 2015;**351**:h3267

[90] Andersson N, Arostegui J, Nava-Aguilera E, Harris E, Ledogar RJ. Camino Verde (the green way): Evidence-based community mobilisation for dengue control in Nicaragua and Mexico: Feasibility study and study protocol for a randomised controlled trial. BMC Public Health. 2017;**17**(S1):407

[91] Arosteguí J, Ledogar RJ, Coloma J, Hernández-Alvarez C, Suazo-Laguna H, Cárcamo A, et al. The Camino Verde intervention in Nicaragua, 2004-2012. BMC Public Health. 2017;**17**(Suppl. 1):406

[92] Ledogar RJ, Hernández-Alvarez C, Morrison AC, Arosteguí J, Morales-Perez A, Nava-Aguilera E, et al. When communities are really in control: Ethical issues surrounding community mobilisation for dengue prevention in Mexico and Nicaragua. BMC Public Health. 2017;**17**(Suppl. 1):410

[93] Morales-Perez A, Nava-Aguilera E, Legorreta-Soberanis J, Paredes-Solís S, Balanzar-Martínez A, Serrano-de los Santos FR, et al. Which green way: Description of the intervention for mobilising against Aedes aegypti under difficult security conditions in southern Mexico. BMC Public Health. 2017;**17**(S1):398

[94] Toledo ME, Vanlerberghe V, Baly A, Ceballos E, Valdes L, Searret M, et al. Towards active community participation in dengue vector control: Results from action research in Santiago de Cuba. Transactions of the Royal Society of Tropical Medicine and Hygiene. 2007;**101**(1):56-63

[95] Baly A, Sanchez I, Ceballos E, Carvajal M, Maso R, La Rosa M, et al. Cost-effectiveness of a community-based approach intertwined with a vertical Aedes control program. American Journal of Tropical Medicine and Hygiene. 2009;**81**(1):88-93

[96] Sanchez L, Perez D, Perez T, Sosa T, Cruz G, Kouri G, et al. Intersectoral coordination in Aedes aegypti control.

A pilot project in Havana City, Cuba. Tropical Medicine & International Health. 2005;**10**(1):82-91

[97] Sánchez L, Pérez D, Cruz G, Silva LC, Boelaert M, Van der Stuyft P. Participación comunitaria en el control de Aedes aegypti: opiniones de la población en un municipio de La Habana. Cuba: Revista Panamericana de Salud Pública; 2004;**15**(1)

[98] Pérez D, Lefèvre P, Sánchez L, Sánchez LM, Boelaert M, Kourí G, et al. Community participation in Aedes aegypti control: A sociological perspective on five years of research in the health area '"26 de Julio"', Havana, Cuba. Tropical Medicine & International Health. 2007;**12**(5):664-672

[99] Pengvanich V. Family leader empowerment program using participatory learning process for dengue vector control. Journal of the Medical Association of Thailand. 2011;**94**(2):7

[100] Sommerfeld J, Kroeger A. Eco-bio-social research on dengue in Asia: A multicountry study on ecosystem and community-based approaches for the control of dengue vectors in urban and peri-urban Asia. Pathogens and Global Health. 2012;**106**(8):428-435

[101] Quintero J, Brochero H, Manrique-Saide P, Barrera-Pérez M, Basso C, Romero S, et al. Ecological, biological and social dimensions of dengue vector breeding in five urban settings of Latin America: A multi-country study. BMC Infectious Diseases. 2014;**14**(1):38

[102] Tana S, Abeyewickreme W, Arunachalam N, Espino F, Kittayapong P, Wai KT, et al. Eco-bio-social research on dengue in Asia: General principles and a case study from Indonesia. In: Charron DF, editor. Ecohealth Research in Practice. New York, NY: Springer New York; 2012. pp. 173-184

[103] Quintero J, García-Betancourt T, Caprara A, Basso C, Garcia da Rosa E, Manrique-Saide P, et al. Taking innovative vector control interventions in urban Latin America to scale: Lessons learnt from multi-country implementation research. Pathogens and Global Health. 2017;**111**(6): 306-316

[104] Wilcox BA, Colwell RR. Emerging and Reemerging infectious diseases: Biocomplexity as an interdisciplinary paradigm. EcoHealth. 2005;**2**(4):244

[105] Meadows DH, Wright D. Thinking in Systems: A Primer. London [u.a.]: Earthscan; 2009. p. 218

[106] Stewart-Ibarra AM. A Socio-Ecological Analysis of Vulnerability to Dengue Fever in Southern Coastal Ecuador. Syracuse, New York, NY: State University of New York; 2012

[107] Stewart-Ibarra AM, Muñoz ÁG, Ryan SJ, Ayala EB, Borbor-Cordova MJ, Finkelstein JL, et al. Spatiotemporal clustering, climate periodicity, and social-ecological risk factors for dengue during an outbreak in Machala, Ecuador, in 2010. BMC Infectious Diseases. 2014;**14**(1):610

[108] Stewart Ibarra AM, Luzadis VA, Borbor Cordova MJ, Silva M, Ordoñez T, Beltrán Ayala E, et al. A social-ecological analysis of community perceptions of dengue fever and Aedes aegypti in Machala, Ecuador. BMC Public Health. 2014;**14**:1135

[109] Stewart-Ibarra AM, Lowe R. Climate and non-climate drivers of dengue epidemics in southern coastal Ecuador. American Journal of Tropical Medicine and Hygiene. 2013;**88**(5):971-981

[110] King B. Political ecologies of health. Progress in Human Geography. 2010;**34**(1):38-55

[111] Harris ML, Carter ED. Muddying the waters: A political ecology of mosquito-borne disease in coastal Ecuador. Health & Place. 2019;**57**:330-338

[112] Bayona-Valderrama A, Acevedo-Guerrero T, Artur C. Cities with mosquitoes: A political ecology of Aedes Aegypti's habitats. Water Alternatives. 2021;**14**(1):19

[113] Gómez Romero SE, Hernández Rodríguez CZ, Corrales Ramírez LC. Bacillus sphaericus: biocontrolador de vectores que producen malaria, fiebre amarilla y dengue. Nova. 2009;**7**(12):161

[114] Ge Y, Hu X, Zheng D, Wu Y, Yuan Z. Allelic diversity and population structure of Bacillus sphaericus as revealed by multilocus sequence typing. Applied and Environmental Microbiology. 2011;**77**(15):5553-5556

[115] Dambach P, Louis VR, Kaiser A, Ouedraogo S, Sié A, Sauerborn R, et al. Efficacy of Bacillus thuringiensis var. israelensis against malaria mosquitoes in northwestern Burkina Faso. Parasites & Vectors. 2014;**7**(1):371

[116] Gowelo S, Chirombo J, Spitzen J, Koenraadt CJM, Mzilahowa T, van den Berg H, et al. Effects of larval exposure to sublethal doses of Bacillus thuringiensis var. israelensis on body size, oviposition and survival of adult Anopheles coluzzii mosquitoes. Parasites & Vectors. 2020;**13**(1):259

[117] Derua YA, Kweka EJ, Kisinza WN, Githeko AK, Mosha FW. Bacterial larvicides used for malaria vector control in sub-Saharan Africa: Review of their effectiveness and operational feasibility. Parasites & Vectors. 2019;**12**(1):426

[118] Hughes GL, Koga R, Xue P, Fukatsu T, Rasgon JL. Wolbachia infections are virulent and inhibit the human malaria parasite plasmodium falciparum in Anopheles Gambiae. PLoS Pathogens. 2011;**7**(5):e1002043

[119] Hughes GL, Dodson BL, Johnson RM, Murdock CC, Tsujimoto H, Suzuki Y, et al. Native microbiome impedes vertical transmission of Wolbachia in Anopheles mosquitoes. Proceedings of the National Academy of Sciences. 2014;**111**(34):12498-12503

[120] Baldini F, Segata N, Pompon J, Marcenac P, Robert Shaw W, Dabiré RK, et al. Evidence of natural Wolbachia infections in field populations of Anopheles gambiae. Nature Communications. 2014;**5**(1):3985

[121] Bian G, Joshi D, Dong Y, Lu P, Zhou G, Pan X, et al. Wolbachia invades Anopheles stephensi populations and induces refractoriness to plasmodium infection. Science. 2013;**340**(6133):748-751

[122] Walker T, Quek S, Jeffries CL, Bandibabone J, Dhokiya V, Bamou R, et al. Stable high-density and maternally inherited Wolbachia infections in Anopheles moucheti and Anopheles demeilloni mosquitoes. Current Biology. 2021;**31**(11):2310-2320.e5

[123] Walker T, Quek S, Jeffries CL, Bandibabone J, Dhokiya V, Bamou R, et al. Genomic and microscopic evidence of stable high density and maternally inherited Wolbachia infections in Anopheles mosquitoes. bioRxiv preprint; 2020. p. 1-43. Available in: https://doi.org/10.1101/2020.10.29.357400 [cited 10 April 2022]

[124] Wong ML, Liew JWK, Wong WK, Pramasivan S, Mohamed Hassan N, Wan Sulaiman WY, et al. Natural Wolbachia infection in field-collected Anopheles and other mosquito species from Malaysia. Parasites & Vectors. 2020;**13**(1):414

[125] Knols BG, Bukhari T, Farenhorst M. Entomopathogenic fungi as the next-generation control agents against malaria mosquitoes. Future Microbiology. 2010;**5**(3):339-341

[126] Jin L, Niu G, Guan L, Ramelow J, Zhan Z, Zhou X, et al. Discovery of mosquitocides from fungal extracts through a high-throughput cytotoxicity-screening approach. Parasites & Vectors. 2021;**14**(1):595

[127] Ghosh SK, Podder D, Mukherjee A. An insight of anopheline larvicidal mechanism of Trichoderma asperellum (TaspSKGN2). Scientific Reports. 2021;**11**(1):16029

[128] Podder D, Ghosh SK. A new application of Trichoderma asperellum as an anopheline larvicide for eco friendly management in medical science. Scientific Reports. 2019;**9**(1):1108

[129] WHO. Data Sheet on the Biological Control Agent. Romanomermis culicivorax (Ross and Smith 1976). Geneva: WHO; 1980. p. 21

[130] Santamarina Mijares A, Bellin AC. Producción masiva de Romanomermis iyengari (Nematoda: Mermithidae) y su aplicación en criaderos de anofelinos en Boa Vista (Roraima). Brasil: Revista Panamericana de Salud Pública; 2000;7(3):151-161

[131] Pérez-Pacheco R, Rodríguez-Hernández C, Lara-Reyna J, Montes-Belmont R, Ruiz-Vega J. Control of the mosquito Anopheles pseudopunctipennis (Diptera: Culicidae) with Romanomermis iyengari (Nematoda: Mermithidae) in Oaxaca. Mexico: Biological Control. 2005;**32**(1):137-142

[132] Rivera Mendoza P, Blanco J, Solis Quant S, Eliseo Astin G, García Avila I, García García I, et al. Romanomermis culicivorax (Nematoda: Mermithidae): una alternativa para el control de vectores de malaria en Nicaragua. Revista Cubana de Medicina Tropical. 2014;**66**(1):101-111

[133] Abagli AZ, Alavo TBC, Perez-Pacheco R, Platzer EG. Efficacy of the mermithid nematode, Romanomermis iyengari, for the biocontrol of Anopheles gambiae, the major malaria vector in sub-Saharan Africa. Parasites & Vectors. 2019;**12**(1):253

[134] Alavo TB, Abagli AZ, Pérez R, Platzer EG. Large-scale production of the malaria vector biocontrol agent Romanomermis iyengari (Nematoda: Mermithidae) in Benin. West Africa: Malaria World Journal. 2015;**6**:1-5

[135] Braks M, van Lenteren JC, Takken W. Human Skin Emanations in the Host-Seeking Behaviour of the Malaria Mosquito Anopheles gambiae. Netherlands and Tanzania: Laboratory of Entomology of the Wageningen University and the Ifakara Health Research and Development Center; 1999. p. 112

[136] Owino EA. Sampling of an Gambiae s.s mosquitoes using limburger cheese, heat and moisture as baits in a homemade trap. BMC Research Notes. 2011;**4**(1):284

[137] Mozūraitis R, Hajkazemian M, Zawada JW, Szymczak J, Pålsson K, Sekar V, et al. Male swarming aggregation pheromones increase female attraction and mating success among multiple African malaria vector mosquito species. Nature Ecology & Evolution. 2020;**4**(10):1395-1401

[138] Oliva CF, Vreysen MJB, Dupé S, Lees RS, Gilles JRL, Gouagna LC, et al. Current status and future challenges for controlling malaria with the sterile insect technique: Technical and social perspectives. Acta Tropica. 2014;**132**:S130-S139

[139] Mashatola T, Ndo C, Koekemoer LL, Dandalo LC, Wood OR, Malakoane L,

et al. A review on the progress of sex-separation techniques for sterile insect technique applications against Anopheles arabiensis. Parasites & Vectors. 2018;**11**(S2):646

[140] Ndo C, Poumachu Y, Metitsi D, Awono-Ambene HP, Tchuinkam T, Gilles JLR, et al. Isolation and characterization of a temperature-sensitive lethal strain of Anopheles arabiensis for SIT-based application. Parasites & Vectors. 2018;**11**(S2):659

[141] Kaiser ML, Wood OR, Damiens D, Brooke BD, Koekemoer LL, Munhenga G. Estimates of the population size and dispersal range of Anopheles arabiensis in northern KwaZulu-Natal, South Africa: Implications for a planned pilot programme to release sterile male mosquitoes. Parasites & Vectors. 2021;**14**(1):205

[142] Benelli G, Beier JC. Current vector control challenges in the fight against malaria. Acta Tropica. 2017;**174**:91-96

[143] Wooding M, Naudé Y, Rohwer E, Bouwer M. Controlling mosquitoes with semiochemicals: A review. Parasites & Vectors. 2020;**13**(1):80

[144] Zoh MG, Bonneville JM, Tutagata J, Laporte F, Fodjo BK, Mouhamadou CS, et al. Experimental evolution supports the potential of neonicotinoid-pyrethroid combination for managing insecticide resistance in malaria vectors. Scientific Reports. 2021;**11**(1):19501

[145] Lwetoijera D, Harris C, Kiware S, Dongus S, Devine GJ, McCall PJ, et al. Effective autodissemination of pyriproxyfen to breeding sites by the exophilic malaria vector Anopheles arabiensis in semi-field settings in Tanzania. Malaria Journal. 2014;**13**(1):161

[146] Kiware SS, Corliss G, Merrill S, Lwetoijera DW, Devine G, Majambere S, et al. Predicting scenarios for successful autodissemination of Pyriproxyfen by malaria vectors from their resting sites to aquatic habitats; description and simulation analysis of a field-Parameterizable model. Vontas J, editor. PLoS One. 2015;**10**(7):e0131835

[147] Elmosaad YM, Elhadi M, Khan A, Malik EM, Mahmud I. Communication for behavioural impact in enhancing utilization of insecticide-treated bed nets among mothers of under-five children in rural North Sudan: An experimental study. Malaria Journal. 2016;**15**(1):509

[148] Barry N, Toé P, Pare Toe L, Lezaun J, Drabo M, Dabiré RK, et al. Motivations and expectations driving community participation in entomological research projects: Target malaria as a case study in Bana, Western Burkina Faso. Malaria Journal. 2020;**19**(1):199

[149] McCann RS, van den Berg H, Diggle PJ, van Vugt M, Terlouw DJ, Phiri KS, et al. Assessment of the effect of larval source management and house improvement on malaria transmission when added to standard malaria control strategies in southern Malawi: Study protocol for a cluster-randomised controlled trial. BMC Infectious Diseases. 2017;**17**(1):639

[150] Ng'ang'a PN, Aduogo P, Mutero CM. Strengthening community and stakeholder participation in the implementation of integrated vector management for malaria control in western Kenya: A case study. Malaria Journal. 2021;**20**(1):155

[151] SantoDomingo AF, Castro-Díaz L, González-Uribe C. Ecosystem research experience with two indigenous communities of Colombia: The Ecohealth calendar as a participatory and innovative methodological tool. EcoHealth. 2016;**13**(4):687-697

Chapter 7

Different Strategies for Mosquito Control: Challenges and Alternatives

Taruna Kaura, Neha Sylvia Walter, Upninder Kaur and Rakesh Sehgal

Abstract

Vector control is an imperative method for the control of vector borne diseases. Over the last few decades, many methods have been developed for their control and the main goal of these strategies is to reduce the number of mosquito populations to overcome the epidemic situations. Though despite continuous efforts of the present interventions being deployed in the vector control programs we are unable to control the disease transmission and outbreaks. Therefore, it highlights the importance of exploring the challenges which are hindering the success of these strategies and also alternative solutions for the same so as to boost the vector control interventions.

Keywords: vector, mosquitoes, challenges for control, alternative strategies

1. Introduction

Diseases transmitted by mosquitoes such as malaria, filariasis, dengue, chikungunya, zika and yellow fever, malaria among many others have global importance. By 2050 approximately half of the world's population is expected to be at risk of arboviral transmission [1]. The rapid increases in the geographic distribution of these mosquitoes and the diseases transmitted by them have contributed significantly to global mortality and morbidity. Vector based interventions are the most common methods to reduce the burden of the most mosquito-borne diseases and a wide range of tools exist which are mainly classified into chemical and non-chemical methods. The chemical methods involve the use of insecticides, Insecticide-treated materials (ITMs) as Insecticide Treated Nets (ITNs), for spraying on indoor surfaces as Indoor Residual Spray (IRS) and among the non-chemical methods, it involves the use of biological and genetic innovations [2]. The basic purpose of vector control is to restrict disease transmission potential by minimizing or eliminating human contact with the vector. To control malaria, in malaria elimination programs the use of Long-Lasting Insecticide Nets (LLINs) and IRS are being used to control the transmission in high malaria endemic areas but due to emerging insecticide resistance, the mosquito vectors does not remain susceptible to these insecticides.

Despite of all these vector control interventions and continuous efforts to control their spread and epidemics, they continue to threat health of billions of people worldwide [3]. However, all these recent vector control methods being used are not able to successfully control the epidemics being spread by different mosquitoes. Thus, the absence of sustainable vector control due to emerging insecticide resistance has led to the development of alternative methods.

2. Vector control strategies for mosquito control

To overcome or reduce the population of the vector species of mosquitoes, various methods are being used in the vector control programmes. Till the development of the insecticides, the only method being adopted is the removal of the breeding sites

Name of the method	Insecticides/active materials used	Description	Target mosquito species	References
Chemical methods				
Indoor residual spraying (IRS)	Carbamates:- Bendiocarb, propoxur Pyrethroids:- Lambda-cyhalothrin; Alpha-Cypermethrin, Etofenprox Organochlorines:- dichloro-diphenyl-trichloroethane (DDT) Organophosphates:- Malathion; Fenitrothion; Pirimiphos-methyl	Kerosene or oil	*An. stephensi; Cx. Quinquefasciatus; Ae. albopictus; Ae. aegypti*	[5, 6]
Insecticidal treated nets (ITNs) [LLINs, ITN–PermaNet]	Pyrethroids:- Deltamethrin, Alphacypermethrin, permethrin, bifenthrin Pyrethroids:- Deltamethrin, permethrin, deltamethrin + Piperonyl butoxide (PBO)	Lasts for 20 washes Coating	*An. stephensi; Cx. quinquefasciatus; Ae. albopictus; Ae. aegypti*	[7]
Repellents	DMP (Dimethyl phthalate) Allethrin	Surface of fabric	*An. stephensi; Cx. quinquefasciatus; Ae. albopictus; Ae. aegypti*	[8]
Ultra-low volume (ULV) spray	Organophospahtes- Malathion, fenitrothion; Pyrethroids	Small droplets that float in the air and kill flying mosquitoes on contact.	*An. stephensi; Cx. quinquefasciatus Ae. albopictus, Ae. aegypti*	[9, 10]
Larval source management				
Chemical method Insect growth regulators (IGRs)	Isostearyl alcohol, petroleum distillates, Spinosad (spinosyn a and spinosyn d) Methoprene, pyriproxyfen, diflubenzuron and triflumeron	Monomolecular surface films Microcapsules, granules or in briquettes form	*An. stephensi; Cx. quinquefasciatus; Ae. albopictus Ae. aegypti; Ae. albopictus*	[11] [12, 13]

Name of the method	Insecticides/active materials used	Description	Target mosquito species	References
Non-chemical methods				
Biological control				
Bacterial larvicides Bacteria Mosquito fish *Gambusia affinis*, Guppies-*Poecilia reticulata* Tilapia-*Oreochromis mossambicus* Giant gourami –*Osphronemus goramy* Carp-*Cyprinus carpio* Mermithid nematodes—*Romanomermis culicivorax* Fungi—*Laegenidium giganteum*	*Bacillus thuringiensis subsp. israelensis (Bti)*, *Bacillus sphaericus* *Wolbachia*	spore-forming bacteria trans-infected into mosquitoes	*Culex* and *Anopheles* but ineffective against *Ae. aegypti* *An. stephensi, Cx. quinquefasciatus, Ae. albopictus, Ae. aegypti* *An. stephensi; Cx. quinquefasciatus; Ae. albopictus, Ae. aegypti*	[14] [15] [16]
Sterile Insect Technique (SIT)	—	Release of these sterile males' mosquitoes into the wild population.	*Ae. albopictus*	[17]
Genetically modified (GM) mosquitoes	—	Express specific genes, which enhance their immunity against the parasite	*An. stephensi; Ae. aegypti*	[18, 19]

Table 1.
Different methods for the mosquito control.

of mosquitoes and use of screens so as to avoid the entry of mosquitoes through doors and windows [4]. Thus, different methods *viz.* chemical methods and non-chemical methods being used by different control programmes are explained in the **Table 1**.

3. Challenges in mosquito control

Controlling vectors of the major diseases constitute an important part of the global disease elimination and control programs, which if implemented successfully can lead towards tremendous reduction in the disease incidence globally. However, there are several challenges to the vector control strategies, which are outlined below:

One of the foremost challenges to the successful implantation of vector control strategies is the prevalence of high levels of insecticide resistance among vectors against the available insecticides [20]. Insecticide resistance can largely impact the control of adult vector mosquitoes, thereby leading to dire health consequences. Moreover, variation in the susceptibility of mosquitoes to different insecticides is another challenge [21]. Though employment of ITNs and IRS have resulted in the decline of some mosquito vector borne diseases such as malaria; however, insecticide resistance and failure to sustain these interventions can result in reversing the achieved goals [22]. Another challenge is to implement disease-specific vector control programs, as some measures for ITNs and IRS have shown promise in malaria control, but are limited for dengue control [23] due to variation in the ecology of *Anopheles* and *Aedes* mosquitoes. Besides these, other challenges include changes in behavior of the mosquitoes, presence of avoidance behavior, the high vector biodiversity etc. Moreover, the impact of the changing environment on the habitat of vectors, rapid urbanization and climate change [24] can have unpredictable and complicated influence on the distribution of the vectors posing other key challenges to the vector control interventions.

In addition to this, other challenges in the implementations of vector control programs include issues arising in public health interventions such as limited amount of funds or fair distribution of funds for vector control. Lack of proper surveillance systems pertaining to insecticide resistance and behavior of vectors can also weaken the vector control interventions. Also, the lack of coordination between governmental and non-governmental organizations may influence vector control interventions. Migration of humans and goods pose challenges for vector control as well as disease emergence [25].

The techniques employing pouring of kerosene oil or chemical larvicides are effective in killing the larvae, but this technique suffers a major drawback i.e. its hazardous impact on the environment. In addition, the techniques to eliminate mosquito breeding sites, though are quite effective but these are not possible in areas having irregular water supply and also if these methods are not implemented at the grass root level, then the effectiveness of these techniques is reduced [26].

BTI (dead spores of the soil bacterium *Bacillus thuringiensis israelensis*) is also a successful technique to reduce the larval populations, but it is effective only against the larval stages. Recent reports have shown that BTI can impact the food chains and pose other potential effects on the environment [27, 28]. Moreover, techniques involving direct introduction of *Tilapia* and mosquito fish into the ecosystems without using a controlled ecosystem can also pose serious hazardous effects on the environment.

Thus, due to the deleterious effect of these chemical larvicides, development of new vector control products with the epidemiological evidence of their impact on public health must be clearly understood and evaluated by WHO before implementing in the field. Therefore, below different alternative vector control strategies and the studies being carried out are discussed. Such as the release of sterile insects by irradiation, use of *Wolbachia* and gene-drive technologies etc. are promising strategies, considered safe but public acceptability and regulatory approval necessitates a thorough risk assessment as well as extensive stakeholder participation.

For genetically engineered species, such barriers are clearly higher than for purely biological control strategies like *Wolbachia*. Secondly, employment of these interventions will place tremendous selection pressures that can result in development of resistance in either the target pathogen (in the case of *Wolbachia* or vector competence gene drive constructs) or the vector (for population suppression genetic constructs and possibly *Wolbachia*). Moreover, *Wolbachia's* long-term phenotypic stability in *Ae. aegypti* is still unknown [29].

Technique involving the use of Genetically Modified (GM) mosquitoes for vector control is also a promising strategy offering distinct advantages such as being non-toxic and also avoids the use of chemicals insecticides. However, there are several ethical concerns in the use of GM mosquitoes [30]. In addition, the potential impact of these organisms on the environment also needs to be taken into consideration [31]. Moreover, the technique to generate GM mosquitoes is quite expensive and may not be sustainable for poor endemic countries. The WHO also recommends and calls for further field trials and assessment of risk to evaluate the impact of this technique on transmission of the disease [32].

Recently, the use of green synthesis of nanoparticles has emerged as cost-effective and simple method for vector control. However, there are certain limitations to the large-scale synthesis and their possible impact on the environment. In addition, there is a large gap between the theoretical and the practical implications of this technology. Also, very little information is available on the impact of these nanoparticles on other aquatic organisms [33, 34]. Moreover, many of these nanoparticles have been tested for their acute toxicity non-target organisms or on other aquatic organisms which occur in the same ecological niche as the vector mosquitoes.

The difficulty of attaining eradication is worsened by heterogeneity and the existence of high-transmission hotspots; yet control in low-transmission areas may be easier than projected based on spatially imprecise transmission intensity projections [35].

Another most difficult task will be to make the best use of limited resources (particularly in low-income areas) to have the largest public health benefit. Extrapolation of clinical trial data to forecast population effect of each intervention in a wider variety of contexts and in conjunction with other control methods would require rigorous epidemiological research and mathematical modeling to ensure such optimal deployment. To assess the real-world effectiveness of treatments, rigorous monitoring and assessment are also required [22]. Concomitantly, the political commitment and employment of collaborative vector control strategies is the key to achieve the goal of vector control, thereby, reducing disease transmission and contributing towards disease eradication.

4. Alternative solutions for mosquito control

Despite continuous efforts to control vector borne diseases by the use of existing intervention methods, we are unable to control these epidemics as almost 4 billion people are at risk of dengue virus transmission alone [36]. Thus, the present scenario necessitates the development of alternative strategies for the control of mosquito vectors. The rapid spread of insecticide resistance and adverse effects of these chemicals on non-target species strengthen the need to employ novel strategies for mosquito control.

Continuous efforts are being done to improve the current interventions and various new strategies and products are under consideration by the World Health Organization Vector Control Advisory Group (WHO VCAG). The following methods are used to as alternative solutions for mosquito control:

4.1 Paratransgenesis: by the use of symbiotic bacteria, entomopathogenic fungi, pyriproxyfen: novel larvicides

It is the process to decrease the vector competence of pathogens by the genetic manipulation of the insect symbiont. The prerequisite of this technique is that symbiotic organisms must be cultivable and can easily propagate in the vectors. The most common species of bacteria which are found to be susceptible to genetic manipulation in mosquitoes are *Asaia* species and Pantoea *agglemorans* [37, 38]. These bacteria have been reported to colonize rapidly in tissues of various mosquito species *viz. An. stephensi*, *An. gambiae*, *Ae. albopcitus*, *Ae. aegypti* and species of *Culex* from *pipiens* complex [39].

In addition to the use of bacteria, in this approach fungal species can be used as it can survive in the environment for months. Moreover it can cause infection in mosquitoes directly through the cuticle and in *Anopheles,* Fang *et al*. used genetically transformed *Metarhizium anisopliae* and antimicrobial toxin scorpine which reduces the mosquito infectivity by interfering with *P. falciparum* development [40]. Pidiyar *et al*. reported the presence of *Aspergillus* and *Streptomyces* spp. in *Cx. Quinquefasciatus* [41]. Hence, using GM bacteria or fungus, paratransgenesis might be utilized to create an environmentally friendly, efficacious and specialized biopesticide.

4.2 Spatial repellents

These are the chemicals which work in vapor phase so as to prevent contact between humans and vector by making the space unsuitable for the insect. It is predicted that by the use of this technique by the diversion of mosquitoes to non-human host and will also decrease the toxic effect of chemicals to humans and other non-target organisms. In this method, the focus remains to prevent biting by the insect instead of killing it, basically a repellent is developed [42]. This method can be improved by the using novel active chemical components which will have new mode of action and affect the vector by altering the normal vector behavioral patterns. Presently, no evidence is reported regarding the epidemiological impact of this technique. To implement the use of spatial repellents as a tool in vector control, many challenges are yet to overcome as they come at very high cost. Moreover, the use of these repellents requires use of electricity and, therefore, makes them less suitable in less developed areas with high transmission rate. To ease the introduction of the use of these deterrents in vector control programs, their cost must be in concurrence with IRS or LLINs [43].

Many preliminary field studies have been carried out to test the efficacy of two spatial repellents allethrin emanators (ThermaCELL) and metofluthrin emanators (OFF! clip-ons or lamps) which have received more than 70% protection in different studies [44]. The use of these deterrents within push-pull systems ultimately helps the mosquito to push away from human host towards the baited traps. Many studies have been carried with the use of different repellents *viz.* PMD, catnip oil and delta-undecalactone.

4.3 Use of plant based (herbal) repellents

Plant-based "natural" smelling repellents are now widely used across the world since plants are regarded as a safe and reliable method to prevent mosquito bites. Because of their high vapor toxicity, many plant volatiles are apt to be insect deterrents or repellents. Phytophagous (plant-eating) insects are protected by compounds found in most of the plants. Repellents, growth regulators, toxins and feeding deterrents are among the substances used [45]. Nitrogenous compounds (mainly alkaloids), terpenoids, proteinase inhibitors, phenolic compounds and growth regulators are the best instances. The volatile components generated by herbivory are currently best recognized for their ability to repel mosquitoes and other biting insects. Volatile odors attach to odorant receptor (OR) proteins on ciliated dendrites of specialist odor receptor neurons (ORNs), which are often found on the antennae and maxillary palps of insects, allowing them to sense smell [46].

The insect repellent qualities of Lemon eucalyptus have been known for millennia and essential oil contains 85 percent citronellal which is significantly more efficient in repelling mosquitoes for many minutes. On the contrary, one of its constituents, para-menthane-3,8-diol, provides excellent protection against a wide variety of insect vectors for a long period of time due to its low vapor pressure. Nanotechnology has lately opened up new possibilities for utilizing eucalyptus extracts successfully [47]. The extract and essential oil of lemongrass are frequently used as repellents, for instance, citronella, at concentrations of 5–10%, and vanillin (5%). Nano-emulsion of citronella oil is prepared to generate stable droplets that promote oil retention and delay the release. Likewise, several field investigations in India have demonstrated that neem-based medicines also have very high effectiveness [48].

4.4 Traps

Adult mosquitoes can be caught using traps. The carbon dioxide generated when propane is broken down into water might be the attractant. Biting insects, such as mosquitoes, are attracted to the warm water vapors containing carbon dioxide. The insecticide octenol, also known as 1-octen-3-ol, has been used to attract mosquitos up to 30 m away from the trap. Mostly zoophagous mosquitoes are attracted to this attractant. A dim light is used as an attractant in some traps. Because mosquitoes are attracted to light, some mosquito traps include a fan that sucks the insects flying close into a gathering chamber or bag. The trap will collect a large number of other flying insects such as beetles, moths, and flies. Traps are most successful when they are put up, maintained, and operated appropriately. A wind may have an impact on their efficacy. If the trap is placed in an inconvenient area, mosquitoes may attack more frequently. The placement of traps, on the other hand, might be considered as one of the mosquito-prevention strategies [49, 50].

There is no adult mosquito killing or catching mechanism in the system. Mosquito traps that employ UV/visible light attract not only mosquitoes, but also beneficial pollinating insects, inflicting collateral harm. To prevent killing undesirable insects, a larvicide medication package is released; however, attracted insects may generate misleading positive image processing findings. Additionally, removing active traps that need actuators can assist to minimize power usage [51].

The BG-Sentinel (Biogents GmbH, Regensburg, Germany) is another trap for mosquitoes that uses visual, olfactory, and chemical attractants to mimic convection currents formed by the human body. Given its usefulness as a collecting technique for medically importante *Aedes* (Stegomyia) species, the BG Sentinel has been shown to gather mosquitoes efficiently in urban environment in Australia and is used extensively globally for mosquito monitoring in metropolitan regions. The BG Gravid *Aedes* Trap (BG-GAT) features no moving components, few total parts, requires no energy, and is less expensive to buy. Attractant signals for ovi-positing female mosquitoes are formed using water and organic material. Adult mosquitoes are killed with residual insecticides, for instance synthetic pyrethroids administered from a propellant can or when attached to an adhesive panel placed into the trap, after being drawn inside the trap. Mosquitoes are unable to access the trap's water and perish on a mesh screen, where they are subsequently collected [52].

4.5 Attractive toxic sugar bait (ATSB)

It is a new and a promising strategy for mosquito control. In this method, mosquitoes are attracted to Attractive Toxic Sugar Bait (ATSB) solution by spraying it either on plants or in bait stations. ATSB solutions consists of an attractant (fruit or flower scent), a feeding stimulant (sugar solution), and an oral toxin to kill the mosquitoes. The field trial of this method has been carried out for controlling the *Anopheline* and *Culicine* mosquito species. Studies on *Culex quinquefasciatus* and *Anopheles gambiae* s.l in Florida, USA and Mali, West Africa has shown success of ATSB field trials [53]. This new method is simple, cost effective and environmentally safe.

The ATSB methods are not only efficacious, easy to perform, and cost-effective but also overcome the drawbacks of contact insecticides [54] by attracting sugar-seeking mosquitoes and utilizing toxins that are non-toxic to humans and safe to the environment for example boric acid.

4.6 Mosquito-repellent controlled-release formulations

Currently available insect repellents, such as lotions, roll-ons and sprays do not provide enough long-term protection. They usually need to be reapplied or updated on a regular basis. Encapsulation and liberation of repellents from a variety of matrices have emerged as a viable approach for the creation of repellent-based systems. Various types of repellent controlled-release formulations have been recently developed which have emerged as novel tools for controlling mosquito-borne diseases. These include polymer microcapsules, polymer micelles, polymer microporous formulations, liposomes, nano-emulsions, solid-lipid nanoparticles and cyclodextrins [55, 56].

Personal protection items have been linked to fewer mosquito bites and illness incidence in previous research [57]. Mosquito bite control can be successfully reduced with repellents such as DEET-based soaps [58]. Rodriguez et al. also evaluated the efficacy of several commercially available repellent based controlled release formulations against *Ae. aegypti* [59]. DEET and PMD are known to be the most efficient and long-lasting insect repellents in the market [60]. In the controlled-release formulations, the regulated release from the formulations is a type of technology that allows the active component to be released to the target at a restricted pace. Moreover, the concentration of the active component in the formulation is maintained within optimal limits for a long time. The major benefits of this technology comprise; activity prolongation over a longer duration, reduced pollution and is inexpensive [60, 61].

4.7 Sterile insect technique (SIT)

The SIT is an ecologically friendly pest management strategy that involves releasing mass-reared sterile males in a particular region to suppress an insect population. There are no progeny when these sterile males mate with females in the wild [62]. The introduction of sterile males in a systematic and recurring manner decreases the target wild insect population over time. The IAEA has been improving the SIT for use against disease-transmitting mosquitoes in collaboration with the Food and Agriculture Organization of the United Nations (FAO), and has tried it on a modest scale in various countries, including Brazil, Cuba, Italy, Mauritius, Mexico, and Germany [17, 63, 64]. Pilot releases on a larger scale are planned as part of International Atomic Energy Agency (IAEA) research and technical cooperation operations, as well as test releases in conjunction with epidemiological studies as part of the IAEA, TDR (Special Programme for Research and Training in Tropical Diseases), and WHO partnership. Female mosquitos bite and thus spread illnesses, whereas male mosquitos do not bite and thus do not pose a risk of disease transmission. The sterile mosquitoes are likewise unable to reproduce, thus they will not contribute to the increase of the mosquito population. Sterile mosquitoes are typically released via ground, although good results were recently obtained in Brazil using a drone release method developed by the IAEA in collaboration with the FAO and others.

This approach has been used to remove the New World screwworm, tsetse fly, Queensland fruit fly, pink bollworm, melon fruit fly, and other insects. The efficiency of this technique can be further improved by creating better strains for mass production and release, identifying molecular markers to detect the released sterile insects in the field, sterilization and genetic sexing. Distinguishing between released wild and sterile insects is crucial for assessing the performance of the SIT programme [65]. The incorporation of a fluorescent transformation marker into a transgenic insect might aid in the simple identification of released insects. In mosquito species such as *Anopheles gambiae* and *Aedes aegypti* fluorescent sperm marking systems have been developed [66].

4.8 Gene drives

This technique utilizes CRISPR gene-editing tool to spread a genetic modification rapidly through a population than normal rate of inheritance. It can be used to insert a new gene or induce alteration or silencing a particular gene. After the entire drive is inserted into the genome the progeny will inherit the drive on one chromosome and the normal gene on partner chromosome. During development the CRISPER portion cuts the other copy which is repaired using the drive and thus the genome contains two copies of the gene drive. This allows passing the alteration to 100% of the progeny than 50% in the usual case. Gene drives have been proposed to be used against mosquito borne diseases and also reverse insecticide resistance. CRISPR-based HEGs (homing endonuclease genes) have shown close to 100% inheritance rates [67] in both *Anopheles gambiae* and *A. stephensi* mosquitoes. The gene drives cause a reduction in the reproductive capacity of the mosquitoes [68] CRISPR-based gene-drives, which are targeting the *doublesex* gene of *Anopheles gambiae* (vector of malaria) have been reported to efficiently suppress mosquitoes in small laboratory cages for a year and were not found to select for resistance to the gene drive [69, 70].

4.9 Resistance management

The main aim of this technique is to prolong the susceptibility of mosquito vectors to insecticides so as to maintain the effectiveness of the vector control interventions. The methods being used under this intervention include rotations, mosaics, mixtures and combinations [71]. Among these methods, rotational use of insecticide is the most common and effective solution for managing insecticide resistance. These methods are still not widely explored for the control of vectors.

4.10 Prediction modeling to control mosquitoes

To predict the spread of VBDs, pathogens, reservoirs, and vector before the onset of transmission season, mathematical and statistical methods are being prepared. These types of models can help in providing information to public health authorities so that they can plan their vector control interventions accordingly [72]. Mainly two different types of model are used viz. prediction model and importation model. To forecast the spread of disease, their vector in correlation with the climatic factors, prediction model is used [73]. Moreover, to investigate the introduction, movement of disease, vector prevalence in endemic and non-endemic region, the importation model is used [74, 75]. It is presumed that these models can be helpful for advance planning and programming in those regions which will be at risk for the disease outbreak according to the prediction of developed model. But these models have to be continuously updated according to the rate of disease transmission, vector prevalence and rapid changing environmental factors [76].

5. Conclusions

Reduction of vector population remains the only key strategy for the control of different mosquito borne diseases. Though various methods like chemical, biological and genetic methods are being used to maintain these vector populations below threshold level, still we are unable to control the disease transmission. Thus, to achieve our target especially malaria elimination, the present scenario suggests the urgent need to develop alternative solutions to tackle the problem of insecticide resistance. Recently, many new strategies such as SIT, GM mosquitoes, paratransgenesis, ATSB, gene drives etc. can be explored for their efficacy and make cost effective so that they can be implemented in the vector control programs for the control of mosquitoes.

Conflict of interest

None.

Acronyms

LLINs	Long lasting insecticide nets
ITN	Insecticide treated nets
IRS	Indoor residual spray
LSM	Larval source management
MMF	Monomolecular surface films
IGRs	Insect growth regulators
BL	Bacterial larvicides
GM	Genetically modified mosquito
SIT	Sterile insect technology
ATSB	Attractive toxic sugar bait

Author details

Taruna Kaura†, Neha Sylvia Walter†, Upninder Kaur and Rakesh Sehgal*
Department of Medical Parasitology, Postgraduate Institute of Medical Education and Research, Chandigarh, India

*Address all correspondence to: sehgalpgi@gmail.com

† The first two authors have equally contributed and must be considered as joint first authors.

References

[1] Bamou R, Mayi MPA, Djiappi-Tchamen B, Nana-Ndjangwo SM, Nchoutpouen E, Cornel AJ, et al. An update on the mosquito fauna and mosquito-borne diseases distribution in Cameroon. Parasit Vectors. 2021;**14**:527. DOI: 10.1186/s13071-021-04950-9

[2] Abeku TA, Helinski MEH, Kirby MJ, Ssekitooleko J, Bass C, Kyomuhangi I, et al. Insecticide resistance patterns in Uganda and the effect of indoor residual spraying with bendiocarb on kdr L1014S frequencies in Anopheles gambiae s.s. Malaria Journal. 2017;**16**:156. DOI: 10.1186/s12936-017-1799-7

[3] Wilson AL, Courtenay O, Kelly-Hope LA, Scott TW, Takken W, Torr SJ, et al. The importance of vector control for the control and elimination of vector-borne diseases. PLoS Neglected Tropical Diseases. 2020;**14**(1):e0007831. DOI: 10.1371/journal.pntd.0007831

[4] WHO. Dengue: Guidelines for Diagnosis, Treatment, Prevention and Control: New Edition. Geneva: World Health Organization; 2009. 3, Vector Management and Delivery of Vector Control Services. Available from: https://www.ncbi.nlm.nih.gov/books/NBK143163/

[5] Pluess B, Tanser FC, Lengeler C, Sharp BL. Indoor residual spraying for preventing malaria. Cochrane Database of Systematic Reviews. 2010;**2010**(4):CD006657. DOI: 10.1002/14651858.CD006657.pub2

[6] WHO. Guidelines for Malaria Vector Control. Geneva: World Health Organization. Licence: CC BY-NC-SA 3.0 IGO. 2019. ISBN 978-92-4-155049-9

[7] Wang Y, Cheng P, Jiao B, Song X, Wang H, Wang H, et al. Investigation of mosquito larval habitats and insecticide resistance in an area with a high incidence of mosquito-borne diseases in Jining, Shandong Province. PLoS One. 2020;**15**(3):e0229764. DOI: 10.1371/journal.pone.0229764

[8] Karunamoorthi K. Vector control: A cornerstone in the malaria elimination campaign. Clinical Microbiology and Infection. 2011;**17**(11):1608-1616. DOI: 10.1111/j.1469-0691.2011.03664

[9] Bonds JAS. Ultra-low-volume space sprays in mosquito control: A critical review. Medical and Veterinary Entomology. 2012;**26**(2):121-130. DOI: 10.1111/j.1365-2915.2011.00992.x

[10] Gunning CE, Okamoto KW, Astete H, Vasquez GM, Erhardt E, Del Aguila C, et al. Efficacy of *Aedes aegypti* control by indoor ultra low volume (ULV) insecticide spraying in Iquitos, Peru. PLOS Neglected Tropical Diseases. 2018;**12**(4):e0006378. DOI: 10.1371/0006378

[11] Nayar JK, Ali A. A review of monomolecular surface films as larvicides and pupicides of mosquitoes. Journal of Vector Ecology. 2003;**28**(2):190-199

[12] Kamal HA, Khater EI. The biological effects of the insect growth regulators; pyriproxyfen and diflubenzuron on the mosquito Aedes aegypti. Journal of the Egyptian Society of Parasitology. 2010;**40**(3):565-574

[13] Lau KW, Chen CD, Lee HL, Norma-Rashid Y, Sofian-Azirun M. Evaluation of insect growth regulators against field-collected Aedes aegypti and Aedes albopictus (Diptera: Culicidae) from Malaysia. Journal of Medical

Entomology. 2015;**52**(2):199-206. DOI: 10.1093/jme/tju019

[14] Derua YA, Kweka EJ, Kisinza WN, Githeko AK, Mosha FW. Bacterial larvicides used for malaria vector control in sub-Saharan Africa: Review of their effectiveness and operational feasibility. Parasites & Vectors. 2019;**12**:426. DOI: 10.1186/s13071-019-3683-5

[15] Hancock PA, Sinkins SP, Godfray HC. Strategies for introducing Wolbachia to reduce transmission of mosquito-borne diseases. PLoS Neglected Tropical Diseases. 2011;**5**(4):e1024. DOI: 10.1371/journal.pntd.0001024

[16] Kamareddine L. The biological control of the malaria vector. Toxins (Basel). 2012;**4**(9):748-767. DOI: 10.3390/toxins4090748

[17] Oliva CF, Benedict MQ, Collins CM, Baldet T, Bellini R, Bossin H, et al. Sterile insect technique (SIT) against Aedes species mosquitoes: A roadmap and good practice framework for designing, implementing and evaluating pilot field trials. Insects. 2021;**12**(3):191. DOI: 10.3390/insects12030191

[18] Catteruccia F, Godfray HC, Crisanti A. Impact of genetic manipulation on the fitness of Anopheles stephensi mosquitoes. Science. 2003;**299**(5610):1225-1227. DOI: 10.1126/science.1081453

[19] Zhang A. Transgenic Mosquitoes: A New Approach to Preventing Malaria? Global Health Review: Harvard college; 2011

[20] Girod R, Guidez A, Carinci R, Issaly J, Gaborit P, Ferrero E, et al. Detection of chikungunya virus circulation using sugar-baited traps during a major outbreak in French Guiana. PLoS Neglected Tropical Diseases. 2016;**10**(9):e0004876. DOI: 10.1371/journal.pntd.0004876

[21] Dale P, Knight J. Mosquito control: Perspectives on current issues and challenges. Annals of Community Medicine and Practice. 2017;**3**(2):1023

[22] Ferguson NM. 2018. Challenges and opportunities in controlling mosquito-borne infections. Nature. 2018;**559**:490-497. DOI: 10.1038/s41586-018-0318-5

[23] Bowman LR, Donegan S, McCall PJ. Is dengue vector control deficient in effectiveness or evidence?: Systematic review and Meta-analysis. PLoS Neglected Tropical Diseases. 2016;**10**(3):e0004551. DOI: 10.1371/journal.pntd.0004551

[24] Bai L, Morton LC, Liu Q. Climate change and mosquito-borne diseases in China: A review. Globalization and Health. 2013;**9**:10. DOI: 10.1186/1744-8603-9-10

[25] World Health Organization. Global Vector Control Response 2017-2030. Geneva: WHO; 2017

[26] World Health Organization. Larval source management: a supplementary measure for malaria vector control. In: An Operational Manual. Geneva: World Health Organization; 2013

[27] Allgeier S, Friedrich A, Brühl CA. Mosquito control based on bacillus thuringiensis israelensis (Bti) interrupts artificial wetland food chains. Science of the Total Environment. 2019;**686**:1173-1184. DOI: 10.1016/j.scitotenv.2019.05.358

[28] Brühl CA, Després L, Frör O, Patil CD, Poulin B, Tetreau G, et al. Environmental and socioeconomic effects of mosquito control in Europe using the biocide bacillus thuringiensis subsp. israelensis (Bti). Science of Total

Environment. 2020;**724**:137800. DOI: 10.1016/j.scitotenv.2020.137800

[29] Wang GH, Gamez S, Raban RR, Marshall JM, Alphey L, Li M, et al. Combating mosquito-borne diseases using genetic control technologies. Nature Communications. 2021;**12**(1):4388. DOI: 10.1038/s41467-021-24654-z

[30] Macer D, Johnson R, UNDP/World Bank/WHO Special Programme for Research and Training in Tropical Diseases. Ethical, Legal and Social Issues of Genetically Modified Disease Vectors in Public Health. Geneva: World Health Organization; 2003

[31] Jamrozik E, de la Fuente-Núñez V, Reis A, Ringwald P, Selgelid MJ. Ethical aspects of malaria control and research. Malaria Journal. 2015;**14**:518. DOI: 10.1186/s12936-015-1042-3

[32] World Health Organization. WHO Issues New Guidance for Research on Genetically Modified Mosquitoes to Fight Malaria and other Vector-Borne Diseases. 2021. Available from: https://www.who.int/news/item/19-05-2021-who-issues-new-guidance-for-research-on-genetically-modified-mosquitoes-to-fight-malaria-and-other-vector-borne-diseases

[33] Murugan K, Benelli G, Ayyappan S, Dinesh D, Panneerselvam C, Nicoletti M, et al. Toxicity of seaweed-synthesized silver nanoparticles against the filariasis vector Culex quinquefasciatus and its impact on predation efficiency of the cyclopoid crustacean Mesocyclops longisetus. Parasitology Research. 2015;**114**(6):2243-2253. DOI: 10.1007/s00436-015-4417-z

[34] Murugan K, Benelli G, Panneerselvam C, Subramaniam J, Jeyalalitha T, Dinesh D, et al. Cymbopogon citratus-synthesized gold nanoparticles boost the predation efficiency of copepod Mesocyclops aspericornis against malaria and dengue mosquitoes. Experimental Parasitology. 2015;**153**:129-138. DOI: 10.1016/j.exppara.2015.03.017

[35] Acevedo MA, Prosper O, Lopiano K, Ruktanonchai N, Caughlin TT, Martcheva M, et al. Spatial heterogeneity, host movement and mosquito-borne disease transmission. PLoS One. 2015;**10**(6):e0127552. DOI: 10.1371/0127552

[36] World Health Organization. 2022. Dengue and Severe Dengue. Available from: https://www.who.int/news-room/fact-sheets/detail/dengue-and-severe-dengue

[37] Wilke AB, Marrelli MT. Paratransgenesis: A promising new strategy for mosquito vector control. Parasites & Vectors. 2015;**8**:342. DOI: 10.1186/s13071-015-0959-2

[38] Wang S, Ghosh AK, Bongio N, Stebbings KA, Lampe DJ, Jacobs-Lorena M. Fighting malaria with engineered symbiotic bacteria from vector mosquitoes. Proceedings of the National Academy of Sciences of the United States of America. 2012;**109**:12734-12739. DOI: 10.1073/pnas.1204158109

[39] Scolari F, Casiraghi M, Bonizzoni M. Aedes spp. and Their Microbiota: A Review. Frontiers in Microbiology. 2019;**10**:2036. DOI: 10.3389/fmicb.2019.02036

[40] Fang W, Vega-Rodríguez J, Ghosh AK, Jacobs-Lorena M, Kang A, St Leger RJ. Development of transgenic fungi that kill human malaria parasites in mosquitoes. Science. 2011;**331**(6020):1074-1077. DOI: 10.1126/science.1199115

[41] Pidiyar VJ, Jangid K, Patole MS, Shouche YS. Studies on cultured and uncultured microbiota of wild Culex quinquefasciatus mosquito midgut based on 16s ribosomal RNA gene analysis. The American Journal of Tropical Medicine and Hygiene. 2004;**70**:597-603. DOI: 10.4269/ajtmh.2004.70.597

[42] Achee NL, Bangs MJ, Farlow R, Killeen GF, Lindsay S, et al. Spatial repellents: From discovery and development to evidence-based validation. Malar Journal. 2012;**11**:164. DOI: 10.1186/1475-2875-11-164

[43] Syafruddin D, Asih PBS, Rozi IE, Permana DH, Nur Hidayati AP, Syahrani L, et al. Efficacy of a spatial repellent for control of malaria in Indonesia: A cluster-randomized controlled trial. American Journal of Tropical Medicine and Hygiene. 2020;**103**(1):344-358. DOI: 10.4269/19-0554

[44] Xue RD, Qualls WA, Smith ML, Gaines MK, Weaver JH, Debboun M. Field evaluation of the off! Clip-on mosquito repellent (metofluthrin) against Aedes albopictus and Aedes taeniorhynchus (Diptera: Culicidae) in northeastern Florida. Journal of Medical Entomology. 2012;**49**(3):652-655. DOI: 10.1603/me10227

[45] Shah G, Shri R, Panchal V, Sharma N, Singh B, Mann AS. Scientific basis for the therapeutic use of Cymbopogon citratus, stapf (lemon grass). Journal of Advanced Pharmaceutical Technology & Research. 2011;**2**(1):3-8. DOI: 10.4103/2231-4040.79796

[46] Pichersky E, Gershenzon J. The formation and function of plant volatiles: Perfumes for pollinator attraction and defense. Current Opinion in Plant Biology. 2002;**5**(3):237-243. DOI: 10.1016/s1369-5266(02)00251-0

[47] Sugumar S, Mukherjee A, Chandrasekaran N. Eucalyptus oil nanoemulsion-impregnated chitosan film: antibacterial effects against a clinical pathogen, Staphylococcus aureus, in vitro. International Journal of Nanomedicine. 2015;**10**(Suppl 1):67-75. DOI: 10.2147/IJN.S79982

[48] Tyagi BK. Advances in vector mosquito control technologies, with particular reference to herbal products. In: Vijay V, Gopalakrishnan R, editors. Herbal Insecticides, Repellents and Biomedicines: Effectiveness and Commercialization. New Delhi: Springer India; 2016. pp. 1-9

[49] Chen YC, Wang CY, Teng HJ, Chen CF, Chang MC, Lu LC, et al. Comparison of the efficacy of CO2-baited and unbaited light traps, gravid traps, backpack aspirators, and sweep net collections for sampling mosquitoes infected with Japanese encephalitis virus. Journal of Vector Ecology. 2011;**36**(1):68-74. DOI: 10.1111/j.1948-7134.2011.00142.x

[50] Wilke ABB, Carvajal A, Medina J, Anderson M, Nieves VJ, Ramirez M, et al. Assessment of the effectiveness of BG-sentinel traps baited with CO2 and BG-lure for the surveillance of vector mosquitoes in Miami-Dade County, Florida. PLoS ONE. 2019;**14**(2):e0212688. DOI: 10.1371/0212688

[51] Kim K, Hyun J, Kim H, Lim H, Myung H. A deep learning-based automatic mosquito sensing and control system for urban mosquito habitats. Sensors (Basel). 2019;**19**(12):2785. DOI: 10.3390/s19122785

[52] Bazin M, Williams CR. Mosquito traps for urban surveillance: Collection efficacy and potential for use by citizen scientists. Journal of Vector Ecology.

2018;**43**(1):98-103. DOI: 10.1111/jvec.12288

[53] Beier JC, Müller GC, Gu W, Arheart KL, Schlein Y. Attractive toxic sugar bait (ATSB) methods decimate populations of Anopheles malaria vectors in arid environments regardless of the local availability of favoured sugar-source blossoms. Malaria Journal. 2012;**11**:31. DOI: 10.1186/1475-2875-11-31

[54] Fiorenzano JM, Koehler PG, Xue RD. Attractive toxic sugar bait (ATSB) for control of mosquitoes and its impact on non-target organisms: A review. International Journal of Environmental Research and Public Health. 2017;**14**(4):398. DOI: 10.3390/ijerph14040398

[55] Islam J, Zaman K, Duarah S, Raju PS, Chattopadhyay P. Mosquito repellents: An insight into the chronological perspectives and novel discoveries. Acta Tropica. 2017;**167**:216-230. DOI: 10.1016/2016.12.031

[56] Sibanda M, Focke W, Braack L, Leuteritz A, Brünig H, Tran NHA, et al. Bicomponent fibres for controlled release of volatile mosquito repellents. Materials Science and Engineering: C. 2018;**91**:754-761. DOI: 10.1016/2018.06.016

[57] Debboun M, Strickman D. Insect repellents and associated personal protection for a reduction in human disease. Medical and Veterinary Entomology. 2013;**27**(1):1-9. DOI: 10.1111/j.1365-2915.2012.01020.x

[58] Kroeger A, González M, Ordóñez-González J. Insecticide-treated materials for malaria control in Latin America: To use or not to use? Transactions of the Royal Society of Tropical Medicine and Hygiene. 1999;**93**(6):565-570. DOI: 10.1016/s0035-9203(99)90048-2

[59] Rodriguez SD, Chung H-N, Gonzales KK, Vulcan J, Li Y, Ahumada JA, et al. Efficacy of some wearable devices compared with spray-on insect repellents for the yellow fever mosquito, Aedes aegypti (L.) (Diptera: Culicidae). Journal of Insect Science. 2017;**17**(1):24

[60] Mapossa AB, Focke WW, Tewo RK, Androsch R, Kruger T. Mosquito-repellent controlled-release formulations for fighting infectious diseases. Malaria Journal. 2021;**20**:165. DOI: 10.1186/s12936-021-03681-7

[61] Dubey S, Jhelum V, Patanjali PK. Controlled release agrochemicals formulations: A review. Journal of Scientific and Industrial Research. 2011;**70**:105-112

[62] Bourtzis K, Vreysen MJB. Sterile insect technique (SIT) and its applications. Insects. 2021;**12**(7):638. DOI: 10.3390/insects12070638

[63] Bellini R, Medici A, Puggioli A, Balestrino F, Carrieri M. Pilot field trials with Aedes albopictus irradiated sterile males in Italian urban areas. Journal of Medical Entomology. 2013;**50**:317-325. DOI: 10.1603/ME12048

[64] Abad-Franch F, Zamora-Perea E, Luz SLB. Mosquito-disseminated insecticide for citywide vector control and its potential to block arbovirus epidemics: Entomological observations and modeling results from Amazonian Brazil. PLoS Medicine. 2017;**14**:e1002213. DOI: 10.1371/1002213

[65] Gupta VK, Jindal V. Chapter 16—Biotechnological approaches for insect pest management. In: Abrol DP, editor. Integrated Pest Management. San Diego: Academic Press; 2014. pp. 311-335

[66] Schetelig MF, Wimmer EA. Insect transgenesis and the sterile insect

technique. In: Vilcinskas A, editor. Insect Biotechnology. Dordrecht, NL: Springer; 2011. pp. 169-194

[67] Champer J, Liu J, Oh SY, Reeves R, Luthra A, Oakes N, et al. Reducing resistance allele formation in CRISPR gene drive. Proceedings of the National Academy of Sciences of the USA. 2018;**115**(21):5522-5527. DOI: 10.1073/pnas.1720354115

[68] Hammond A, Galizi R, Kyrou K, Simoni A, Siniscalchi C, Katsanos D, et al. A CRISPR-Cas9 gene drive system targeting female reproduction in the malaria mosquito vector Anopheles gambiae. Nature Biotechnology. 2016;**34**(1):78-83. DOI: 10.1038/nbt.3439

[69] Kyrou K, Hammond AM, Galizi R, Kranjc N, Burt A, Beaghton AK, et al. A CRISPR-Cas9 gene drive targeting doublesex causes complete population suppression in caged Anopheles gambiae mosquitoes. Nature Biotechnology. 2018;**36**(11):1062-1066. DOI: 10.1038/nbt.4245

[70] Hammond A, Pollegioni P, Persampieri T, North A, Minuz R, Trusso A, et al. Gene-drive suppression of mosquito populations in large cages as a bridge between lab and field. Nature Communications. 2021;**12**(1):4589. DOI: 10.1038/s41467-021-24790-6

[71] Dusfour I, Vontas J, David JP, Weetman D, Fonseca DM, Corbel V, et al. Management of insecticide resistance in the major Aedes vectors of arboviruses: Advances and challenges. PLoS Neglected Tropical Diseases. 2019;**13**(10):e0007615. DOI: 10.1371/journal.pntd.0007615

[72] Parham PE, Michael E. Modelling climate change and malaria transmission. Advances in Experimental Medicine and Biology. 2010;**673**:184-199. DOI: 10.1007/978-1-4419-6064-1_13

[73] Tavecchia G, Miranda M, Barcelo DBC, Paredes-Esquivel C, Schwarz C. Modelling the range expansion of the tiger mosquito in a Mediterranean island accounting for imperfect detection. Frontiers in Zoology. 2017;**14**(39). DOI: 10.1186/s12983-017-0217-x

[74] Gardner L, Sarkar S. A global airport-based risk model for the spread of dengue infection via the air transport network. PLoS One. 2013;**8**(8):e72129

[75] Bogoch II, Brady OJ, Kraemer MUG, German M, Creatore MI, Brent S, et al. Potential for Zika virus introduction and transmission in resource-limited countries in Africa and the Asia-Pacific region: A modelling study. The Lancet Infectious Diseases. 2016;**16**(11):1237-1245. DOI: 10.1016/S1473-3099(16)30270-5

[76] Sadeghieh T, Waddell LA, Ng V, Hall A, Sargeant J. A scoping review of importation and predictive models related to vector-borne diseases, pathogens, reservoirs, or vectors (1999-2016). PLoS One. 2020;**15**(1):e0227678. DOI: 10.1371/0227678

Chapter 8

The Potential for Wolbachia-Based Mosquito Biocontrol Strategies in Africa

Femi Ayoade and Tosin S. Ogunbiyi

Abstract

The three foremost medically important mosquito species of public health importance belong to the genera Anopheles, Aedes, and Culex. The Anopheles mosquito is the most important in the transmission of human malaria, while members of the genera Culex and Aedes are more important in the transmission of arboviruses. Reducing the number of competent vectors has been identified as a logical method for the control of malarial and arboviral vector-borne diseases. This chapter provides an update on the potentials of biological vector control, specifically the release of endosymbionts to help limit the reproductive capability of mosquitoes, thereby reducing the population of the disease vectors in Africa. There are examples of successful suppression of mosquito-borne diseases by the establishment of Wolbachia in mosquito populations elsewhere, however, there has been no such report from the African continent. Although the establishment of stable maternally transmissible Wolbachia in natural mosquito populations is yet to be achieved in Africa, this area of research is experiencing unprecedented progress within the past decade. Many of the research efforts are hereby highlighted, including the problems and prospects of establishing a Wolbachia-based biocontrol program in Africa.

Keywords: Wolbachia, cytoplasmic incompatibility, integrated vector control, paratransgenesis

1. Introduction

Of the three foremost medically important mosquito genera of public health significance, namely, *Anopheles*, *Aedes,* and *Culex*, the *Anopheles* mosquito is most important in the transmission of human malaria while members of the genera *Culex* and *Aedes* are more important in the transmission of arboviruses [1]. Since it is impractical to eliminate mosquitoes, reducing the number of competent vectors is a logical target for controlling malaria and arboviral vector-borne diseases. For some mosquito-borne arboviruses such as West Nile, chikungunya, dengue, Zika, and so on that lack licensed vaccines or viable therapeutics, in addition to the problems posed by the ever-plastic plasmodium parasite that continues to exhibit resistance to even the most potent combined therapeutic agents, this may actually be the only option left [2].

IntechOpen

The present chapter is focused on the potential of using a proven biological vector control method, specifically the release of mosquitoes infected with endosymbionts that help to limit the reproductive capability of mosquitoes to reduce the population of the disease vectors in Africa. Many insect species are infected by intracellular bacteria, and these are known to sometimes exert deleterious effects on the host insects. *Wolbachia* is perhaps the best-known example of intracellular bacteria that can drastically reduce the reproductive capability of several insect species, particularly disease-bearing mosquitoes. *Wolbachia* is an alpha proteobacterium first described in *Culex pipens* by *Wolbachia* and for this reason, was named *Wolbachia pipientis* [3]. Similarly, *Wolbachia* has been isolated from *Drosophila*, *Aedes albopictus*, and other insect species; in fact, reports have shown that these bacteria only infect invertebrate hosts and are naturally found in more than 50% of all arthropod species and in several nematodes [4].

Today, *Wolbachia* is still relevant in biological control programs due to its potential as a safe vector for spreading cytoplasmic incompatibility and other means of reproductive isolation among disease-bearing vectors, such as induction of parthenogenesis, feminization, and male-killing [5, 6]. In recent times, there are notable examples of successful establishment of *Wolbachia* in mosquito populations aimed at suppressing mosquito-borne diseases [7–10]. Remarkably, the Australian *Wolbachia* project tagged "eliminate dengue" (www.eliminatedengue.com) has shown that *Wolbachia* bacteria can prevent Dengue virus (DENV) transmission in mosquitoes without high fitness costs. Moreover, a virulent *Wolbachia* strain in Drosophila melanogaster fruit flies (named *w*MelPop) is known to lower the lifespan of its host significantly. It has been shown to shorten the lifespan of mosquitoes [11].

In addition, a closely related avirulent *w*Mel strain was found to protect their native hosts, Drosophila fruit flies, against infection by pathogenic RNA viruses [12, 13]. Recent reports indicate that such strains that provide similar or better characteristics deployable in preventing the capacity of viruses to replicate in the vector or the ability to incapacitate the vector (such as *w*MelPop and *w*Mel strains) exist in Africa. An example is a report by the insect vector research group at the African Centre of Excellence for the Genomics of Infectious Diseases (ACEGID) laboratory recently reported finding *Wolbachia* in Ede (Osun State), which is the first report from Nigeria [14].

Wolbachia has been reported from countries in West Africa and even from *Anopheles* species initially thought not to be naturally infected by *Wolbachia*. African countries from which natural mosquito infections by *Wolbachia* have been reported include Burkina Faso [15]; Ghana, the Democratic Republic of the Congo (DRC) [5, 16], and Mali [17]. Since success rates of *Wolbachia* infections have been attributed to the relatedness of the donor and recipient hosts [16], the present chapter focuses on the great potential in developing indigenous strains of *Wolbachia* that might be used in artificial infections that can reduce the capacity of wild mosquito populations to reproduce and transmit human pathogens in Nigeria and possibly elsewhere in Africa. Moreover, the artificial infection of mosquitoes may produce inhibitory effects on arboviruses and *Plasmodium* parasites as observed in Australia and elsewhere in Asia [18, 19].

2. The microbiome of mosquitoes

As a result of their interactions with biotic and abiotic factors in their ecosystem, mosquitoes internalize diverse consortia of microbes, which have been shown to have a significant effect on this insect's physiology. Microbes belonging to diverse life forms (bacteria, protists, viruses, and yeasts) have been identified and characterized as established or occasional members of the mosquito microbiome. Some members of this symbiotic microbiota can either be beneficial (e.g. dietary supplementation, enhancement of digestive mechanisms, tolerance of environmental perturbations, protection from parasites and pathogens, and maintenance and/or enhancement of host immune system homeostasis) or detrimental (reducing the fitness or life span of

Diseases	Mosquitoes	Global Burden
Dengue	*Aedes aegypti, Aedes albopictus*	• More than 2.5 billion people (over 40% of the world's population) are at risk. • More than 100 million dengue infections are reported yearly. • An estimated 500,000 people with severe dengue require hospitalization each year. • About 2.5% of those affected died.
Yellow fever	*A. aegypti* and *Haemagogus*	• About 200,000 cases of illness and 30,000 deaths are reported yearly. • Number of reported cases has been on the increase for the past two decades due to declining population immunity and deforestation.
Chikungunya	*A. aegypti* and *A. albopictus*	• In 2005–2006, an outbreak in Reunion Island (a French territory in the Indian Ocean) affected about one-third of the population (266,000 of 775,000 inhabitants). • The 2006 outbreak spread to other countries in South-East Asia resulting in 1.4 million reported cases. • In December 2013, the first cases of local transmission of Chikungunya were detected in the WHO Region of the Americas, the Caribbean island of Saint Martin.
Zika virus	*A. aegypti*	No information on global disease burden (as at 28th of April, 2018).
Japanese encephalitis (Found in Asia)	*Culex tritaeniorhynchus*	Causes an estimated 50,000 cases and 10,000 death yearly, mostly in children less than five.
West Nile Virus	*A. albopictus, Culex*	No information on global disease burden (as at 28th of April, 2018).
Malaria	*Anopheles* (more than 60 known species can transmit diseases)	• Malaria transmission occurs in 91 countries. • In 2016, an estimated 216 million cases were reported with an estimated 445,000 deaths. • About 3.4 billion people are at risk.
Lymphatic Filariasis (LF)	*Anopheles* (more than 60 known species can transmit diseases)	• More than 120 million people are currently infected. • 40 million of those infected are disfigured and incapacitated by the disease. • LF afflicts more than 25 million men with the genital disease and more than 15 million people with lymphoedema.

Source: WHO [19]; Available from: www.who.int/news-room/fact-sheets/detail/malaria [Accessed on: 12 December, 2021].

Table 1.
Diseases transmitted by various mosquito species and their global disease burden.

their host); while other members of this community are of medical significance to the host on which the insect feeds on [20–28].

The microbes that constitute the microflora of the mosquito are the causal organisms of infectious diseases of global public health importance. Consequently, the process of diseases vectoring by a mosquito may not be viewed as a deliberate act but rather an accidental act that happens during a normal blood meal, necessary for reproduction. Interestingly, the selective feeding pattern seen in mosquitoes creates a possibility of having infectious agents from an "unusual host" introduced into a completely susceptible new host. This is the basis for most emerging infectious diseases that are of zoonotic origin; mosquito, once infected, remains infectious for life [29]. According to the World Health Organization, the infectious diseases of public health importance that are vectored by mosquitoes include dengue, yellow fever, chikungunya, zika virus, japanese encephalitis, west nile virus, malaria, and lymphatic filariasis [19]. A list of these diseases, the global disease burden, and their mosquito vectors are presented in **Table 1**.

3. Vector control as a means of disease control

In the early twentieth century, vector control emerged as one of the main methods of disease control. During this era, environmental management of breeding sites, including larviciding, was employed in the reduction of mosquito vectors. Around the 1950s, insecticides (most especially DDT) were introduced and used extensively. Interestingly, by the 1970s most mosquitoes had developed resistance to these insecticides, and on discovering the environmental hazard these chemical agents place on the ecosystem, its continuous use was frowned upon [30]. This new development led to the re-evaluation of vector control programs. In 1982, WHO recommended an integrated vector control (IVC) program based on the Axtell principle of integrated pest management [30]. The Axtell principle is founded upon the combination of biological control methods such as the introduction of exotic natural enemies, larvivorous fish, microbial agents with source reduction methods such as intermittent irrigation, water level management, landfilling, channeling, and draining in combination with the use of chemicals, including insect growth regulators, adulticide, and larvicides integrated with the use of personal protection methods, such as bed nets and repellents, concurrently with health education in the various communities at the schools, on television and mass media. Of all the mosquito control components highlighted in the IVC strategy, only biological control has not been implemented successfully in Africa, although some baseline data necessary for implementation are recently being generated. Most of the problems preventing the incorporation of biological control methods in IVC strategies in Africa are due to limited capacity, as the implementation of biocontrol methods requires a high level of technical capability. Moreover, since other control measures like chemical control have inherent limitations of environmental toxicity and the emergence of resistant strains of the vector, IVC programs in Africa have not been so successful, largely due to the lack of mastery of the biological control component.

4. Biocontrol in IVC programs

Biological control methods employ the use of natural enemies like fish, insects, protozoa, fungi, bacteria, and viruses to reduce the population of mosquitoes or reduce their vectorial competence. The two most widely employed mosquito biological vector control methods include larvicides and larvivorous fish. The use of small-sized fishes that feed on mosquito larvae has the advantages of being cost-effective, environmentally safe, and long-term effective control measures against different varieties of mosquito species. On the other hand, this has some limitations such as it requires a large number, takes about 2 months (not suitable for quick intervention), less effective in waters with floating garbage or vegetation. Sometimes birds and in some African communities, humans prey on the fishes as some of the larvivorous species are delicacies in these African communities. Examples of larvivorous fish include *Gambusia spp* and *Poecilia spp* (Guppy) [31]. On the other hand, the use of bio-larvicides involves the use of bacteria for the control of mosquito larvae. *Bacillus sphaericus* and *Bacillus thuringiensis* H 14 are the two most widely used bio-larvicide usually available as granules and wettable powder, which contain lyophilized bacteria, spores, and toxic crystals. The mechanism of biolarvicide control employed by *B. thuringiensis* H 14 and *B. sphaericus* involves the production of endotoxins (Cry4A, Cry4B, and Cry11A) which result in gut paralysis and leakage of gut contents into the body cavity, which finally results in death due to osmotic shock. Toxins of *B. sphaericus* have been shown to be more effective in polluted water (polluted water is characteristic of *Culex* breeding sites). They are environmentally safe and do not pose any threat to humans and their livestock but are expensive [31–33].

The third mosquito biological vector control method is paratransgenesis involving the use of native bacteria flora in disease vectors to express effector molecules capable of interfering with pathogen transmission. Paratransgenesis begins by the screening of internal microbiota of the vector to isolate symbiotic bacteria that are genetically modified to express effector molecules, after which they are again reintroduced into the vector that is now introduced into the wild where they produce the desired effect [34–36]. Understanding bacteria diversity in mosquitoes is the bull's eye in paratransgenic control of mosquitoes, and this requires a detailed knowledge base of the biology of the local mosquitoes and their microflora. To be effective, the bacterial population in the local mosquito populations are screened in order to identify bacteria that are consistent and persistent in all generations and across a variety of mosquito species. For this reason, a bacterium is considered suitable as a paratransgenesis agent when it has an effector molecule that produces the desired effect; an exocytotic mechanism to discharge the effector molecule on its cell surface; and ability to survive long enough to produce the expected amount of effector molecules in the mosquito [37–39].

Gaio et al. [40] investigated the contribution of midgut bacteria to blood digestion and egg production in *Ae. aegypti*. Findings from this study showed that eradication of gut bacteria resulted in a slower growth rate and decline in fecundity. The researchers concluded that alteration of gut flora should be further investigated as a new approach for preventing the transmission of pathogens and controlling mosquito populations.

Paratransgenic management of infectious disease and their insect vector is considered to have advantages of increased bacteria number after ingestion of blood (by the vector), which will invariably cause an increase in the secretion of effector molecules by the genetically modified bacteria. The expected outcomes of paratransgenesis include a reduction in mosquito's vectorial competence; obstruction of pathogen transmission; loss of fecundity in mosquito (non-viable eggs and alteration of embryogenesis); and eventual death of the mosquito [41–45].

5. *Wolbachia*: a paratransgenic agent

Wolbachia is an obligate intracellular gram-negative bacterium belonging to the family Rickettsiales; it is known to be part of the microbiota of insects, isopods, nematodes, and mites (**Figures 1** and **2**). As an obligate parasite, they infect the cytoplasmic vacuoles of their host cell, including gonads. *Wolbachia* can be vertically transmitted or maternally inherited and are therefore considered as potential targets for paratransgenic systems [48, 49]. Many mosquito species (especially those

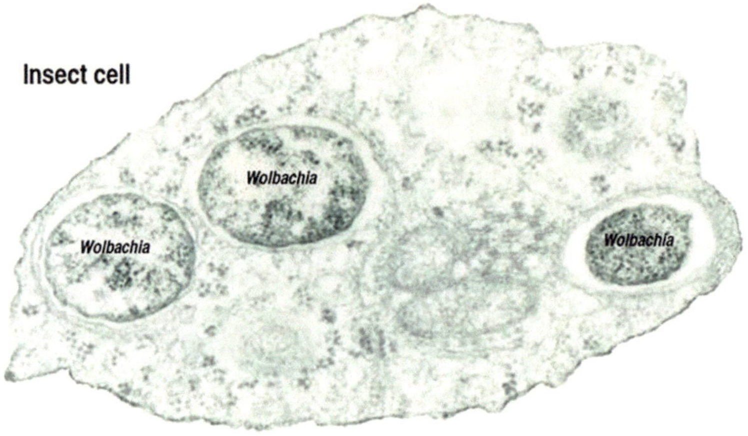

Figure 1.
Electron micrograph of Wolbachia *within an insect cell [46].*

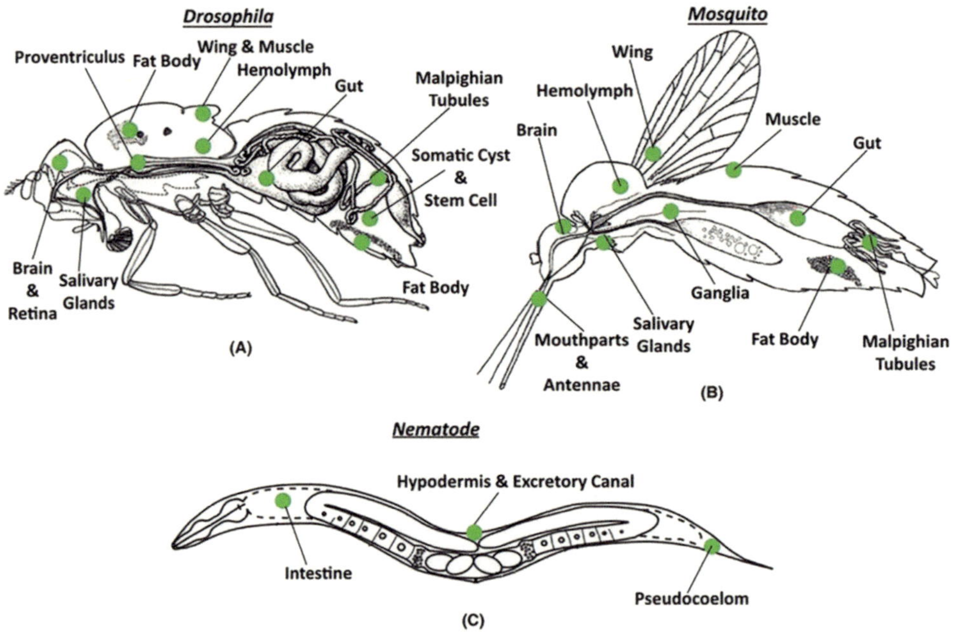

Figure 2.
Distribution of Wolbachia *(in green) in somatic tissues of various hosts as detected by PCR and fluorescent cytology [47].*

of epidemiological importance) are known to be susceptible to *Wolbachia* infection; however, the prevalence of this bacterium is notably high in wild *Ae. albopictus* and *Cx. pipiens* population. Different phylogenetic strains of *Wolbachia* induce distinct extended phenotypes in the mosquito they infect; the effect induced by this bacterium in their host can be cytoplasmic compatibility, incompatibility or compatibility in only one direction [50]. The persistence of *Wolbachia* population through the generation of mosquitoes is known due to the bacterium's ability to induce a severe selective pressure that rapidly drives its transovarial transmission [51, 52].

Basic approaches to using *Wolbachia* for paratransgenic control of vectors of infectious diseases include:

1. Direct insertion of the transgene into the bacterium's genome and the use of cytoplasmic incompatibility to suppress the targeted vector population.

2. Fixing the transgene on cytoplasmic elements of the host that are co-inherited with the bacterium; and

3. Transformation of the host genome coupled with the use of the bacterium's cytoplasmic incompatibility mechanism to insert this gene into other members of the target population [48].

The ability of *Wolbachia* to induce transovarian transmission of itself is considered a major boost in paratransgenic systems. This means once the bacterium has been introduced into the host, they can persist for several generations in the insect; hence, once introduced, there is no need for subsequent re-introduction [53, 54]. Interestingly, the effect induced by *Wolbachia* is species-dependent [55]. For example, infected *Aedes aegypti* with different strains of *Wolbachia* resulted in three outcomes: shortened lifespan [54]; reduced susceptibility to dengue or chikungunya virus and *Plasmodium* infection [18]; and, depending on the infecting strain, cytoplasmic incompatibility was observed, with apparent high horizontal transmission and no high fitness cost [54]. The foregoing underscores the importance of capacity development in the areas of research and laboratory-based surveillance systems in ensuring the successful introduction, establishment, and maintenance of *Wolbachia* populations wherever paratransgenesis is used as a biocontrol method as part of an integrated vector control strategy.

6. Wolbachia in Africa

The presence of *Wolbachia* in wild *Anopheles gambiae* mosquitoes was first demonstrated by Baldini et al. [15] in Burkina Faso. Hughes et al. [56] demonstrated that a stable maternally transmissible *Wolbachia* population can be achieved in *An. gambiae* and *An. stephensi* by suppressing other members of the insect microbiota with the use of antibiotics. Furthermore, Shaw et al. [5] demonstrated the ability of the *wAnga* strain to stably infect reproductive tissues (ovaries), and certainly somatic tissues where the *Plasmodium* development occurs, with the potential to effectively compete for resources or upregulate the immune response to kill the malaria parasite. Similar results were reported in Mali with a new anopheline *Wolbachia* strain (*wAnga*-Mali) [17]. Moreover, reports have shown that there are native *Wolbachia* infections in 16 out of 25 wild African *Anopheles* species, including both vectors and non-vectors of malaria

[16, 57]. These reports and more recent reports [58] confirm that natural *Wolbachia* infection in anopheline mosquitoes is more common than expected and underscores the need for further studies in the diversity of anopheline *Wolbachia* strains towards identifying suitable strains that may serve to impede the development of *Plasmodium* parasites in mosquitoes and other *Wolbachia* strains associated with non-malaria vectors that are responsible for other infectious agents of health importance.

7. Conclusions and recommendations

The fact that more researchers in Africa in recent years are looking and finding *Wolbachia* [14, 15, 17, 58] in African mosquito populations is a welcomed change, unlike previously when there was no activity in this area of research in Africa. However, none of these strains are yet to be found to confer Cytoplasmic Incompatibility (CI), a condition needed to spread rapidly in natural populations and as such disrupt disease transmission. In laboratory experiments, environmental factors such as temperature and availability of food have been shown to affect the expression of CI. For example, rearing males at temperatures higher than 25°C and low levels of nutrition was found to lead to increases in cytoplasmic incompatibility [59], although the environmental factors were found to be mediated by bacterial density. On the other hand, it may be expedient to consider developing a genetically modified *Wolbachia* to induce CI or to select *Wolbachia* strains that can spread efficiently in natural mosquito populations.

Five strategic areas of development have been identified as critical to the establishment of impactful IVM programs in Africa; enhanced advocacy, intra, and inter-collaboration, integrated approach, capacity building, particularly human resource development [60]. Apart from these strategic areas, basing decisions increasingly on local evidence, and community involvement and empowerment to ensure sustainability have also been identified as key components of successful IVM programs in Africa [61]. There are wide variations to the extent of adoption and promotion of these prerequisites to successful IVM among the African countries with the consequent variations in success rates. While some countries are still grappling with the consolidation of strategic and operational frameworks, others have advanced to the point of adopting IVM as a national policy, and have implemented its key elements in different measures of success [61].

Using IVM strategies, progress has been achieved with increased intervention coverage, reduced risk of transmission, and reduced VBD burden, particularly for malaria, in some African countries, including, Namibia [62], Swaziland [63], Botswana [64], Zambia and Zimbabwe [65]. These successes however may not be entirely attributed to vector control alone but also to effective case management, community mobilization, and sensitization, including changing climatic and environmental factors. These kinds of successes can be replicated in Africa if the best practices are adopted by more countries in Africa.

Developing the required technical capacity and infrastructure for entomological surveillance is another area of focus that needs to be developed in Africa, particularly, sub-Saharan Africa. This has been identified as a major challenge for most African countries [62]. Although it may take some time to develop this capacity, reports show that in countries where targeted training of entomological technicians have been conducted, such as Burundi, Eritrea, Guinea, and Zambia, the corresponding reduction in the malaria burden by up to 99% was achieved in some cases [60].

Moreover, since vector control of mosquito-borne diseases, must rely on insecticides as its backbone, particularly via long-lasting insecticidal nets (LLIN) and indoor residual spraying (IRS), the development of insecticide resistance has been identified as a potentially limiting factor in IVM programs [66]. On the other hand, combination innovative approaches including genetically modified or transinfected mosquitoes (Wolbachia-based), durable wall linings, mosquito traps such as eave tubes and entomopathogenic bacteria traps, odor-baited traps, attractive toxic sugar baits, spatial repellents, and entomopathogenic fungus-impregnated targets are expected to be effective when used in support of the application of insecticides "backbone" [62].

In conclusion, a great potential for IVM has been demonstrated in various regions of Africa, particularly in the area of malaria vector control [67, 68]. However, deploying IVM strategies for effective vector control in Africa will require sustained funding, removal of governmental bureaucracy, strategic planning and human resource development, and synergy among stakeholders, including community-based groups and their collaboration with nongovernmental organizations, international and national research institutes, and various government ministries.

Author details

Femi Ayoade[1,2*] and Tosin S. Ogunbiyi[3]

1 Department of Biological Sciences, College of Natural Sciences, Redeemer's University, Ede, Osun State, Nigeria

2 African Center of Excellence for the Genomics of Infectious Diseases (ACEGID), Redeemer's University, Ede, Osun State, Nigeria

3 Department of Biological Sciences, Mountain Top University, Prayer City, Ogun State, Nigeria

*Address all correspondence to: ayoadef@run.edu.ng

References

[1] Baskar K, Sudha V, Nattudurai G, Ignacimuthu S, Duraipandiyan V, Jayakumar M, et al. Larvicidal and repellent activity of the essential oil from Atalantia monophylla on three mosquito vectors of public health importance, with limited impact on non-target zebra fish. Physiological and Molecular Plant Pathology. 2018;**101**:197-201

[2] Hunter P. Challenges and options for disease vector control:The outbreak of zika virus in South America and increasing insecticide resistance among mosquitoes has rekindled efforts for controlling disease vectors. EMBO Reports. 2016;**17**(10):1370-1373

[3] Ricci I, Cancrini G, Gabrielli S, D'Amelio S, Favi G. Searching for Wolbachia (Rickettsiales: Rickettsiceae) in mosquitoes (Diptera: Culicidae): Large polymerase chain reaction survey and new identifications. Journal of Medical Entomology. 2002;**39**:562-567

[4] Zug R, Hammerstein P. Still a host of hosts for Wolbachia: Analysis of recent data suggests that 40% of terrestrial arthropod species are infected. PLoS One. 2012;7:e38544

[5] Shaw WR, Marcenac P, Childs LM, Buckee CO, Baldini F, Sawadogo SP. Wolbachia infections in natural anopheles populations affect egg laying and negatively correlate with plasmodium development. Nature Communications. 2016;**7**(11172): 1-7

[6] Zug R, Hammerstein P. Bad guys turned nice? A critical assessment of Wolbachia mutualisms in arthropod hosts. Biological Reviews. 2015;**90**(1):89-111

[7] Hoffmann AA, Ross PA, Rašić G. Wolbachia strains for disease control: Ecological and evolutionary considerations. Evolutionary Applications. 2015;**8**(8):751-768

[8] Jeffries CL, Walker T. Wolbachia biocontrol strategies for arboviral diseases and the potential influence of resident Wolbachia strains in mosquitoes. Current Tropical Medicine Reports. 2016;**3**(1):20-25

[9] Rossi P, Ricci I, Cappelli A, Damiani C, Ulissi U, Mancini MV, et al. Mutual exclusion of Asaia and Wolbachia in the reproductive organs of mosquito vectors. Parasites & Vectors. 2015;**8**(1):278

[10] Schultz MJ, Connor JH, Frydman HM. Group B Wolbachia strain-dependent inhibition of arboviruses. DNA and Cell Biology. 2018;**37**(1):2-6

[11] Benelli G, Jeffries CL, Walker T. Biological control of mosquito vectors: Past, present, and future. Insects. 2016;**7**(4):52

[12] Hedges LM, Brownlie JC, O'Neill SL, Johnson KN. Wolbachia and virus protection in insects. Science. 2008;**322**(5902):702-702

[13] Teixeira L, Ferreira Á, Ashburner M. The bacterial symbiont Wolbachia induces resistance to RNA viral infections in Drosophila melanogaster. PLoS Biology. 2008;**6**(12):e1000002

[14] Ogunbiyi TS, Eromon P, Oluniyi P, Ayoade F, Oloche O, Oguzie JU, et al. First report of Wolbachia from field populations of culex mosquitoes in South-Western Nigeria. African Zoology. 2019;**54**(3):181-185

[15] Baldini F, Segata N, Pompon J, Marcenac P, Shaw WR, Dabiré RK, et al. Evidence of natural Wolbachia infections in field populations of Anopheles gambiae. Nature Communications. 2014;**5**:3985

[16] Jeffries CL, Lawrence GG, Golovko G, Kristan M, Orsborne J, Spence K, et al. Novel Wolbachia strains in anopheles malaria vectors from sub-Saharan Africa. Welcome Open Research. 2018;**3**:485

[17] Gomes FM, Hixson BL, Tyner MD, Ramirez JL, Canepa GE, e Silva TLA, et al. Effect of naturally occurring Wolbachia in Anopheles gambiae sl mosquitoes from Mali on plasmodium falciparum malaria transmission. Proceedings of the National Academy of Sciences. 2017;**114**(47):12566-12571

[18] Moreira LA, Iturbe-Ormaetxe I, Jeffery JA, Lu G, Pyke AT, Hedges LM, et al. A Wolbachia symbiont in *Aedes aegypti* limits infection with dengue, chikungunya, and *plasmodium*. Cell. 2009;**139**:1268-1278

[19] WHO. A Global Brief on Vector-Borne Diseases. Geneva: World Health Organization; 2014. Available from: https://apps.who.int/iris/handle/10665/111008 [Accessed: 24th January, 2022]

[20] Azambuja P, Garcia ES, Ratcliffe NA. Gut microbiota and parasite transmission by insect vectors. Trends in Parasitology. 2005;**21**:568-572

[21] Degnan P, Moran N. Diverse phage-encoded toxins in a protective insect endosymbiont. Applied and Environmental Microbiology. 2008;**74**:6782-6791

[22] Dillon RJ, Dillon VM. The gut bacteria of insects: Non-pathogenic interactions. Annual Review of Entomology. 2004;**49**:71-92

[23] Engel P, Moran NA. The gut microbiota of insects-diversity in structure and function. FEMS Microbiology Reviews. 2013;**37**:699-735

[24] Gendrin M, Christophides GK. The *anopheles* mosquito microbiota and their impact on pathogen transmission. In: Manguin S, editor. Anopheles Mosquitoes - New Insights Into Malaria Vectors. London: INTECH; 2013

[25] Minard G, Mavingui P, Moro CV. Diversity and function of bacterial microbiota in the mosquito holobiont. Parasites and Vectors. 2013;**6**:146

[26] Nartey R, Owusu-Dabo E, Kruppa T, Baffour-Awuah S, Annan A, Oppong S, et al. Use of *bacillus thuringiensis* var *israelensis* as a viable option in an integrated malaria vector control Programme in the Kumasi Metropolis, Ghana. Parasites and Vectors. 2013;**6**:116

[27] Ng TFF, Willner DL, Lim YW, Schmieder R, Chau B, Nilsson C, et al. Broad surveys of DNA viral diversity obtained through viral metagenomics of mosquitoes. PLoS One. 2011;**6**(6):e20579

[28] Weiss B, Aksoy S. Microbiome influences on insect host vector competence. Trends in Parasitology. 2011;**27**:514-522

[29] Xi Z, Joshi D. Genetic control of malaria and dengue using Wolbachia. In: Genetic Control of Malaria and Dengue. Cambridge, Massachusetts, United States: Academic Press; 2016. pp. 305-333

[30] World Health Organization. Manual on Environmental Management for Mosquito Control, with Special Emphasis on Malaria Vectors. World Health Organization; 1982. Available

from: https://apps.who.int/iris/handle/10665/37329 [Accessed: 24th January, 2022]

[31] Huang Y, Higgs S, Vanlandingham DL. Biological control strategies for mosquito vectors of arboviruses. Insects. 2017;**8**(21):1-25

[32] Federici BA. The future of microbial insecticides as vector control agents. Journal of the American Mosquito Control Association. 1995;**11**(2):260-268

[33] Wilke ABB, Marrelli MT. Genetic control of mosquitoes: Population suppression strategies. Revista do Instituto de Medicina Tropical de São Paulo. 2012;**54**(5):287-292

[34] Gonzalez-Ceron L, Santillan F, Rodriguez MH, Mendez D, Hernandez-Avila JE. Bacteria in midguts of field-collected *Anopheles albimanus* block *plasmodium vivax* sporogonic development. Journal of Medical Entomology. 2003;**40**:371-374

[35] Hurwitz I, Fieck A, Read A, Hillesland H, Klein N, Kang A, et al. Paratransgenic control of vector borne diseases. International Journal of Biological Sciences. 2011;**7**(9):1334-1344

[36] Wilke ABB, Marrelli MT. Paratransgenesis: A promising new strategy for mosquito vector control. Parasites & Vectors. 2015;**8**:342

[37] Pidiyar VJ, Jangid K, Patole MS, Shouche YS. Studies on cultured and uncultured microbiota of wild *Culex quinquefasciatus* mosquito midgut based on 16s ribosomal RNA gene analysis. The American Journal of Tropical Medicine and Hygiene. 2004;**70**:597-603

[38] Riehle MA, Jacobs-Lorena M. Using bacteria to express and display anti-parasite molecules in mosquitoes: Current and future strategies. Insect Biochemistry and Molecular Biology. 2005;**35**:699-707

[39] Riehle MA, Moreira CK, Lampe D, Lauzon C, Jacobs-Lorena M. Using bacteria to express and display anti-plasmodium molecules in the mosquito midgut. International Journal for Parasitology. 2007;**37**:595-603

[40] Gaio AO, Gusmão DS, Santos AV, Berbert-Molina MA, Pimenta PF, Lemos FJ. Contribution of midgut bacteria to blood digestion and egg production in *Aedes aegypti* (Diptera: Culicidae). Parasites and Vectors. 2011;**14**:4-105

[41] Aksoy S, Weiss B, Attardo G. Paratransgenesis applied for control of tsetse transmitted sleeping sickness. Advances in Experimental Medicine and Biology. 2008;**627**:35-48

[42] Briones AM, Shililu J, Githure J, Novak R, Raskin L. *Thorsellia anophelis* is the dominant bacterium in a Kenyan population of adult *Anopheles gambiae* mosquitoes. The ISME Journal. 2008;**2**:74-82

[43] Coutinho-Abreu IV, Zhu KY, Ramalho-Ortigao M. Transgenesis and paratransgenesis to control insect-borne diseases: Current status and future challenges. Parasitology International. 2009;**59**:1-8

[44] Favia G, Ricci I, Damiani C, Raddadi N, Crotti E, Marzorati M, et al. Bacteria of the genus *Asaia* stably associate with *Anopheles stephensi*, an Asian malarial mosquito vector. Proceedings of the National Academy of Sciences of the United States of America. 2007;**104**:9047-9051

[45] Sayler GS, Ripp S. Field applications of genetically engineered microorganisms for bioremediation

processes. Current Opinion in Biotechnology. 2000;**11**:286-289

[46] O'Neill S. Wolbachia bacteria in insect cell. In: How common are Wolbachia and other bacteria in Insect cells? 2019. Available from: https://entomologytoday.org/2019/01/28/how-common-wolbachia-bacterial-endosymbionts-insects/wolbachia-bacteria-in-insect-cell/ [Accessed 27th March, 2022

[47] Pietri JE, DeBruhl H, Sullivan W. The rich somatic life of Wolbachia. Microbiology Open. 2016;**5**(6):923-936

[48] Townson H. *Wolbachia* as a potential tool for suppressing filarial transmission. Annals of Tropical Medicine and Parasitology. 2002;**96**:117-127

[49] Yoshida S, Ioka D, Matsuoka H, Endo H, Ishii A. Bacteria expressing single chain immuno-toxin inhibit malaria parasite development in mosquitoes. Molecular and Biochemical Parasitology. 2001;**113**:89-96

[50] Atyame CM, Pasteur N, Dumas E, Tortosa P, Tantely ML, Pocquet N, et al. Cytoplasmic incompatibility as a means of controlling *Culex pipiens quinquefasciatus* mosquito in the islands of the South-Western Indian Ocean. PLoS Neglected Tropical Diseases. 2011;**5**:e1440

[51] Calvitti M, Moretti R, Skidmore AR, Dobson SL. *Wolbachia* strain wPip yields a pattern of cytoplasmic incompatibility enhancing a *Wolbachia*-based suppression strategy against the disease vector *Aedes albopictus*. Parasites and Vectors. 2012;**5**:254

[52] Werren JH, Baldo L, Clark ME. *Wolbachia*: Master manipulators of invertebrate biology. Nature Reviews. Microbiology. 2008;**6**:741-751

[53] Walker T, Johnson PH, Moreira LA, Iturbe-Ormaetxe I, Frentiu FD, McMeniman CJ, et al. The wMel *Wolbachia* strain blocks dengue and invades caged *Aedes aegypti* populations. Nature. 2011;**476**:450-453

[54] Weiss BL, Mouchotte R, Rio RV, Wu YN, Wu Z, Heddi A, et al. Interspecific transfer of bacterial endosymbionts between tsetse fly species: Infection establishment and effect on host fitness. Applied and Environmental Microbiology. 2006;**72**:7013-7021

[55] Zimmer C. *Wolbachia*, a tale of sex and survival. Science. 2001;**292**:1093-1095

[56] Hughes GL, Rivero A, Rasgon JL. *Wolbachia* can enhance *plasmodium* infection in mosquitoes: Implications for malaria control? PLOS Pathogens. 2014;**10**(9):e1004182

[57] Ayala D, Akone-Ella O, Rahola N, Kengne P, Ngangue MF, Mezeme F, et al. Natural Wolbachia infections are common in the major malaria vectors in Central Africa. Evolutionary Applications. 2019;**12**(8):1583-1594

[58] Walker T, Quek S, Jeffries CL, Bandibabone J, Dhokiya V, Bamou R, et al. Stable high-density and maternally inherited Wolbachia infections in anopheles moucheti and anopheles demeilloni mosquitoes. Current Biology. 2021;**31**(11):2310-2320

[59] Clancy DJ, Hoffmann AA. Environmental effects on cytoplasmic incompatibility and bacterial load in Wolbachia-infected Drosophila simulans. Entomologia Experimentalis et Applicata. 1998;**86**(1):13-24

[60] Chanda E, Ameneshewa B, Bagayoko M, Govere JM, Macdonald MB.

Harnessing integrated vector management for enhanced disease prevention. Trends in Parasitology. 2017;**33**(1):30-41

[61] Sande S, Zimba M, Nyasvisvo D, Mukuzunga M, Kooma EH, Mberikunashe J, et al. Getting ready for integrated vector management for improved disease prevention in Zimbabwe: A focus on key policy issues to consider. Malaria Journal. 2019;**18**(1):1-8

[62] Chanda E, Mzilahowa T, Chipwanya J, Mulenga S, Ali D, Troell P, et al. Preventing malaria transmission by indoor residual spraying in Malawi: Grappling with the challenge of uncertain sustainability. Malaria Journal. 2015;**14**(1):1-7

[63] Cohen JM, Dlamini S, Novotny JM, Kandula D, Kunene S, Tatem AJ. Rapid case-based mapping of seasonal malaria transmission risk for strategic elimination planning in Swaziland. Malaria Journal. 2013;**12**(1):1-12

[64] Chihanga S, Haque U, Chanda E, Mosweunyane T, Moakofhi K, Jibril HB, et al. Malaria elimination in Botswana, 2012-2014: Achievements and challenges. Parasites & Vectors. 2016;**9**(1):1-12

[65] Chanda E, Phiri FN, Ch J, Ramdeen V, Kamuliwo M, Baboo KS. Impact of entomological interventions on malaria vector bionomics in low transmission settings in Zambia. Journal of Public Health and Epidemiology. 2012;**4**(7):189-196

[66] Rivero A, Vezilier J, Weill M, Read AF, Gandon S. Insecticide control of vector-borne diseases: When is insecticide resistance a problem? PLoS Pathogens. 2010;**6**(8):e1001000

[67] Mutero CM, Schlodder D, Kabatereine N, Kramer R. Integrated vector management for malaria control in Uganda: Knowledge, perceptions and policy development. Malaria Journal. 2012;**11**(1):1-10

[68] Van den Berg H, Takken W. Evaluation of integrated vector management. Trends in Parasitology. 2009;**25**(2):71-76

Chapter 9

Community Engagement and Social Assessment for *Wolbachia*-Based Suppression of Natural Populations of *Aedes aegypti*: The Mexican Experience

Josué Villegas-Chim, Abdiel Martin-Park, Henry Puerta-Guardo, María Eugenia Toledo-Romaní, Norma Pavía-Ruz, Yamili Contreras-Perera, Silvia Pérez-Carrillo, Azael Che-Mendoza, Jorge Palacio-Vargas, Fabián Correa-Morales, Héctor Gómez-Dantés and Pablo Manrique-Saide

Abstract

The *Wolbachia*-based approach is under evaluation as a control strategy against *Aedes aegypti* in Mexico. From 2017 to 2019, we performed a pilot study to evaluate an open-field mass-release of *w*AlbB-infected *Ae. aegypti* male mosquitoes, as part of an integrated vector management (IVM) plan led by the Ministry of Health in Mexico to suppress natural populations of *Ae. aegypti* in southern Mexico. Community engagement and social evaluation were part of the key activities conducted. Overall, results showed the positive benefits of this *Wolbachia*-based method in the reduction of *Aedes* mosquitoes (90%). Mosquito's nuisance at bedtime and the increasing circulation of mosquitoes during the releasing days were reported as the negative perceptions of this method. Importantly, participants understood the difference between wild mosquitoes and those released as part of the project, as well as the importance of the IVM. A significant number of the population accepted and supported the project, and feedback was given to improve future mosquito-releasing activities. The social license was a key factor in the success of the intervention and should be part of innovative paradigms for mosquito-vector control strategies involving community engagement. We outline the Mexican experience of community engagement and social assessment in implementing a *Wolbachia*-based strategy.

IntechOpen

Keywords: *Wolbachia*-based vector control, community engagement, social assessment, mosquito-borne diseases

1. Introduction

Mosquito-borne diseases remain as one of the major challenges for public health and vector control programs at global and local levels. Up-to-date, there is not a 100% effective vaccine or therapy for dengue, chikungunya, or Zika virus. Hence, traditional mosquito-vector control strategies are among the most common ways to combat these diseases, with proven efficacy [1]. Integrated vector management has been the approach recommended by the World Health Organization [2, 3] to reinforce the vector control programs.

As a result of new biotechnologies for pest control, innovative approaches have been developed for the suppression and/or replacement of mosquito populations. The "rear and releases" is the new change of paradigm in this agenda and social assessment must be a key aspect to consider. A novel strategy to suppress vector populations based on the endosymbiotic bacterium *Wolbachia pipientis* is a promising complementary strategy that potentially reduces mosquito populations and the risk of mosquito-borne disease transmission [3–12]. This approach known as the incompatible insect technique (IIT), consists of the release of male mosquitoes infected with maternally inhered *Wolbachia*. The mating between *Wolbachia*-infected males and urban/wild-type female mosquitoes in the environment (not infected with *Wolbachia*) produced non-viable eggs due to a phenomenon called cytoplasmic incompatibility (CI) [4]. However, IIT approaches can combine additional measures, such as the sterile insect technique (SIT) to minimize the unintentional release of fertile *Wolbachia*-infected female mosquitoes (IIT-SIT approach) (**Figure 1**) [7–9]. In this low-dose irradiation is used to sterilize residual pupae females after the sex sorting process, thus preventing the stable establishment of field populations derived from released *Wolbachia*-infected males [6]. The IIT-SIT approach to suppress *Ae. aegypti* populations have been tested in two recent successful pilot trials in Thailand [10] and Mexico [13] and *Ae. albopictus* in China [11]. Furthermore, the circulation of *Wolbachia* strains in native populations of *Ae. albopictus* have been already identified in the southern region of Mexico [13, 14].

Currently, the *Wolbachia*-based approach that combines both incompatible and sterile insect techniques (IIT-SIT) is under evaluation as a control strategy against *Ae. aegypti* in Mexico. From 2017 to 2019 a pilot study was performed to evaluate an open-field mass-release of *w*AlbB-infected *Ae. aegypti* males (*Wolbachia* strain *w*AlbB from *Ae. albopictus* [donor host] and successfully established in *Ae. aegypti* [novel host]), as part of an integrated vector management (IVM) plan led by the Ministry of Health in a semi-urban community called San Pedro Chimay, Yucatan, Mexico, with the collaboration of the autonomous university of Yucatan, to suppress natural populations of *Ae. aegypti* in southern Mexico [12]. In this pilot study, a protocol for the implementation of a *Wolbachia*-based biocontrol aiming to suppress *Ae. aegypti* mosquito population was designed. At first, anthropological research seeking community engagement and cultural sensitization was conducted, followed by an entomological baseline survey. Secondly, the Ministry of Health carried out an attack phase with vector control routines followed by a suppression phase, including male-mosquito releasing activities and the social assessment of the entire project [12].

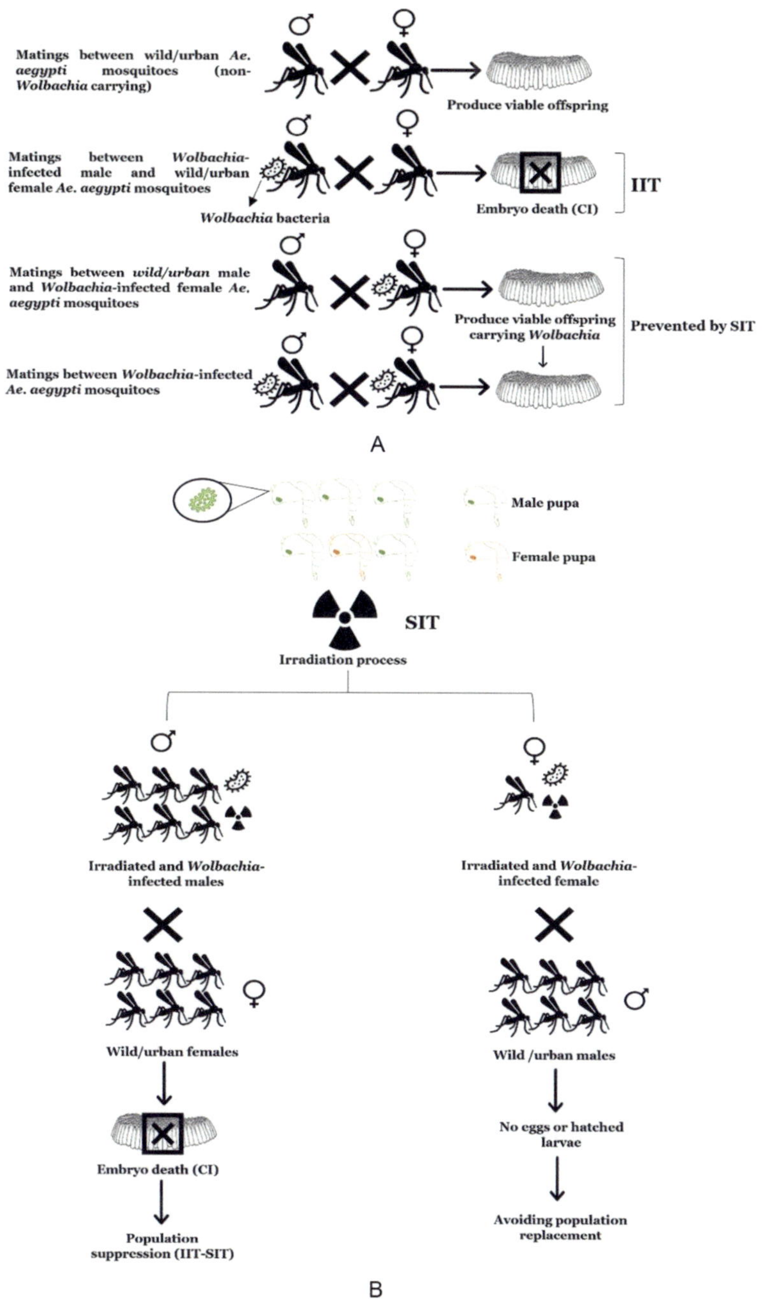

Figure 1.
The combined IIT-SIT approach is depicted schematically: (A) The four types of possible crosses between wild/ urban Aedes aegypti *mosquitos and* Wolbachia-*infected* Ae. aegypti *mosquitos; and (B) Irradiation of residual* Wolbachia-*infected females (SIT) to prevent them from reproducing in the wild; mass-production, irradiation, and release of* Wolbachia-*infected males with residual females, as well as mating crosses with wild/urban populations.*

For the pilot study, community engagement and social evaluation were part of the key activities conducted [15, 16]. Throughout the suppression phase, we observed significant reductions in the adult females collected at the release site in comparison to control sites, with the greatest effect observed on the number of indoor *Ae. aegypti* females collected per house (90% of reduction efficacy) [12].

In this chapter, we outline the Mexican experience, including community engagement and social assessment, in implementing a *Wolbachia*-based strategy intended to suppress the natural population of *Ae. aegypti* in San Pedro Chimay, a Mayan indigenous location situated in Yucatan, Mexico.

2. Principles of community engagement

Projects based on IIT-SIT require models or frameworks for the community engagement process and activities. Every approach has its own strengths and limitations, but they offer guidance for the implementation of the plan of action. The center for disease control and prevention has developed a guideline that provides an interesting system that integrates steps for a successful engagement [17].

Before the intervention: (1) Establish clear purposes and goals; (2) address the main characteristics of the community (culture, economics, politics, norms, and values) and the experiences with other projects in the past or present.

For engagement to occur: (1) Establish a bond of trust with the community and their formal and informal leaders, as well as other local organizations; and (2) respect the self-determination of the community.

For engagement to succeed: (1) Build partnership with the community in order to create changes and improve topics related to health; (2) acknowledge the internal diversity of the community and the relations during the whole process of community engagement; (3) the engagement can be sustainable by the appropriation of the community; (4) the community must be involved from the beginning, be prepared, and develop decisions capacity in order to the sustainability of the engagement; and (5) the community collaboration demands wider commitment by the engaging of all sort of interested actors.

Therefore, the community engagement of the project, based on those principles for community engagement, was divided into four phases (**Table 1**), each one addressed in a transversal way the guidelines to express the social inclusion of the community targeted. Detailed information of each phase was already published elsewhere [12].

I. Preparation of the community	II. Prereleasing activities	III. Releasing activities	IV. Postreleasing activities
Rapid social assessment of the feasibility of the community	Social research on mosquito-borne diseases and social acceptance of the project.	Social license of the leaders and community through workshops.	Follow-up educational activities and social assessment of the perceived benefits.
Surveillance of social impact for the implementation of the intervention.			

Table 1.
Community engagement and social evaluation.

3. The mosquitoes in the Mayan culture

The very presence of the mosquitoes in the Mayan culture had been represented with ambivalence, as an unpleasant pest, a hero, and an ally. Archeological evidence in both pre-Columbian pottery and Codex portrayed the mosquito sucking women's breasts [18], while she tried to swat it (**Figure 2**). However, the narratives and interpretations are far from the current conception of the mosquito (transmitter of diseases). The plot is associated with the mythological personification of a disguised god (as a mosquito) that tries to marry the maiden represented, against the will of the father-in-law.

In the Mayan sacred book called Popol Vuh, there is a narrative about a mythic journey to the Xibalbá (Mayan underworld) led by the mythical twins Hunahpú and Ixbalanqué. In their trek, they needed to figure out the name of all the gods and gave the mosquito a mission in this plot, to push them to reveal their names, that says:

> *"Bite them one by one; first bite the one sitting on the foreground and end up biting them all, because that is the part that corresponds to you, sucking the blood of man on the road." [19]*

Although no associations were linked to mosquitoes as the transmitter of diseases in pre-Columbine documents, there are historical mentions of a plague called in the Mayan language "xekik" (vomiting blood) that was associated with yellow fever [20, 21], but once again no mentions of the mosquito as the carrier of any pathogens were proposed.

In the Mayan culture, there is a worldview classification of the arthropods associated with medicine, economics, food, and religion [22]. The mosquito does not seem to be included here, but only in contemporary studies [23–26] we can identify the association with diseases, such as dengue.

Social research on cultural understanding of mosquito-borne diseases is as important as the study of the perceptions toward their vectors. Local taxonomies and

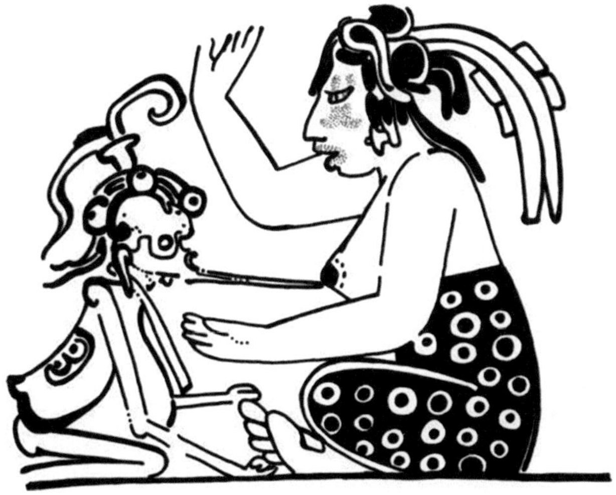

Figure 2.
Mosquito biting a maiden's breast [18].

ethnoecological approaches that frame the political, historical, and cultural context of this topic, shape the way people learn, think, represent, and take action for preventing practices [27–30].

4. Uts k'oxol: a cross-cultural approach for IIT-SIT

In Yucatan, Mexico, 43.8% of the population are Mayan speakers and most of them live in Merida and the surrounding villages because of the urbanization, immigration, and economic changes [31–34]. The releasing site of *Wolbachia*-infected mosquitoes, San Pedro Chimay, is part of those communities and the indigenous knowledge of the relationship between society and nature plays a key role in the community. Hence, a cross-cultural approach was considered to design strategies and materials for the engagement and social assessment [15, 16].

In the formative stage of the project (phases I and II, see **Table 1**), anthropological diagnosis and research were performed which aims to validate the feasibility of the community for the activities and the social acceptance of the whole process [15, 16]. To pursue the change of paradigm "from kill to release mosquitoes", the necessity to transform scientific speech of the IIT-SIT methods into more appropriate local linguistic frames, meetings were organized to discuss the best way to achieve this goal. Most of the attendants, elders, and community leaders, acknowledged the value of using the Mayan language to communicate the main messages and goals of the project itself. During extensive discussion sessions about the challenges and benefits, they came out with the idea in the Mayan language of "Uts k'oxol" (translation: uts = good; k'oxol = mosquito) as a cultural-sensitive brand. The novelty of this achievement is that the team and the local leaders, created a new word, even for the indigenous worldview, to introduce IIT-SIT strategy in Yucatan, Mexico.

5. Social assessment of perceived benefits and disadvantages

The social assessment study was conducted in the sub-urban and Mayan indigenous community of San Pedro Chimay, which belongs to the municipality of Merida (capital city), the capital of the state of Yucatan located in the southern region of Mexico. This locality comprises 1246 inhabitants, 646 men and 615 women, and 305 houses [35]. However, the scientific team identified that only 150 dwellings were occupied by families able to participate in the project.

A semi-structured interview was applied to 70 participants heads of family of the community (December 2019 – February 2020). The design included both quantitative and qualitative questions that addressed several topics, such as profile of participants, reasons for participation in the activities, perceived characteristics of both wild and released mosquitoes, and the perception of the benefits and disadvantages of the project. In addition, an ethnographic approach was performed to gather information about the cultural contexts of the social assessment.

The information from the interviews was analyzed in two steps described as follows: quantitative data was processed using Microsoft Excel™ spreadsheets (2019), and qualitative data were explored in MaxQda software (2020). Both results were compared to create categories related to each aspect of the interview. In addition, ethnographic data were systematized within the emerged categories identified in the interviews.

5.1 Profile of participants

The semi-structure interview was applied to 70 heads of family in the community, 74.3% (52/70) were women and 25.7% (18/70) were men. 77.1% (54/70) were married, 11.4% (7/70) divorced, 11.4% (8/70) single, and 8.6% (6/70) were widow. About the education level, 57.1% (40/70) had elementary school level, 21.4% (15/70) had middle school, 8.6% (6/70) had high school level, 2.9% (2/70) had bachelor's degree, and 10% (7/70) never went to school. All the participants (100%, 70/70) were both Spanish and Mayan speakers. Spanish was mostly used at workplaces, for traveling, and for business or education activities. In turn, Mayas were used more for domestic and private conversations among adults.

5.2 Engagement and participation in activities

As part of the engagement process, since the very beginning of the project, people were invited to several activities, such as workshops, community meetings, and educational demonstrations (**Figures 3** and **4**) [15, 16]. However, as expected, not all the families could participate in every phase of the intervention. A 42.9% (30/70) of the interviewed participants reported to be actively involved, while 57.1% (40/70) did not. Here, qualitative data help us to understand this divergence. For the people that embraced the actions and events, they said to recognize the importance of mosquito-borne diseases and they liked to participate in the project. The primary obstacles that the second set of members encountered were a lack of time, health problems, domestic issues, and the fact that they worked all week outside of the community.

This evidence framed a critical situation to achieve the engagement of a whole community, where families just cannot take part in it, regardless of the reasons. This is perhaps the main reason people interviewed asked for more house-to-house visits and the distribution of brochures because for them it is the best mechanism to be informed about the goals, processes, and benefits of the intervention. In words of a housewife and domestic worker woman interviewed, she said:

> *"To go to workshops is a luxury of time that I don't have. My family must eat, my kids need to go to school, and this is not an easy thing for me and my family. Here in San Pedro [release-site], there are more women like me, this is real life."*

5.3 Perceived characteristics of wild mosquitoes

People were asked about the characteristics of the wild mosquitoes that they knew before the project started. 52.9% (37/70) reported that those mosquitoes are transmitters of diseases, 22.9% (16/70) said that mosquitoes do not transmit any disease, and 24.3% (17/70) were not sure about this aspect. A 45.7% (32/70) of participants reported that the female mosquito is responsible for this transmission of diseases, 4.3% (3/70) said the male mosquito, 5.7% (4/70) told both male and female, and 44.3% (31/70) were not sure.

In addition, people's narratives and descriptions of experiences reflected a qualitative pattern emerged, such as "they are black with white stripes on their legs," "it's a big mosquito," "it is called *Ae. aegypti,*" "they are black mosquitoes," "there are female mosquitoes," and "they bite."

A 57.1% (40/70) reported that the female mosquitoes presented a blood-feeding behavior, 7.1% (5/70) identified the male mosquitoes with the same feeding pattern,

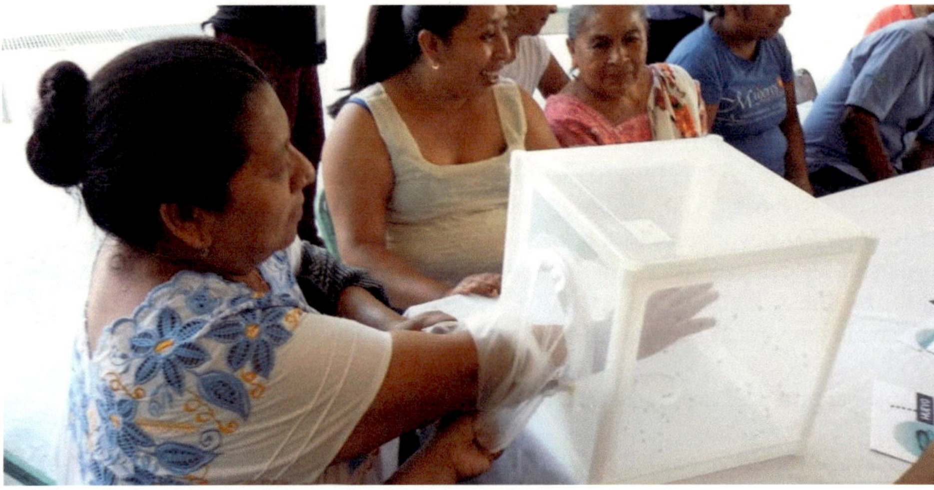

Figure 3.
Demonstration activity "hand-cage".

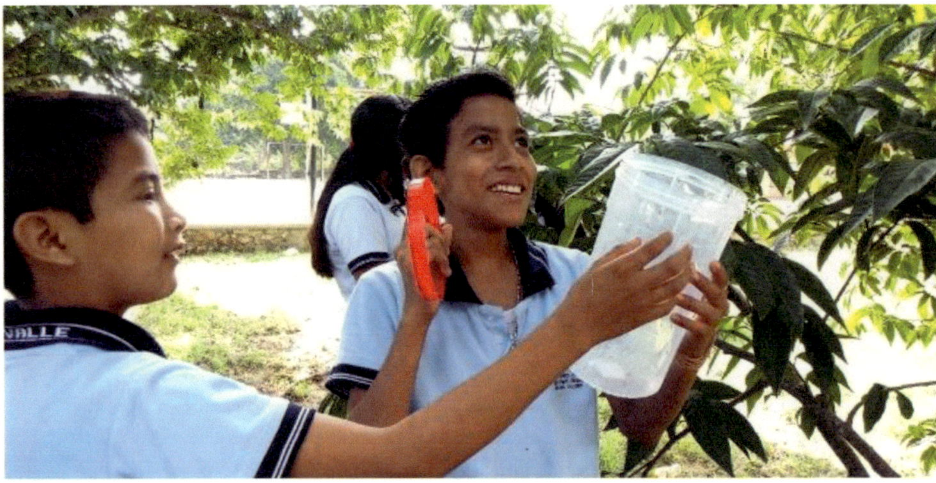

Figure 4.
Male mosquito releasing activities with school children.

5.7% (4/70) believed that both male and female bite for human blood, and 30% (21/70) did not know about it. The information presented is a portrait of the general feature of the *Ae. aegypti*, the main mosquito in the community.

5.4 Perceived characteristics of released mosquitoes

Overall, 55.7% (39/70) reported that the mosquitoes released by the scientific team were females, 5.7% (4/70) told that they were male mosquitoes, 7.1% (5/70) both male and female mosquitoes, and 31.4% (22/70) did not know. To obtain a deep understanding of lay knowledge, people were asked to give their daily narratives of the presence and co-habitations of the released mosquitoes. Categories were developed to structure the verbatim provided by the participants, as shown in the following **Table 2**, top-down in order of most frequently mentioned.

Categories	Narratives
Feeding-behavior	"Male mosquitoes that do not bite"
Mating-behavior	"They are male mosquitoes that when mating with local females, their eggs will not hatch"
Wolbachia-references	"They are mosquitoes with *Wolbachia*" "They have a chemical substance for the female mosquito to die"
Block-transmission	"They are mosquitoes that do not transmit Dengue, Chikungunya or Zika"
Reduce-mosquitoes	"They are mosquitoes that will help to reduce mosquitoes that transmit diseases" "They are mosquitoes to hunt or kill female mosquitoes" "The released mosquitoes will eat the bad mosquitoes" "To catch other mosquitoes"
Name-*Aedes aegypti*	"They are *Aedes aegypti* mosquitoes"

Table 2.
Narrative descriptions of the released mosquitoes.

5.5 Perceived benefits and disadvantages

Overall, the majority of the interviewed perceived a positive benefit of the intervention, although there were people that did not acknowledge any advantage of this (**Table 3**).

In addition, the participants related their experiences about the advantages and benefits of the project.

> *"The truth is that it is a great benefit to reduce the risk of diseases in San Pedro. There are not too many mosquitoes that bite." (Man interviewed, 22 years old)*

> *"It is about preventing mosquito biting. Is the benefit that we learnt." (Women interviewed, 60 years old)*

> *"You must keep informed to avoid misunderstandings and gossip and the people will understand and acknowledge what you are doing." (Women interviewed, 36 years old)*

> *"We have to work with the people that believe those released mosquitoes are the bad ones because they are stubborn." (Women interviewed, 67 years old)*

Description	%/n
Reduction of mosquitoes	43% (30/70)
Help to prevent mosquito-borne diseases	26% (18/70)
Does not know	16% (11/70)
No benefits perceived	10% (7/70)
Learnings about mosquito-borne diseases	5% (4/70)
Total	100% (70/70)

Table 3.
Perceived benefits of the project.

On the other hand, 64.3% (45/70) of the participants reported no complaints about the released mosquitoes, while 35.7% (25/70) did. In-deep questions were asked to the last group about the reasons for the disadvantages and that must be addressed with a specific context. The two main reasons were identified here, mosquito's nuisance at bedtime (35.5%, 25/70) and an increase of mosquitoes during the releasing days (37.2%, 26/70). In the community, families usually keep the doors and windows open during the day and rarely use bed nets or house-screening [15]. Thus, this facilitates the entrance of mosquitoes at any time given.

During the fieldwork, ethnographic data collected evidenced the concern of the elders of the community about the transmission of the *Wolbachia* to other organisms, such as bees and humans. In San Pedro Chimay, there is a strong presence of peasants that work in corn fields and beekeeping. In their experience, crop pests and diseases for bees are a huge problem. Therefore, they were worried about the unknown organism carried by released male mosquitoes.

5.6 Social acceptance of the project

At the beginning of the project (2017), a study was carried out addressing cultural barriers, strengths, and social acceptance of the intervention [15]. At the end of the project (2020), people were asked again if they would be interested in continuing to participate. 94.3% (66/70) of participants agreed, 4.3% (3/70) said no, and 1.4% (1/70) were not sure. The positive perception of the interviewed were supported by many experiences such as that the project was helping to improve the community's health, other general benefits perceived (knowledge about domestic prevention against mosquitoes), and they were very interested in the main effect perceived, the reduction of the mosquitoes in their houses.

6. Conclusion

This research was conducted to evaluate the perceived benefits and disadvantages of an IVM control of the *Ae. aegypti* that included the release of male mosquitoes for the suppression of the mosquito population in Yucatan, Mexico. Previous studies reported a good social acceptance [15] and the educational approach regarding this innovative method [16]. As main conclusion, the population interviewed for this chapter, considered that the intervention is an important initiative, and as with every new strategy it comes with some challenges to be addressed.

6.1 Mosquitoes: Friend or foe?

For decades the purpose of the vector control programs was focused on killing the mosquitoes rather than increasing their number. The change of paradigm, from "kill to rear and release" demands a strong community engagement [36–43]. Hence, the main challenge is not only the social acceptance of the early stages but the community support and social license until the closure of the projects based on these new biological vector control methods.

In Yucatan, Mexico, there are socio-anthropological studies about diseases, such as dengue, chikungunya, and Zika virus [23, 24, 25, 28, 29]. However, more research is required with an ethno-entomological approach, that is, focused on the local cultural understandings of the mosquitoes besides the learned knowledge from the government campaigns [27, 30]. Research conducted in Australia, based on innovative biological control methods, showed important perceived differences in the characteristics of wild mosquitoes [38]. Although education activities about the taxonomic differences between male and female mosquitoes were explained to participants at the release site, still residents mentioned the similar appearance among different species of mosquitoes. In our study, ethnographic data evidenced that the participants identified at least one or two characteristics of the *Ae. aegypti*; however, residents that could not be involved in the project (workshops and demonstrative release activities), hardly reported the basic aspects of the mosquitoes [16]. This is a very important issue because the strategic discourse of "reduce *Ae. aegypti* mosquitoes" can be confused with "reduce all the species of mosquitoes" in the community, and, as a result, misunderstandings on the efficacy of the method might arise.

6.2 Community engagement for IIT-SIT: Challenges and experiences

According to the CDC's principles for community engagement, the transversal path is key to all the phases, processes, and actions for the implementation of the project. All three steps of this model had to be reinforced along the development of the activities.

The goals need to be presented in different formats and for several audiences (adults, children, and elders) and languages (Mayan-Spanish). Also, unexpected political scenarios took place during the beginning, such as political elections at national and local level, which required changes in the leader-engagement strategies because the whole municipal committee was new, and all the political landscape changed. Therefore, the bound of trust initially constructed demanded the inclusion of other informal actors in the arena, and with this unrepresented groups of the community emerged.

To respect the self-determination of the community, there was a flexible partnership collaboration to build that could include more social groups, even with political and cultural differences, to become part of the decision-making process. The very sustainability of the project was once again challenged by another unexpected situation, that is, the COVID-19 pandemic. We conducted an additional social evaluation addressing if the leaders will be agreeing that the project could be continued, with minimal activities (entomological surveillance and mosquito-releasing activities following the proper preventive measures), but the result was that they preferred to put it in stand by the project until the pandemic event ends.

Finally, it is important to highlight that social license was a key factor for the success of the intervention and should be part of innovative paradigms for mosquito-vector control strategies involving community engagement. In this chapter, we outlined the Mexican experience of community engagement and social assessment in implementing a *Wolbachia*-based strategy intended to suppress the natural population of *Ae. aegypti*.

Acknowledgements

Abdiel Martin-Park is supported by the Catedras-CONACYT program. Research funding was provided by Fondo Mixto Consejo Nacional de Ciencia y Tecnología (CONACYT) (México)–Gobierno del Estado de Yucatán (project YUC-2017-2103-01-556) and U.S. Agency for International Development (USAID) (project

AID-OAA-F-16-00082). In addition, special thanks to the people of San Pedro Chimay and the personnel of the Ministry of Health for supporting during the project and field activities.

Conflict of interest

The authors declare no conflict of interest.

Author details

Josué Villegas-Chim[1], Abdiel Martin-Park[1*], Henry Puerta-Guardo[1], María Eugenia Toledo-Romaní[2], Norma Pavía-Ruz[1], Yamili Contreras-Perera[1], Silvia Pérez-Carrillo[1], Azael Che-Mendoza[1], Jorge Palacio-Vargas[3], Fabián Correa-Morales[4], Héctor Gómez-Dantés[5] and Pablo Manrique-Saide[1]

1 Autonomous University of Yucatan, Merida, Yucatan, Mexico

2 Institute of Tropical Medicine "Pedro Kourí" (IPK), Habana, Cuba

3 Ministry of Health, Yucatan, Mexico

4 National Center for Preventive Programs and Disease Control (CENAPRECE), Mexico

5 National Institute of Public Health, Cuernavaca, Mexico

*Address all correspondence to: ampark27@gmail.com

References

[1] World Health Organization. World Malaria Report. Geneva: World Health Organization; 2015

[2] World Health Organization. Global Strategic Framework for Integrated Vector Management. Geneva: World Health Organization; 2004. p. 14

[3] Pan-American Health Organization, World Health Organization. El manejo integrado de vectores: una respuesta integral a las enfermedades de transmisión vectorial, Resolución Consejo Directivo OPS/OMS, CD48.R8. 2008

[4] Brelsfoard C, Dobson S. *Wolbachia*-based strategies to control insect pests and disease vectors. Asia-Pacific Journal of Molecular Biology and Biotechnology. 2009;**17**:55-63

[5] Bourtzis K, Dobson SL, Xi Z, Rasgon JL, Calvitti M, Moreira LA, et al. Harnessing mosquito-*Wolbachia* symbiosis for vector and disease control. Acta Tropica. 2014;**132**(Suppl):S150-S163

[6] Lees RS, Carvalho DO, Bouyer J. Potential impact of integrating the Sterile Insect Technique into the fight against disease-transmitting mosquitoes. In: Dyck VA, Hendrichs J, Robinson AS, editors. Sterile Insect Technique – Principles and Practice in Area-Wide Integrated Pest Management. Second ed. Boca Raton, Florida, USA: CRC Press; 2021. pp. 1081-1118

[7] Dobson SL, Fox CW, Jiggins FM. The effect of Wolbachia-induced cytoplasmic incompatibility on host population size in natural and manipulated systems. Proceedings of the Biological Sciences. 2002;**269**(1490):437-445. DOI: 10.1098/rspb.2001.1876

[8] Xi Z, Khoo CC, Dobson SL. *Wolbachia* establishment and invasion in an *Aedes aegypti* laboratory population. Science. 2005;**310**:326-328. DOI: 10.1126/science.1117607

[9] Dyck VA, Hendrichs J, Robinson AS, editors. Sterile Insect Technique – Principles and Practice in Area-Wide Integrated Pest Management. Second ed. Boca Raton, FL, USA: CRC Press; 2021. p. 1200

[10] Kittayapong P, Ninphanomchai S, Limohpasmanee W, Chansang C, Chansang C, Mongkalangoon P. Combined sterile insect technique and incompatible insect technique: The first proof-of-concept to suppress *Aedes aegypti* vector populations in semi-rural settings in Thailand. PLoS Neglected Tropical Diseases. 2019;**13**:e0007771

[11] Zheng X, Zhang D, Li Y, Yang C, Wu Y, Liang X, et al. Incompatible and sterile insect techniques combined eliminate mosquitoes. Nature. 2019;**572**(7767):56-61. DOI: 10.1038/s41586-019-1407-9

[12] Martín-Park A, Che-Mendoza A, Contreras-Perea Y, Pérez-Carrillo S, Puerta-Guardo H, Villegas-Chim J, et al. Pilot trial using mass field-releases of sterile males produced with the incompatible and sterile insect techniques as part of integrated *Aedes aegypti* control in Mexico. PLOS Neglected Diseases. 2022;**16**(4):e0010324. DOI: 10.1371/journal.pntd.00103

[13] Roblero-Andrade AE, RosalesRamírez G, Torres-Monzón JA, López-Ordóñez T, Avendaño-Rabiell A, Casas-Martínez M. Distribución de la infección por *Wolbachia* sp. en

mosquitos de cementerios del sur de Chiapas, México. Entomología Mexicana. 2019;**6**:484-489

[14] Puerta-Guardo H, Contreras-Perera Y, Pérez-Carrillo S, Che-Mendoza A, Ayora-Talavera G, Vazquez-Prokopec G, et al. *Wolbachia* in native populations of *Aedes albopictus* (Diptera: Culicidae) from Yucatan peninsula, Mexico. Journal of Insect Science. 2020;**16**:20(5). DOI: 10.1093/jisesa/ieaa096

[15] Martínez-Cruz C, Villegas-Chim J, Barrera-Fuentes GA, Espinosa-Lizama F, Toledo-Romaní ME, Pavía-Ruz N, et al. Barreras y fortalezas para la introducción del control biológico de *Aedes aegypti* con *Wolbachia* y liberación de mosquitos macho como parte del manejo integrado de vectores en México 2017-2018. Salud Colectiva. Forthcoming

[16] Martínez-Cruz C, Gómez-Dantés H, Villegas-Chim J, Barrera-Fuentes GA, Pavía-Ruz N, Che-Mendoza A, et al. Intervención educativa basada en PRECEDE-PROCEDE para la adopción comunitaria de control de *Aedes aegypti* basado en *Wolbachia* en Mérida, Yucatán, México. RCSP. Forthcoming

[17] Centre for Disease Control and Prevention. Principles of Community Engagement. Second ed. National Institutes of Health, U.S; 2011

[18] Mazariegos O. Of birds and insects: The hummingbird myth in ancient Mesoamerica. Ancient Mesoamerica. 2010;**21**(1):45-61. DOI: 10.1017/S0956536110000155

[19] Recinos A, Vuh P. Las antiguas historias del Quiché. Mexico: Fondo de Cultura Económica; 1993

[20] Barrera-Vásquez A, Rendón S. El libro de los libros de Chilam Balam. México: Fondo de la Cultura Económica; 1948. pp. 21-43

[21] De Landa D. Relación de las Cosas de Yucatán. México: Editorial Porrúa; 1978. pp. 19-20

[22] Pinkus RM. El hombre y los artrópodos: un vínculo inalienable. Península. 2010;**5**(2):81-100

[23] Winch P, Lloyd L, Godas MD, Kendall C. Beliefs about the prevention of dengue and other febrile illnesses in Mérida, Mexico. Journal of Tropical Medicine and Hygiene. 1991;**94**(6):377-387

[24] Lloyd L, Winch P, Ortega-Canto J, Kendall C. Results of a community-based *Aedes aegypti* control program in Merida, Yucatan, Mexico. The American Journal of Tropical Medicine and Hygiene. 1992;**46**(6):635-642

[25] Chávez Arias NP, Villegas Chim JE, Wejebe Shanahan M, Barrera Buenfil D, Rafful Ceballos MJ, Ramos Valencia JE, et al. Studying Sociocultural Factors Associated with Dengue Fever in Elementary School Children in Yucatán. Mexico: SAGE Research Methods; 2017

[26] Villegas-Chim J, Gómez-Dantés H, Pavía-Ruz N, Vera-Gamboa L, Rafful-Ceballos MJ, Ramos-Valencia JE, et al. Arboviruses in Yucatan, Mexico: Anthropological challenges, multidisciplinary views and practical approaches. In: Bardosh K, editor. Locating Zika Social Change and Governance in an Edge of Mosquito Pandemics. Taylor & Francis Group. 2019;**1847**:152-170

[27] Whiteford LM. The ethnoecology of dengue fever. Medical Anthropology Quarterly. 1997;**11**(2):202-223

[28] Torres López TM, Caballero Hoyos R, Barraza Salas JH, Romero PJ. Cultural conceptions about dengue in Nayarit, Mexico. Dengue Bulletin. 2006;**30**

[29] Torres López T, Gerrero Cordero JL, Salazar Estrada JG. Dimensiones culturales del dengue que favorecen o dificultad su prevención en México. Revista Panamericana de Salud Pública. 2012;**31**(3):197-203

[30] Suarez M, Olarte S, Gonzalez A. Is what I have just a cold or is it dengue? Addressing the gap between the politics of dengue control and daily life in Villavivencio, Colombia. Social Science and Medicine. 2005;**61**:495-502

[31] Güemez PM. La lengua maya en el contexto sociolingüístico peninsular. In: Krotz E, editor. Yucatán ante la Ley General de Derechos Lingüísticos de los Pueblos Indígenas. México: Universidad de Oriente; 2008. pp. 115-148

[32] Güemez Pineda M. La lengua maya en Yucatán: una perspectiva sociodemográfica [Internet]. Available from: https://www.mayas.uady.mx/articulos/miguel.html. [Accessed: December 23, 2021]

[33] Pfeiler B, Sánchez I, Villegas-Chim J. La vitalidad lingüística del maya en cuatro localidades de la zona metropolitana d Mérida. In: Santillán RL, editor. Crecimiento urbano y cambio social: escenarios de transformación de la zona metropolitana de Mérida. Mexico: CEPHCIS- UNAM; 2016

[34] Baños O. La península de Yucatán en la ruta de la modernidad (1970-1995). Revista Mexicana del Caribe. 2000;**9**:164-190

[35] Instituto Nacional de Estadística, Geografía e Informática. Censo Nacional de Población y Vivienda. 2010

[36] Popovici J, Moreira LA, Poinsignon A, Iturbe-Ormaetxe I, McNaughton D, O'Neill SL. Assessing key safety concerns of a *Wolbachia*-based strategy to control dengue transmission by *Aedes* mosquitoes. Memórias do Instituto Oswaldo Cruz. 2010;**105**(8):957-964

[37] McNaughton D, Clough A, Johnson P, Ritchie S, O'Neill S. Beyond the 'back yard': Lay knowledge about *Aedes aegypti* in northern Australia and its implications for policy and practice. Acta Tropica. 2010;**116**(1):74-80

[38] McNaughton D. The importance of long-term social research in enabling participation and developing engagement strategies for new dengue control technologies. PLOS Neglected Tropical Diseases. 2012;**6**(8):e1785

[39] McNaughton D, Duong TTH. Designing a community engagement framework for a new dengue control method: A case study from Central Vietnam. PLOS Neglected Tropical Diseases. 2014;**8**(5):e2794

[40] Costa GB, Smithyman R, O'Neill SL, Moreira LA. How to engage communities on a large scale? Lessons from World Mosquito Program in Rio de Janeiro, Brazil. Gates Open Research. 2020;**4**:109

[41] Liew C, Soh LT, Chen I, Ng LC. Public sentiments towards the use of *Wolbachia-Aedes* technology in Singapore. BMC Public Health. 2021;**21**:1417

[42] O'Neill SL, Ryan PA, Turley AP, Wilson G, Retzki K, Iturbe-Ormaetxe I, et al. Scaled deployment of Wolbachia to protect the community from *Aedes* transmitted arboviruses. Gates Open Research. 2018;**2**:36

[43] Kolopack PA, Parsons JA, Lavery JV. What makes community engagement effective?: Lessons from the eliminate dengue program in Queensland Australia. Plos Neglected Tropical Diseases. 2015;**9**(4):e0003713

Chapter 10

Low-Cost Materials for Do-It-Yourself (DIY) Installation of House Screening against *Aedes aegypti*

Josué Herrera-Bojórquez, Josué Villegas-Chim, Daniel Adrian, Azael Che-Mendoza, Juan Navarrete-Carballo, Anuar Medina-Barreiro, Miguel Xcaer, Hugo Delfín-González, Norma Pavía-Ruz, Henry Puerta-Guardo, María Eugenia Toledo-Romaní, Héctor Gómez-Dantés, Gonzalo Vazquez-Prokopec and Pablo Manrique-Saide

Abstract

House-screening (HS) using fixed-aluminium frames to reduce the risk of indoor infestation with *Aedes aegypti* mosquitoes as well as the risk of *Aedes*-transmitted diseases in communities living in endemic areas. However, the success of this approach has been hindered by the elevated cost of the aluminium-based materials as well as their professional installation, which cannot be afforded by people living under vulnerable conditions. Cost-saving strategies such as the use of low-cost materials including wood, PVC, and Velcro are within the list of HS options available and offered by HS businesses and/or Do-it-yourself (DIY) packages *verbi gratia* ready-made and ready-to-install mosquito-screens. Here, we evaluated the efficacy of low-cost frames constructed with different materials to protect against *Ae. aegypti* indoor infestation using experimental huts. The efficacy of protection in preventing female mosquito passing inside the huts of any of the options of frames was high (>93%) compared to the control with no-screen. People's perceptions on the different materials showed the most "popular" alternative was the frame made of wood (62%). All the prototype-frames of HS made of different materials were effective at blocking *Ae. aegypti* entering-mosquitoes particularly, low-cost options like magnets and Velcro.

Keywords: house-screening, *Ae. aegypti*, low-cost materials, Zika, dengue, chikungunya

1. Introduction

"Building the vector out" and "keeping the vector out" are principles encouraged by the world health organisation (WHO) [1–3] to promote effective and sustainable housing interventions for the prevention of vector-borne diseases. Covering doors and windows with insect mesh, known as house-screening (HS), is one such intervention to "build-out" vector-borne diseases [4–7]. The WHO has historically recommended HS as a method of environmental management [8] to prevent the entry of disease-transmitting vectors into human habitations and to reduce human-vector-pathogen contact. Unfortunately, HS has been underutilised [4] and overlooked by policies & programs for the prevention and control of *Aedes*-transmitted diseases (ATDs), namely dengue, chikungunya, and Zika [9–12]. In 2017, HS was finally cited as a promising vector management approach for preventing and controlling dengue and ATDs in a research-to-policy forum convened by tropical disease research (TDR)/WHO [13–19].

HS on doors and windows, the most common entry points of mosquitoes into a house, works as a physical barrier that reduces the access and subsequent contact of humans with "hungry" female mosquitoes searching for blood within houses. We recently evaluated the efficacy of HS permanently fixed with aluminium frames to reduce *Ae. aegypti* mosquitoes and the risk of ATDs in a cluster randomised controlled trial in the Mexican city of Merida, Mexico [20–23]. Compared to unprotected households located in the control arm, houses with HS showed a lower risk (OR≈0.50) of finding indoor *Ae. aegypti* female mosquitoes. On the note, compared to those unprotected households, the presence of *Ae. aegypti* infected with dengue and Zika viruses was reduced in clusters with HS by 71%.

Although HS can be considered an effective and, more importantly, an "available" method to reduce mosquito contact with humans in the households of Merida, the cost of the house-installing of HS is high. Thus, no HS was installed prior to the intervention [22]. The current cost for the professional installation of HS by "aluminium & mosquito-screens" (A&MS) establishments in Merida with aluminium frames in an average house is ~$ 140 USD (two doors and 7 windows). Although the price per m^2 of a regular fibber-glass net used for HS is ~$ 0.85 USD, most of the cost for protecting a house with HS is due to the cost of frames and hardware (72.5% of the total cost) and hand labor (18% of the total cost) if installed by an A&MS professional.

Potential solutions to increase community access and make HS more affordable identified in a previous phase of implementation [22, 23] included introducing low-cost strategies such as the use of less-expensive materials rather than using the aluminium frames offered by A&MS companies and/or the commercialised Do-it-yourself (DIY) packages v.gr. ready-made and ready-to-instal mosquito screens with low-cost materials. Here we described some evidence of the use of inexpensive materials for the installation of HS as additional options used by households and/or small businesses in increasing HS affordability, HS efficacy and acceptance, and ultimately, HS access to the community.

2. Potential options for frame materials other than aluminium, prototype design and manufacturing

The study involved different research topics/components related to using different materials rather than aluminium to instal HS. First, our team searched, reviewed, and selected different materials to replace aluminium frames, then designed and constructed prototypes with those materials. Using Google and other shopping platforms such as Amazon, eBay, and Mercado Libre, from March to April 2019 we sought "mosquito screens", "insect screens", "window screens", and "door screens" in order to identify different potential models and materials that were different from aluminium. As the inclusion criteria, we considered availability in the market, less expensive than aluminium, and suitability for housing structures, such as the ability to keep mosquito nets fixed on doors and windows. After the online review, the team visited local suppliers to check for the availability of the materials in the local-regional-national market.

In the initial phase, we designed and built small-scale prototypes (1: 5 of a window and 1:10 of a door) and real-sized versions (average size of 2.20 × 0.95 m for doors and 1.20 × 0.80 m for windows found in houses from different neighbourhoods in Merida) (**Figure 1**). All materials required for installation including rivets, adhesives, screws, nails, fabric, locks, among others, along with some additional information such as handling, time for manufacturing per square meter, were identified, evaluated, and recorded, information later used to calculate the total costs based on the different options (**Table 1**, **Figure 1**). A regular fibber-glass net (brand Herralum®)

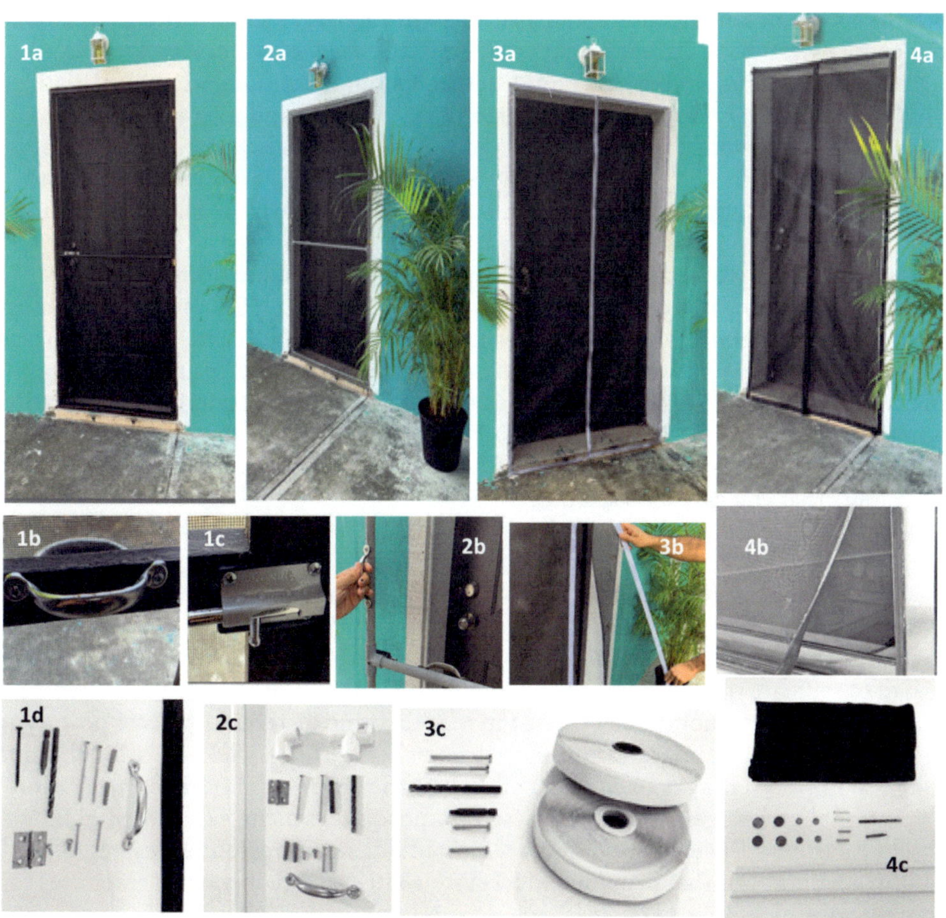

Figure 1.
Different options and materials for the installation of house screening other than aluminum: (1a–1d) wood, (2a–2c) polyvinyl chloride plastic (PVC), (3a–3c) velcro and (4a–4c) magnets.

Material	Materials	Costs in USD
Aluminum	28 pcs aluminum frame for windows, 5 pcs of aluminum for doors, 28 galvanized frame corners, 18 m of fiberglass net (1.50 m of width), 45m of spline #10, 15 screws round head $1^{1/2}$ × 8", 8 screws round head 1 × 8".	91.00
Wood	33 Wood strips (4 width × 1.8 thickness cm), 1 pc of glue, 18m fiberglass net, 8 wood screws, 25 staples.	43.00
PVC	33 PVC strips, 1 pc of glue, 18m fiberglass net, 6 PVC frame corners, 3 pcs silicone sealer.	39.00
Magnet	20 m of polyester cloth, 66 small magnets, 18m fiberglass net, 14 pcs of wooden rod, 3 pcs of thread? rows, 2 sewing needles	34.00
Velcro	33 velcro strips, 18m fiberglass net, 3 pcs row, 2 sewing needles	30.00

Table 1.
Costs associated with different materials that can be used for the construction of frames for house-screening. Costs for installing house-screening per house: including seven windows and two doors. Costs only consider materials and exclude cost of installation (1 USD = $23.00 MX PESOS).

with the following dimensions and features: 30 m length × 1.50 m width rolls, colour grey, mesh light 0.6 × .07 mm, density 0.32 mm was used to as blocking barrier.

To replace aluminium for HS frames, several potential options were identified as follows: wood, polyvinyl chloride plastic (PVC), Velcro, and magnets. All these materials can be installed in doors and windows and are less expensive than aluminium. In fact, magnets and Velcro were the less costly options, followed by PVC and wood. Additionally, these were available within local and national markets, and more importantly, easily accessible to the population.

Several options were identified for the installation of HS, including fixed (not mobile), retractable, and removable HS frames. Fixed insect HS screens are the most common insect screens, not mobile and held by a stable frame. Like fixed HS, retractable screens are also fixed, but they can be opened/closed with a "rolling" system. Finally, removable screens use adhesive or magnetic elements, contain a temporarily fitting system, and are usually an "easy DIY installation". All of these options are versatile and functional with an enriched market, including numerous accessories and colours that you can choose from.

3. Evaluation of prototypes in experimental huts

On March 2019, a trial following a 6 × 6 Latin-square experimental design was performed to evaluate the HS installation in experimental huts at the unidad colaborativa para bioensayos entomologicos (UCBE) in Merida using different low-cost prototype options vs. the gold standard (aluminium frames) (**Figure 2**). We quantified the entomological impact (entry or exclusion) of each of the different materials/installation as a physical barrier against female *Ae. aegypti* mosquitoes using experimental huts as testing systems. Experimental huts are simplified, standardised representations of human habitations that provide model systems to evaluate mosquito responses to different control methods [24, 25].

Mosquito screens (with regular fibber-glass net, brand Herralum®) with each of the different framing materials were made as real-sized doors (2.20 × 0.95 m) and fixed on an entrance located within the release tunnel of experimental huts (**Figure 2**).

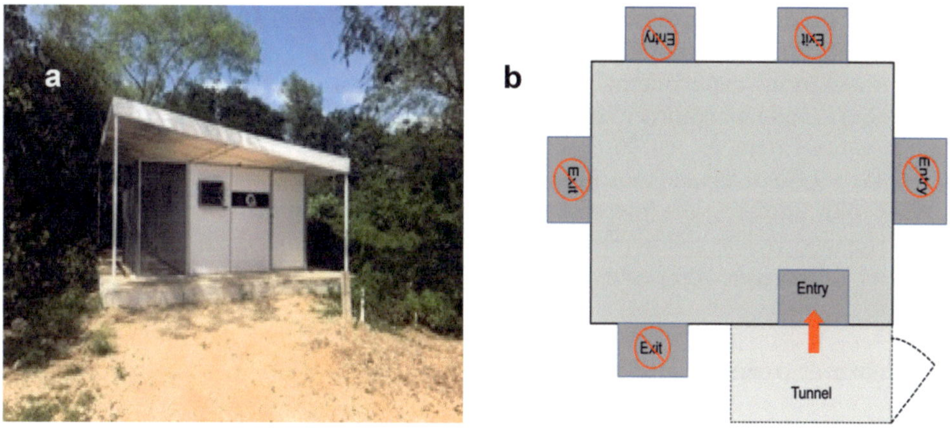

Figure 2.
(a and b) Experimental huts and (c–f) experimental layout of the different options and materials tested.

All the other entries-exits of the hut were sealed. The mosquito-door-screens of each material were fixed with its corresponding method of installation (**Figure 1**) and evaluated for a 24-hour period, and next day swapped of the hut until a total of six replicates were completed following the Latin-square experimental design. One of the huts was always left without protection as control.

Groups of 2–5 days-old and non-fed female *Ae. aegypti* mosquitoes (New Orleans F3 strain reared at UCBE) (n = 100), were released in the tunnel of the experimental huts in the morning (8:30 a.m) and collected 24 hours later. A BG-sentinel mosquito trap [26] with its bait (weight 1.7 kg, Dimension 38 × 47, ventilator 12 V dc 3.6 watt.) added with CO_2 (generation rate of 200 ml/min) [10, 27], was set inside the hut and active for collections for the whole 24-h period. In addition, the interior of the hut was revised, and any mosquito found was collected with Prokopack aspirators [10]. Mosquitoes that did not enter were collected (from the tunnel and outside the hut) with Prokopack aspirators. The collected mosquitoes were kept in a recovery bottle and then stored at −20°C for counting. Data was computed as the difference between initial mosquito abundance (adult) and the values at 24 hours post-release.

Frame material	Mean No. *Ae. aegypti* females entering after 24 h (95% C. I.)	% Protection (95% C. I.)	Incidence rate ratio (95% C. I.)	SE (mean)	P value
Aluminum	0.7 (0.4–1.7)	99.2 (97.9–100.5)	0.01 (0.003–0.02)	0.004	<0.001
Wood	1.7 (0.1–3.2)	97.9 (95.9–99.9)	0.02 (0.01–0.04)	0.01	<0.001
PVC	2 (0.7–3.3)	97.6 (96.0–99.2)	0.02 (0.01–0.04)	0.01	<0.001
Magnets	5.7 (2.6–8.7)	93.1 (89.6–96.7)	0.07 (0.05–0.10)	0.01	<0.001
Velcro	5.7 (2.6–8.8)	92.9 (88.9–97.0)	0.07 (0.05–0.10)	0.01	<0.001
Control	82.3 (77.9–86.7)	17.7	—		

Table 2.
Efficacy of protection (relative to the control treatment) against Aedes aegypti *(entry of mosquitoes) with frames constructed from different materials in the experimental huts. A total of 100 adult female* Ae. aegypti *mosquitoes were released into entry chamber in each treatment (n = 6 huts): Control, velcro, Magnet, PVC, Wood, and Aluminum.*

Table 2 presents the comparative results of the efficacy of frames constructed from different materials and their protection against *Ae. aegypti* (entry of female mosquitoes) in the experimental huts. All HS options had a high efficacy (>93%) in preventing female mosquitoes from passing inside the huts once compared with the control huts with no-screen. The aluminium-based HS showed the highest protection by blocking 99% of female mosquitos going inside the households (IRR = 0.01, C.I. 0.003–0.02); however, the low-cost options which cost is 60% lower than aluminium, also performed well as follow: magnets (Average protection = 93.1%, 95% CI = 89.6–96.7) and Velcro (Average protection = 92.9%, 95% CI = 88.9–97.0).

4. Consumer opinion and small company's perspective on HS prototypes

Here, to investigate people's perception of low-cost materials to replace aluminium frames, we applied a questionnaire (**Table 3**) to 55 families that had previously received the installation of HS with aluminium frames (July–August 2019) as part of the cohort project [22, 23]. In this survey, participants were asked about the distinct material options as if they would be hypothetically installed on their houses to replace aluminium frames. Questions included whether they have any previous knowledge or experience with the alternative materials/frames, perception of the cost of the materials, durability, aesthetics, the installation process, and their preferences (if any) for a specific type of frame. During this process, small-scale prototypes constructed were shown as well as the pictures of the real-sized prototypes installed in a house (**Figure 1**) to people, but no other explanation was given to avoid bias in answers.

A high percentage of the participants interviewed were women (76.36%, 42/55) with ages ranging between 30 and 50 years old (54/55); all of them were married and heads of families from houses that had received the HS installation previously as part of the cohort project. Frames made of wood (62%, 34/55) were the most "popular" alternative among the participants, followed by magnets (45%, 25/55), PVC (45%, 25/55), and Velcro (29%, 16/55). People acknowledged the existence of wood frames, but the other materials v.gr. PVC, Velcro, and magnets were "uncommon" to them; although some participants recalled having seen the other options on the Internet, magazines, or TV programs. Regarding the cost, 45–60% of participants believed that the prices of the four different frames were between 5 and 50 USD, and they thought Velcro and magnets were expensive. The expected durability of the materials was associated with weather conditions, but most participants thought that all materials were highly resistant (which could last 1–5 years). On the aesthetics, which is the perception of "how beautiful" the frames can be seen on the houses, the wood option got the best scores (73%, 40/55), followed by magnets (56%, 31/55). More than 50% of the interview participants thought all the options were easy to instal; however, many of them disagreed on how easy to maintain them. All materials were seen as an acceptable positive improvement of the house except for PVC.

We also investigated the perspective of A&MS businesses on the prototypes/materials (November–December 2020). To do so, A&MS companies located in Merida, Yucatan were identified (n = 100) by searching on Yellow pages. Because of COVID-19 pandemic, person-to-person contact was avoided, so telephone calls were used to reach them. Forty companies dedicated to the assemblage of HS in the city of Merida were surveyed (**Table 4**). Participants were asked about costs, durability, aesthetics,

Previous knowledge/experience with alternative materials for HS				
Responses	**Wood**	**PVC**	**Velcro**	**Magnets**
Yes	(39/55) 71%	(7/55) 13%	(5/55) 9%	(1/55) 2%
No	(16/55) 29%	(47/55) 85%	(50/55) 91%	(54/55) 98%
Do not know	0%	(1/55) 2%	0%	0%
Cost perceived				
5–50 USD	(25/55) 45%	(28/55) 51%	(33/55) 60%	(28/55) 51%
50–100 USD	(19/55) 35%	(26/55) 29%	(12/55) 22%	(12/55) 22%
Up to 100 USD	(5/55) 9%	(2/55) 4%	(1/55) 2%	(5/55) 9%
Do not know	(6/55) 11%	(9/55) 16%	(9/55) 16%	(19/55) 18%
Expectation of durability				
Less than a year	(3/55) 5%	(6/55) 11%	(11/55) 20%	(1/55) 2%
1–2 years	(22/55) 40%	(16/55) 29%	(20/55) 36%	(17/55) 31%
2–5 years	(18/55) 33%	(21/55) 38%	(22/55) 40%	(20/55) 36%
More than 5 years	12/55) 22%	(12/55) 22%	0%	(7/55) 13%
Do not know	0%	0%	(2/55) 4%	(10/55) 18%
Aesthetics				
Yes	(40/55) 73%	(15/55) 27%	(23/55) 42%	(31/55) 56%
No	(15/55) 27%	(35/55) 64%	(28/55) 51%	(21/55) 38%
Do not know	0%	(5/55) 9%	(4/55) 7%	(3/55) 5%
Easy to install				
Yes	(37/55) 67%	(29/55) 53%	(36/55) 65%	(36/55) 65%
No	(15/55) 27%	(14/55) 25%	(10/55) 18%	(9/55) 16%
Don't know	(3/55) 5%	(12/55) 22%	(9/55) 16%	(10/55) 18%
Easy maintenance				
Yes	(27/55) 49%	(21/55)38%	(29/55) 53%	(25/55) 45%
No	(23/55) 42%	(22/55) 40%	(15/55) 27%	(17/55) 31%
Do not know	(5/55) 9%	(12/55) 22%	(11/55) 20%	(13/55) 24%
Preferences and acceptance				
Yes	(34/55) 62%	(25/55) 45%	(16/55) 29%	(25/55) 45%
No	(12/55) 22%	(20/55) 36%	(28/55) 51%	(21/55) 38%
Do not know	(9/55) 16%	(10/55) 18%	(11/55) 20%	(9/55) 16%

Table 3.
Results recorded from householders about alternative frame materials other than aluminum for the installation of house-screening in Merida, Mexico.

perceived comfort, acceptance, and an open section on the customer preferences from entrepreneurs' perspectives, and the production-manufacturing process of the HS (**Table 4**). Small-scale prototypes and a photographic catalog of the different prototypes (**Figure 1**) were also employed.

	Aluminum	Wood	PCV	Velcro	Magnets
Material preferred (N = 31)	96.77% (30/31)	3.23% (1/31)	0% (0/31)	0% (0/31)	0% (0/31)
Material most requested by consumers (N = 31)	100% (30/31)	43.3% (13/31)	10% (3/31)	0% (0/31)	0% (0/31)
Perceived cost (N = 40)	Expensive (97.5%, 39/40)	Cheap (7.5%, 3/40)	Cheap (12.5%, 5/40)	Cheap (52.5%, 21/40)	Cheap (57.5%, 23/40)
Duration of materials perceived/expected (N = 40)	8.5 years	21.85 months	21.24 months	8.44 months	9.56 months
Opinion but aesthetic (N = 40)	NA	57.5% (23/40)	20% (8/40)	12.5% (5/40)	47.5% (19/40)
Easy to manufacture	NA	96% (26/27)	92% (23/25)	100% (23/23)	100% (25/25)
Easy to maintain	NA	89% (24/27)	96% (23/24)	100% (19/19)	95% (20/21)

Table 4.
Perspectives of professional small companies dedicated to the installation of house-screening about potential low-cost alternatives to replace aluminum frames.

We identified "producers", those who manufacture and instal HS, and "distributors" who only sell materials for HS. Fifty-five percent of (22/40) the companies declared to be in the formal sector and the remaining 45% (18/40) were informal. Of those in the formal sector, 59.09% (13/22) were producers, the remaining 40.90% (9/22) were distributors, and the informal ones were only producers. Only one producer (1/31) made mosquito nets with one of the alternative materials (wood).

The interviewed producers declared that the alternative material most requested by consumers after aluminium was wood (41.93% [13/31]) (**Table 4**) and that few of them had received requests for PVC (9.67% [3/31]); and recalled that customers had never requested them for Velcro or magnets. Respondents considered aluminium to be an expensive material (97.5% [39/40]); despite not working with alternative materials, some considered wood and PVC were cheaper (7.5% [3/40], 12.5% [5/40], respectively), and considered that Velcro and magnets were the less expensive options (52.5% [21/40], 57.5% [23/40]) (**Table 4**). Regarding the duration of the alternative materials, they expected an average extent of 21.9 months for wood, 21.2 months for PVC, 8.4 months for Velcro, and 9.6 months for magnets (**Table 4**). Wood and magnets (57.5% [23/40], 47.5% [19/40]) were considered the most aesthetical alternative materials for the elaboration of HS (**Table 4**). Regarding whether alternative materials are easy to manufacture and maintain, many of the interviewees could not answer because they do not know enough about the material to give a real opinion (**Table 4**). However, those who responded considered that the alternative materials were easy to manufacture and maintain.

Although alternative materials are considered cheaper, aesthetic, easy to maintain and instal by A&MS small companies, they declared not willing to use this type of materials and rejected the use of Velcro (97.5% [39/40]), PVC (90% ([36/40]), magnets (82.5% [33/40]) and wood (77.5% [31/40]). Nevertheless, they acknowledged that consumers could request these materials, with wood being the material with the highest potential to be requested (43.1%), followed by PVC and magnets (22.5%) and finally Velcro (14.4%).

5. Conclusions

In this study, we examined the efficacy of low-cost frames built using different materials (e.g. wood, PVC, Velcro) to protect against *Ae. aegypti* getting inside experimental huts. All HS frame prototypes described here were highly effective in blocking the entry of *Ae. aegypti* mosquitoes (>93%), and even without "total" protection, entry was lower compared to no netting. Of note, all the prototype frames of HS made of different materials rather than aluminium, were low-priced. For instance, HS made with magnets and Velcro performed very well against mosquitoes and had a 54–68% lower cost than aluminium. Thus, it was estimated that protecting a house (with seven windows and two doors) using these no-aluminium materials costs about US$35 [22].

Additionally, we investigated people's perceptions of using different materials to build HS. The most "popular" and more commonly used alternative was the wooden-made frame (62%) compared to magnets, Velcro, and PVC-based frames; this latter was considered the "least popular" material as it was not considered a positive improvement to the houses. To mention, aluminium is usually associated with quality and aesthetics, as well as an improvement of the home, which poses an enormous burden on using low-cost materials as these must be aesthetically accepted by the community to be perceived as an improvement in the quality of their housing and living conditions. On top of this, little or no information on the characteristics, effectiveness, cost, and availability of the different materials used to build HS rather than aluminium are available; therefore, this latter is considered the only option to build HS, limiting people's perspective on installing not-aluminium-based HS in their houses, instead leaving them unprotected.

During the interviews, people learned about these low-cost options through demonstration prototypes and expressed their doubts; expanding their options to request from A&MS or to assemble and instal themselves in their homes. Small A&MS businesses, being more accessible, provide an important service to the population, especially the low-income population. Therefore, producers and consumers need information and alternatives to evaluate. Thanks to the companies surveyed, we know that they tend to produce 30 units of aluminium mosquito nets (for one window) per month, costing on average USD 14.83 each and with an approximate profit of 40%. It will last almost 10 years and the professional service, if any, is only to change the broken/damaged ones. It would be useful to show the benefits of all the different alternatives for established producers; for example, Velcro and magnets are the materials with the highest benefits, derived mainly from the short lifetime, which increases the frequency of purchases. However, they are also easy for users to instal themselves at home.

Overall, these results support the possibility of using alternative, accessible, and less expensive materials such as wood, PVC, Velcro, and magnets, instead of aluminium-based HS to protect people's houses against *Ae. aegypti* invasion inside households. This study changes the paradigm between the A&MS seeking to maximise their profit and the consumers seeking cheaper costs. According to the A&MS, the quality and durability of aluminium are unmatched, and they do not have the "social benefit" of consumers as a policy. Low-income people are constrained by the cost of conventional house screens and the labor involved; unaware of alternative models, their households lack protection against *Ae. aegypti*. Therefore, this study suggests strategies involving the government, the private sector, and academia for disseminating and accessing these low-cost alternative materials, either through micro-credits, vouchers for people at risk (e.g., pregnant women), or partial or monthly payments.

Author details

Josué Herrera-Bojórquez[1], Josué Villegas-Chim[1]*, Daniel Adrian[1], Azael Che-Mendoza[1], Juan Navarrete-Carballo[1], Anuar Medina-Barreiro[1], Miguel Xcaer[1], Hugo Delfín-González[1], Norma Pavía-Ruz[2], Henry Puerta-Guardo[1,2], María Eugenia Toledo-Romaní[3], Héctor Gómez-Dantés[4], Gonzalo Vazquez-Prokopec[5] and Pablo Manrique-Saide[1]

1 Autonomous University of Yucatan, Merida, Mexico

2 Regional Research Center "Dr. Hideyo Noguchi", Autonomous University of Yucatan, Merida, Mexico

3 Institute of Tropical Medicine "Pedro Kourí" (IPK), Habana, Cuba

4 National Institute of Public Health, Cuernavaca, Mexico

5 Department of Environmental Sciences, Emory University, Atlanta, USA

*Address all correspondence to: jovich.etnos@gmail.com

References

[1] WHO, editor. Keeping the Vector Out - Housing Improvements for Vector Control and Sustainable Development. Geneva: WHO, editor; 2017

[2] WHO. Global Strategy for Dengue Prevention and Control 2012-2020. Geneva: World Health Organisation; 2012

[3] WHO. Inception meeting for the pilot-study project on sustainable management of long-lasting insecticidal nets throughout their life-cycle. 2011. Available from: http://www.who.int/malaria/publications/atoz/who_htm_gmp_2011_1/en/index.html. [Accessed: 12 October 2011]

[4] Lindsay S, Wilson A, Golding N, Scott TW, Takken W. Improving the built environment in urban areas to control *Aedes aegypti*-borne diseases. Bulletin of the World Health Organization. 2017;**95**:607-608

[5] Tusting LS, Willey B, Lines J. Building malaria out: Improving health in the home. Malaria Journal. 2016;**15**:320. DOI: 10.1186/s12936-016-1349-8

[6] Vazquez-Prokopec G, Lenhart A, Manrique-Saide P. Housing improvement: A renewed paradigm for urban vector-borne disease control? Transactions of the Royal Society of Tropical Medicine and Hygiene. 2016;**110**(10):567-569

[7] Wilson AL, Courtenay O, Kelly-Hope LA, Scott TW, Takken W, Torr SJ, et al. The importance of vector control for the control and elimination of vector-borne diseases. PLoS Neglected Tropical Diseases. 2020;**14**(1):e0007831

[8] WHO. Manual on Environmental Management for Mosquito Control. Geneva: WHO; 1982

[9] Dekker T, Geier M, Cardé RT. Carbon dioxide instantly sensi- tizes female yellow fever mosquitoes to human skin odours. The Journal of Experimental Biology. 2005;**208**:2963-2972

[10] Vazquez-Prokopec GM, Galvin WA, Kelly R, Kitron U. A new, cost-effective, battery-powered aspirator for adult mosquito collections. Journal of Medical Entomology. 2009;**46**(6):1256-1259

[11] WHO. Handbook for Integrated Vector Management. World Health Organisation 2012. ISBN 9789241502801. Available from: http://apps.who.int/iris/bitstream/10665/44768/1/9789241502801_eng.pdf

[12] WHO. Dengue Guidelines for Diagnosis, Treatment, Prevention and Control: New Edition. Geneva: World Health Organisation; 2009. Available from: http://www.who.int/iris/handle/10665/44188

[13] Bowman LR, Donegan S, McCall PJ. Is dengue vector control deficient in effectiveness or evidence?: Systematic review and meta-analysis. PLoS Neglected Tropical Diseases. 2016;**10**(3):e0004551

[14] Che-Mendoza A, Guillermo-May G, Herrera-Bojórquez J, Barrera-Pérez M, Dzul-Manzanilla F, Gutierrez-Castro C, et al. Long-lasting insecticide treated house screens and targeted treatment of productive breeding-sites for dengue vector control in Acapulco, Mexico. Transactions of the Royal Society of Tropical Medicine and Hygiene. 2015;**109**(2):106-115

[15] Grietens KP, Muela RJ, Soto V, Tenorio A, Hoibak S, Rosas AA, et al. Traditional nets interfere with the uptake of long-lasting insecticidal nets in the Peruvian Amazon: The relevance of net

preference for achieving high coverage and use. PLoS One. 2013;**8**(1):e50294

[16] Herrera-Bojórquez J, Trujillo-Peña E, Vadillo Sánchez J, Riestra-Morales M, Che-Mendoza A, Delfín-González H, et al. Efficacy of long-lasting insecticidal nets with declining physical and chemical integrity on *Aedes aegypti*. Journal of Medical Entomology. 2020;**57**(2):503-510

[17] Jones C, Benítez-Valladares D, Barrera-Pérez M, Selem-Salas C, Chablé-Santos J, Dzul-Manzanilla F, et al. Use and acceptance of long-lasting insecticidal nets for dengue prevention in Acapulco, Guerrero, Mexico. BMC Public Health. 2014;**14**(1):846

[18] Olliaro P, Fouque F, Kroeger A, Bowman L, Velayudhan R, Santelli AC, et al. Improved tools and strategies for the prevention and control of arboviral diseases: A research-to-policy forum. PLoS Neglected Tropical Diseases. 2018;**12**(2):e0005967

[19] Quintero J, Brochero H, Manrique-Saide P, Barrera-Perez M, Basso C, Romero S, et al. Ecological, biological and social dimensions of dengue vector breeding in five urban settings of Latin America: A multi-country study. BMC Infectious Diseases. 2014;**14**:38

[20] Che-Mendoza A, Medina-Barreiro A, Koyoc-Cardeña E, Uc-Puc V, Contreras-Perera Y, Herrera-Bojórquez J, et al. House screening with insecticide-treated netting provides sustained reductions in domestic populations of *Aedes aegypti* in Merida, Mexico. PLoS Neglected Tropical Diseases. 2018;**12**(3):e0006283

[21] Manrique-Saide P, Che-Mendoza A, Barrera-Pérez M, Guillermo-May G, Herrera Bojorquez J, Dzul-Manzanilla F, et al. Use of insecticide-treated house screens to reduce infestations of dengue virus vectors, Mexico. Emerging Infectious Diseases. 2015;**21**(2):308-311

[22] Manrique-Saide P, Herrera-Bojórquez J, Medina-Barreiro A, Trujillo-Peña E, Villegas-Chim J, Valadez-González N, et al. Insecticide-treated house screening protects against Zika-infected *Aedes aegypti* in Merida Mexico. PLoS Neglected Tropical Diseases. 2021;**15**(1):e0009005. DOI: 10.1371/journal.pntd.0009005

[23] Manrique-Saide P, Herrera-Bojórquez J, Villegas-Chim J, Puerta-Guardado H, Ayora-Talavera G, Parra-Cardeña M, et al. Protective effect of house screening against indoor *Aedes aegypti* in Mérida, Mexico: A cluster randomised controlled trial. Tropical Medicine & International Health. 2021;**26**:1677-1688

[24] Massue DJ, Kisinza WN, Malongo BB, Mgaya CS, Bradley J, Moore JD, et al. Comparative performance of three experimental hut designs for measuring malaria vector responses to insecticides in Tanzania. Malaria Journal. 2016;**15**:165

[25] Okumu FO, Moore J, Mbeyela E, Sherlock M, Sangusangu R, Ligamba G, et al. A modified experimental hut design for studying responses of disease-transmitting mosquitoes to indoor interventions: The Ifakara experimental huts. PLoS One. 2012;**7**(2):e30967

[26] Biogents. Instrucción manual for Bg- sentinel2. Regenburg, Germany: Biogents AG. 2017. Available from: https://eu.biogents.com/wp-content/uploads/BG-Sentinel-2-Manual-EN-web.pdf

[27] Tessa MV, Marieke PC, Helene H, Merril W, Neil OV, JMK C. Optimisation and field validation of odour-baited traps for surveillance of *Aedes aegypti* adults in Paramaribo, Suriname. Parasites & Vectors. 2020;**13**:121

Chapter 11

Effect of the Mass Distribution of ITNs in an Endemic Area with a High Entomological Index, the Case of Bandundu-City, Kwilu, DRC

Emery Metelo-Matubi, Josue Zanga, Victoire Nsabatien, Aimé Mbala, Solange Ngamukie, Fiacre Agossa, El Hadji Amadou Niang, Jean Maniania-Nguya-Kalenga and Mulenda Basimike

Abstract

The bio-efficacy of Yorkol-branded ITNs collected from Bandundu-city was assessed on the Kisumu strain and wild specimens of *Anopheles gambiae*. The susceptibility of the wild *An. gambiae s.l.* was tested to select insecticides. Adult *An. gambiae s.l.* sampled by PSC and HLC were screened for the presence of *Plasmodium falciparum*. Blood samples were diagnosed by microscopy and RDTs. ITN distributed in Bandundu-city were fully effective on the Kisumu strain, but on wild *An. gambiae s.l.* population (22.3 ± 11.5%). *Anopheles gambiae s.l.* was the main vector in Bandundu. No significant difference was observed between the entomological indices before and after the deployment of nets (OR = 0.8; p = 0.39). Wild *An. gambiae s.l.* populations were resistant to pyrethroids and DDT, with the restoration of the susceptibility to pyrethroids post pre-exposure to PBO. *Plasmodium falciparum* was the main parasite species and was found alone or mixed with. *P. malariae* or *P. ovale*. The confirmation rates by microscopy and RDT were respectively 57.9% and 53.6%. Nets deployed in Bandundu-city were not effective on wild *An. gambiae s.l.* populations. This operational failure is likely explained by the observed resistance to pyrethroids. In the future only PBO-net should be deployed Bandundu-city.

Keywords: *Anopheles gambiae* s.l, ITN, entomological indices, Bandundu-city, DRC

1. Introduction

Anopheles gambiae s.l. is a primary vector of *Plasmodium falciparum* across sub-Saharan African countries causing malaria that continues to be a leading cause of morbidity and mortality across the continent [1]. Malaria is the world's number one parasitic disease, threatening more than 1 billion people [2]. According to the World Health Organisation (WHO), 241 million cases and 62,700 deaths due to malaria were reported in 2020 [3]. Of these cases, 95% occur in sub-Saharan Africa. Globally, nearly 95% of deaths were recorded in 31 countries, of which 3 in Africa accounted for nearly 39% (Nigeria 23%; DRC 11%, Tanzania 5% [2]. More than 200 million cases of malaria are recorded annually in DRC [3]. This high prevalence of malaria reflects a situation of poverty and inadequate health services [4–6]. Moreover, malaria itself and its consequences contribute to keeping populations in a state of poverty. Malaria costs sub-Saharan African countries more than US$ 12 billion each year through lost income, foreign investment and tourism resources [4–6]. International agencies (WHO, UNDP, UNICEF and the World Bank) launched the Roll Back Malaria (RBM) programme, which set out to combat malaria with the aim of reducing malaria mortality by 50% in 2010, 30% in 2015 and 20% in 2025. In its technical strategy for malaria control, WHO has set the goal of eliminating malaria by 2030 [7]. Thus, by the year 2030, malaria should cease to be a major cause of morbidity, mortality, and socio-economic loss [8].

To achieve its objectives, the DRC has developed malaria control strategies based on preventive measures centred on targeted chemoprophylaxis offered to high-risk or vulnerable populations such as infants, pregnant women and migrants; early case management, which implies diagnosis and rapid recourse to appropriate care; and finally, vector control which must remain accessible to malaria-endemic populations [9]. Regarding preventive measures, the WHO gives an important place to vector control. To respond favourably to both international and national strategies, approaches and recommendations aimed at eliminating malaria, the DRC has been committed for at least 7 years through the NMCP and its partners to scale up high-impact malaria control interventions [10]. These interventions include universal distribution of ITNs, chemoprevention of malaria in pregnant women, administration of artemisinin-based combination therapies (ACTs) and strengthening of epidemiological surveillance [11, 12].

Following the evaluation of malaria control interventions, with reference to the implementation framework of the Global Technical Strategy for Malaria Control 2016–2030 in the African Region, WHO has launched the High Burden High Impact (HBHI) approach [13, 14] aiming to reduce malaria morbidity and mortality in countries with a high burden of malaria, including the DRC. It is based on four main pillars: i) political will in favour of the fight against malaria, ii) strategic information that can increase the impact of malaria tenfold, iii) improved support for policies and strategies and iv) coordination of the national response [13, 14].

The significant progress made in malaria control over the past decade in endemic countries is largely attributable to the mass coverage of insecticide-based vector control interventions, such as long-lasting insecticidal nets (ITNs) and indoor residual spraying (IRS) [7, 13, 14].

Long-lasting insecticidal nets are one of the main malaria control tools recommended by WHO and adopted by DRC NMCP through mass and routine distributions channels [15, 16]. Several field studies have demonstrated the effectiveness of its large-scale use [15, 16] showing they can reduce morbidity by 50% and overall mortality by 20–30% in children under 5 years of age [10, 16, 17].

Based on these observations, the promotion of ITNs among the population is an essential component of the NMCP in DRC. Several studies have shown that the combined action of insecticides and the physical barrier is an effective means of controlling malaria vectors [15–17]. Nevertheless, the disease remains endemic in the country, with a worrying prevalence of 32%, despite this large-scale promotion [3, 10]. Counteracting the effectiveness of ITNs are two major handicaps: the increasingly widespread mosquito resistance to pyrethroids used for impregnation of ITNs; and the low recorded durability of ITNs compared to the expected duration of 3 years [10, 13]. The number of *Anopheles* species resistance to insecticides has increased and affects nearly two-thirds of the countries where transmission persists. Resistance to pyrethroids in *An. gambiae* s.l. was first observed in Côte d'Ivoire in followed by other West African countries (Benin and Burkina Faso) and first reported in the DRC in 2012 [12, 18]. Pyrethroid resistance in *An. gambiae* has now been reported in all the DRC NMCP's sentinel sites, where it has the potential to cause the operational failure of the vector control tools put in place by the malaria control programmes [12, 18].

The DRC, like all the countries of sub-Saharan Africa, pays a heavy price for malaria. However, its geographical location and the diversity of its climates make it unique among its neighbours [2, 10, 19]. Spread over an area of approximately 2,345,000 km^2, this country has almost all the epidemiological facies found in Africa, from the Sahelian savannahs to the equatorial forests [10, 19, 20]. Moreover, 97% of the population lives in the stable malaria zones characterised by the equatorial and tropical facies [13, 14]. Three plasmodial species are present (*Plasmodium falciparium* (*P.f*) 95%, *Plasmodium ovale* (*P.o*) and *Plasmodium malariae* (*P.m*)). Currently, *Plasmodium vivax* infections are present in some areas of the country, but in very small numbers [9, 19, 20]. The most common vectors in the DRC are *An. gambiae*, 92%, *An. funestus*, *An. nili*, *An. moucheti* and *An. paludis* [9, 21, 22]. These *Anopheles* can have highly variable vectorial capacities and behaviours [23, 24].

However, this heterogeneity does not allow us to understand malaria in the DRC in its entirety. Knowledge of the different Congolese geographical areas (territories, districts, etc.) and the description of the local epidemiology of malaria in these different environments are initial conditions for a good understanding of the malaria endemicity in this country [13, 14, 18].

Work carried out in a few sites in the DRC, such as Kingasani, Bolenge, Kimpese and Katana by Watsenga and collaborators, has shown that pyrethroid resistance was associated with the presence of the kdr mutation [25]. However, the problem of *Anopheles* resistance to insecticides seems to be growing in the DRC, according to the PMI entomological surveillance report and the DRC Malaria Control Strategic Plan 2013–2015 [26, 27]. Therefore, it is not only necessary to regularly monitor the susceptibility of vectors to these insecticides and to understand the mechanisms of this resistance, but also to consider the actual impact of this resistance on vector control [27, 28].

Our study focused on Kwilu province (ex-Bandundu) where the prevalence of malaria was 18%, sporozoite index 5.6%. *A. gambiae* s.l. is the major malaria vector with 8.86 anopheles per house, 1.55 bites per man per night and entomological stability index 6.512 [29]. On this basis, it was necessary to assess and determine the response of *An. gambiae* s.l. to insecticides and test the hypothesis that the selection of a resistance gene in malaria vectors is associated with the widespread use of insecticides [12, 15].

The aim of this study was to examine the status of *An. gambiae* s.l. resistance to pyrethroids and to determine the mechanism of this resistance in several locations in Kwilu province, once the country's agricultural heartland where different farming systems were used [2, 30, 31]. In addition, this province has long been the focus of vector control interventions through the distribution of ITNs [32]. The results from this study will serve as a basis for decision-makers to properly orientate resistance management policy in the DRC particularly considering the recrudescence and outbreak of malaria cases noted in 2019, and the lack of documentation of *Anopheles* resistance in this part of the country.

2. Effect of the mass distribution of ITNs in an endemic area with a high entomological index, the case of Bandundu-city, Kwilu, DRC

2.1 Methodology

2.1.1 Study site

The town of Bandundu was once considered a city in the territory of Bagata, before it was made the capital of the province. It is located between 17°22′43″E longitude, 3°21′05"S latitude and at an altitude of 324 m to the West. This area is bounded to the north by the NIOKI health zone, to the south by the Nkutu health zone in the province of Maï-Ndombe, to the east by the Bagata health zone and to the west by the Kwamouth health zone (province of Maï-Ndombe). It is located 432 km from Kikwit, 200 km from Kenge and 400 km from Kinshasa, the capital of the DRC [19, 20]. Kwilu province is located in a low altitude climate, characterised by a humid tropical climate, constant heat throughout the year and two well-marked seasons. The rainy season is characterised by heavy rainfall, and the dry season lasts 4 months and rainfall drops to zero [23, 24]. The average annual temperature is 26.9°C, annual rainfall ranges from 800 to 1500 mm and the average annual humidity is 77% [24].

Bandundu city experiences a humid tropical climate with two well-marked seasons: a long rainy season and a short (4-month) dry season, as shown [23, 24]. A short dry period is often noted in January-February, followed by a short rainy period in March-April. Climatological data obtained from the meteorological department of Bandundu-City (METELSAT/BDD). The mass distribution campaign of ITNs (Yorkol) was carried out between 17 and 29 December 2018.

The Town has developed in order to promote Pisco-agricultural activities (ponds, flowerbeds, etc.). The plots constitute the traditional dwelling unit for a family with one or more houses with dry earth walls and roofs usually made of corrugated iron and/or straw. Such dwellings are permeable to mosquito ingress and egress. Cattle, sheep, goats, pigs and poultry are well represented. All of these animals roam and spend the night in the plots. These eco-climatic conditions are favourable to the development of Anopheles vectors of malaria and the multiplication of breeding sites [24–32, 33]. Its surface area is 291 km^2 with approximately 285,411 inhabitants, i.e. a population density of 980.79 inhabitants/Km^2 sites [19, 20, 33].

2.1.2 Data collection

ITNs distributed in Bandundu-city in December 2018 were collected to evaluate their effectiveness with *An. gambiae* s.l. strain Kisumu reared in the insectarium of the Bioecology laboratory of the School of Public Health (BIOLAV/ESP) and wild strains collected in the different sites of Bandundu. The WHO sensitivity test was carried out on collected *An. gambiae* specimens and blood samples taken from the inhabitants of the households for the preparation of thick drops and thin smears in search of plasmodium parasites. Mosquitoes were also captured by morning house spraying with pyrethrum (PSC) and human bait (HLC).

a. Bio-efficacy of ITNs

All ITNs were carefully inspected for physical integrity, date of manufacture and batch number. The ITNs were coded according to the order of analysis: Y1, Y2, Y3... Y30. Five 30 x 30 cm samples were taken from each ITN: a sample from the short side at the bottom (C1), a sample from the long side at 30 cm from the bottom edge (L1), a sample from the short side at 60 cm from the bottom edge (C2), a sample from the long side at its top edge (L2) and a sample from the roof (T). Individual samples were wrapped in aluminium foil and placed inside plastic bags to avoid possible cross-contamination between sub-samples [15].

Five female *An. gambiae* s.l., not gorged from 2 to 5 days old, were collected using the mouth aspirator and introduced into each cone. After 3 minutes, the mosquitoes were sucked out of the cones with a mouth glass aspirator and moved to the disposable cups covered with the net, fitted with cotton wool soaked in 10% glucose solution according to the sample code ITN. Each subsample was tested once, giving a total of 20 mosquitoes tested per subsample, or 100 mosquitoes tested per ITN. The behaviour of the tested mosquitoes was observed for 1 hour. The number of mosquitoes shocked after 3′, 5′, 10′, 15′, 20′, 25′, 30′, 35′, 40′, 45′, 50′, 55′ and 60′ of observation was recorded to calculate the percentage of mosquitoes shocked after 60 minutes of observation, the Kdt50 and Kdt95, which represent the times after which 50% and 95% of mosquitoes were stunned, respectively. The final mortality rate was determined at 24 hours post-exposure [34, 35]. These tests were conducted at room temperature and relative humidity of 25–27°C and 78–80%, respectively. Cone bioassays were also conducted on the *An. gambiae* s.l. population of the Kisumu strain maintained at the BIO-LAV laboratory. Cone bioassays were also conducted with control mosquitoes that were exposed to non-insecticide-impregnated tissue as a control for the test.

The test results were deliberated according to WHO criteria [36]. An ITN is considered effective if it results in a Kd rate of 95% or greater and/or a mortality rate of 80% or greater [36].

b. Susceptibility testing

Larvae and pupae of *A. gambiae* s.l. were collected at different sites identified in each study site (Bandundu-city). The collected specimens were kept in tanks containing water in CDC cages and reared in the laboratory.

The larvae were fed daily with fish food at a rate of 4 g per day per tank. The temperature and humidity of the laboratory were taken daily by thermo-hygrometer. Pupae were harvested daily and placed in CDC/Atlanta cages and adults were fed with 10% glucose solution [36].

Females aged 2–5 days were selected and tested for susceptibility according to the WHO protocol [36]. The tests were carried out with insecticide-impregnated papers, WHO Kit composed of 4 types of insecticides and the synergist PBO in the following concentrations: Deltamethrin 0.05%, Permethrin 0.75%, Bendiocarb 0.1%, DDT 4% and PBO 5% [36].

The first susceptibility test was performed only for the 4 insecticides. The behaviour of *An. gambiae* s.l. subjected to the insecticide was observed for 60 minutes. The second test was carried out with anopheles pre-exposed to PBO for 60 minutes and then tested with insecticides [36–38]. PBO was used only for pyrethroids

(Deltamethrin and Permethrin), because of its action on the cytochrome P450 mono-oxygenase, which plays an important role in the resistance of anopheles to its insecticides [36, 38]. These two pyrethroid insecticides are authorised for use in the impregnation of mosquito nets used in DR Congo [31, 35].

The behaviour of *An. gambiae* s.l. in contact with insecticides was observed for 1 hour; the number of *An. gambiae* s.l. shocked at each, 3′ 5′ 10′ 15′ 20′ 25′ 30′ 35′ 40′ 45′ 50′55′ and 60′ contact with the insecticide was recorded 20–25 *An. gambiae* s.l were used per trial (replication), in total 4 trials were conducted and one control by each type of insecticide following the WHO protocol [36, 37]. This contact time was used to calculate the knockdown time (KDT) and mortality of *An. gambiae* s.l. observed 24 hours later [36]. The KDT has two components, KDT_{50} and KDT_{95} represent the knockdown times after which 50% and 95% of *An. gambiae* s.l are stunned. The two KDTs were determined according to the type of insecticide [28, 36]. The tests were carried out under conditions of temperature ranging from 25 to 27°C and relative humidity from 78 to 80%. The mortality observed 24 hours after contact time, according to WHO, is used to elaborate the criteria for deliberation of susceptibility test results; Susceptible (S), all *An. gambiae* s.l. with a mortality of 98–100% 24 hours after contact with insecticides; Resistant (R) if the mortality of *An. gambiae* s.l. is less than 90%; Probable Resistant (PR), if the mortality of *An. gambiae* s.l. is between 90 and 97% [36].

c. Mosquito collection

A total of 108 houses were visited during the study from 15 July 2018 to 15 June 2019. All sampled houses had mud walls and had tin or thatched roofs. Each month, nine houses were selected at random for mosquito sampling, with different houses selected for each monthly sampling event. Adult mosquitoes were collected between 06:00 and 10:00 am using pyrethrum spray catches [39, 40]. All openings of the house were closed and white sheets were laid on the floor. A commercially available pyrethroid spray (Baygon, Bayer) was sprayed in the house and doors were closed for 15 minutes. The sheets were carefully removed from the house and inspected for mosquitoes, which were collected and placed individually into labelled tubes [39, 40].

Human landing catches (HLCs) were done primarily to determine malaria vector species composition, the location of biting (indoors or outdoors) and times of biting. Mosquitoes were collected monthly from nine houses by two volunteers in six-hour shifts, from 18:00 h to 0:00 h and from 0:00 h to 6:00 h. Two collectors were posted inside the house in the living room and two outside the house, less than five meters from the front door. Different houses were used for each night. Each collector sat on a stool with his lower legs and feet exposed for mosquitoes to land on. The collector monitored mosquitoes as they landed and captured them with small glass tubes that were sealed with cotton wool. The latter were then placed in a sealed bag and labelled according to the hour of collection. These data were used to calculate the nightly human biting rate (HBR) based on eight person-nights of collection indoors and outdoors for each sampling period. The mosquito collectors for HLCs were recruited from the community and provided with requisite training. Collectors showing any signs of illness up to 3 weeks following collections were screened for malaria at a local health centre. There were no positive cases.

A. gambiae s.l. mosquito larvae were collected from breeding sites and transferred to pans containing water from the site and were reared until adult stage in a field insectary. Larvae were not fed and survived from the nutrients in the site water. Adults were identified to species according to morphological identification keys [41, 42].

d. Entomological inoculation rates

Entomological inoculation rates (EIR) are used to estimate the risk of transmission by looking at the number of infectious bites people can be exposed to if prevention methods are not used. EIR pre- and post-ITN distribution were calculated by multiplying the proportion of mosquitoes found to be infective (sporozoite rate) by the average number of females collected by HLCs.

The rate corresponds to the number of infected bites at a location per unit time. It is the only way to truly assess malaria transmission. EIR = entomological inoculation rate per night. This rate is referred to as the number of infectious bites, per person, per night;

- BR: daily number of bites (human biting rate) referred to as the number of bites per person per night. The rate corresponds to the number of bites per man per night (p/h/n). It was calculated in two ways depending on the method of capture. By PSC the number of bitten females captured in a neigh hour hood or commune, divided by the total number of people who spent the night in these houses on the day of capture (indirect aggression). And by HLC the number of anopheles captured per man per night, i.e. the number of mosquitoes captured divided by the number of captors and divided by the number of hours of capture (direct aggression).

- SI = Sporozoite index, refers to the percentage of anephelines carrying Plasmodium sp. Sporozoïtes. After morphological identification, mosquitoes captured by PSC were dissected into head-thorax-abdomen complexes and legs and wings under an AmScope entomological microscope. These head-thorax complexes of *An. gambiae* s.l. females were ground up for analysis by CSP Pf ELISA following the protocol of Wirtz et al. 1991 [43] for the determination of the sporozoite index (SI).

e. Determination of human infectivity by microscopy.

Simultaneously with the capture of the mosquitoes, blood samples were taken from the inhabitants of the houses where the vectors were captured. A peripheral drop of blood from the fingertip was taken on a slide to make thick drops and blood smears for microscopic diagnosis of *Plasmodium* sp. As well as the SD Bioline RDT was performed for the rapid diagnosis of malaria [44–46].

Parasite data collection was carried out by laboratory technicians who were part of the study team. They obtained informed consent, completed a questionnaire, prepared blood slides and performed RDTs, under the supervision of the researchers. The purpose of this supervision was to ensure that the study procedures were followed and to verify the interpretation of the RDTs. A one-day training workshop was held on the study's standard operating procedures (SOPs). The expert microscopists were senior laboratory technicians from the university clinics in Kinshasa.

Blood for thick/thin smears and RDTs was collected from the same finger prick and prepared on the same slide with the patient identification code. Approximately 5 μl of blood was collected by the study team using a loop provided with the RDT device. Test preparation and interpretation were performed according to the manufacturer's instructions. Tests were considered positive when the antigen and control lines were visible in their respective windows, negative when only the control band was visible and invalid when the control band was not visible. In case of an invalid result, the RDT was repeated.

Blood smears were stained with 10% Giemsa for 10 minutes. Thin smears were fixed with methanol before staining. The slides prepared by the study team were first examined by field laboratory technicians, blinded to the RDT results and using the WHO semi-quantitative method [28]. Their results were recorded on cards. All slides were stored in secure slide boxes and read by two expert microscopists from the university clinics in Kinshasa. The expert microscopists were blinded to the results of the field microscopy and RDT. In case of discrepancies >15%, the judgement of a senior laboratory technician was required. And the final result was the mean parasite density. The thin smear was used for species identification.

The results of these slides were used to calculate the parasitological indices, the incidences and the relative risk of malaria. The RDT (SD Bioline) was evaluated on the basis of a contingency table to calculate the sensitivity (Se), specificity (Sp), negative (NPV) and positive (PPV) predictive value, as well as the overall value (AG) of the test.

The sample was taken from the digital pulp to make the Blood for thick and the Blood smears on the same slide. Staining was done with 10% Giemsa working solution for 10 minutes, according to WHO instructions [44–46]. The Blood smears were fixed with methanol prior to staining. The reading was carried out at the Bandundu General Referral Hospital and at the parasitology department of the University clinics in Kinshasa.

At the Bandundu General Referral Hospital, only the microscopy was read and the technicians used the semi-quantitative cross method [44–46]. The reading was performed using an ordinary Olympus CX21 microscope at 1000X magnification (objective 100 and eyepiece 10).

The results of these analyses were used to estimate the prevalence of malaria by calculating the parasite or plasmodium index. This index corresponds to the proportion of subjects carrying plasmodium in a location. This cross-sectional indicator remains the most widely used to quantify and classify malaria endemicity.

2.2 Statistical analysis

The times required in minutes to obtain 50% and 95% of knockdown mosquitoes (KdT_{50} and KdT_{95}) were calculated according to WHO criteria, using log probit with the Polo Plus software version 1.0 [35, 36]. The Chi-square test was used to compare the mortality of A. gambiae sl between the insecticide-only trials and after pre-exposure to the synergist (PBO) at the 0.05 significance level. The effect of synergists was calculated with effective values above 10% [34–36, 38]. Thick drop, thin smear and RDT were performed on 190 individuals for the determination of the plasmodium index. The prevalence of malaria, the sensitivity and specificity of each test, and their positive and negative predictive values were calculated [44, 45].

The odds ratio (OR) was used to determine the risk of exposure to malaria parasite infectivity. The 95% confidence interval or Chi-square test at a significance level of 0.05 was used to measure the association between presumptive diagnosis based on fever history and microscopic diagnosis. The sensitivity, specificity (s), positive predictive value (PPV) and negative predictive value (NPV) of SD Bioline were calculated on the basis of contingency tables.

2.3 Results

Sensitivity tests carried out on populations of *A. gambiae* s.l. from Kisumu at the BIOLAV/ESP laboratory and on wild populations collected in Bandundu in DRC, have allowed us to better understand the levels of sensitivity of this vector to the two pyrethroids (Permethrin and Deltamethrin) commonly used in public health for impregnating nets. The efficacy of these compounds was compared to that of DDT (organochlorine) and Bendiocarb (carbamate), to detect the existence or not of cross-resistance between the three chemical families.

And this insecticide efficacy was measured by their knock down effect and the mortality they caused after 24 hours of observation. This analysis determined the KDT50 and KDT95, the value of these 2 parameters KDT (knock-down time) corresponds to the time after which respectively 50% and 95% of *An. gambiae* s.l. were knocked down. The results are presented in **Table 1**.

The shock time of *An. gambiae* s.l. was variable depending on the type of insecticide used in the test. The reaction of anopheles after contact with deltamethrin was very rapid compared to other insecticides. This insecticide was very active against anopheles compared to permethrin and DDT. The shock effect of anopheles was very low compared to permethrin and DDT. Only deltamethrin reached the Kdt_{50}. No effect of Kdt_{50} and Kdt_{95} was observed in anopheles tested with permethrin and DDT. These anopheles showed a very high resistance to these two insecticides with low mortality. Wild An. gambiae were resistant to deltamethrin, permethrin and DDT. Pre-exposure to PBO fully restored the efficacy of deltamethrin and partially of permethrin. Bendiocarb still remains effective.

Kdt50 and Kdt95 were too early for *An. gambiae* s.l. Kisumu, tested with deltamethrin, 8.45 minutes with 95% CI (7.09–9.79) and 30.34 (25.41–38) minutes. The shock effect of *An. gambiae* s.l. Kisumu tested with DDT did not reach Kdt_{95}.

These *An. gambiae* s.l. Kisumu were sensitive to all insecticides used (deltamethrin and permethrin 100% and DDT 99%) in **Table 2**.

Anopheles gambiae s.l.	Insecticides	N	KdT_{50} (minute)	KdT_{95} (minute)	Mortality 24 h	Statut
wild Souches Bandundu-city	Deltaméthrine 0.05%	100	43.8 (39.9–47.9)	n/a	52	R
	Deltaméthrine 0.05% + PBO 5%	100	16.5 (15–17.8)	38.5 (35–43)	98	S
	Permethrine 0.75%	100	n/a	n/a	17	R
	Permethrine 0.75% + PBO 5%	100	n/a	n/a	88	R
	Bendiocarb 0.1%	100	—	—	100	S
	DDT 4%	100	n/a	n/a	2	R
Kisumu	Deltaméthrine 0.05%	100	8.45 (7.09–9.79)	30.34 (25.41–38)	100	S
	Permethrine 0.75%	100	17.6 (13.58–21.49)	60.5 (45.57–96.37)	100	S
	DDT 4%	100	32.5 (25.68–41.19)	n/a	99	S

KdT50: Knockdown time (min) 50%; KdT95: Knockdown time (min) 95%; 95% CI: confidence interval; S: susceptible, R: resistant; n/a = no available "Knockdown" (< 15% of mosquitoes killed after 1 h exposure).

Table 1.
Insecticide susceptibility, expressed as KDT50, KDT95, and 24 hour mortality, of an. Gambiae s.l.

ITN	*n An. gambiae* s.l. wild strain					*Anopheles gambiae* s.l. Kisumu				
		Kdt50	Kdt95	Mortality(%)	Statut	n	Kdt50	Kdt95	Mortality(%)	*Status
ITN	100	n/a	n/a	20	R	100	5.4(4,1–6.8)	44.4(35,6–59.2)	100	S
ITN	100	n/a	n/a	27	R	100	5.9(4,7–7.0)	35.9(29,8–45.2)	100	S
ITN	100	n/a	n/a	30	R	100	5.6(4,6–6,6)	35.5(30,0–43.6)	100	S
ITN	100	n/a	n/a	27	R	100	6.1(5,3–7.0)	39.8(34,6–47.0)	100	S
MILD5	100	n/a	n/a	32	R	100	6.1(5,1–7.1)	39.3(33,5-47.7)	100	S

**Status: S (Sensitivity) = 24 hr mortality ≥ 80%; R (Resistance) = 24 hr mortality < 80%.*

Table 2.
Efficacy of LLINs against Anopheles gambiae s.l. *wild strain and Kisumu.*

From **Table 2**, it can be seen that low mortality of *A. gambiae* s.l. wild strain was observed in relation to ITNs shot in Bandundu-city, with an average of 22.3 ± 11.5% mortality 24 hours later. The Kdt_{50} and Kdt_{95} were not reached with *A. gambiae* s.l. wild strain. These wild anopheles unanimously showed a very strong resistance to the insecticide used for ITN impregnation. Concerning the sensitive strain, the Kdt_{50} was reached early at 5.8 ± 0.3 minutes and Kdt_{95} was observed early at 39.0 ± 3.6 minutes and mortality was 100 ± 0% 24 hours later. This indicates a high sensitivity to the insecticide.

From **Table 3**, Kdt_{50} and Kdt_{95} were highly variable depending on the type of insecticide and the test period.

Bendiocarb and Deltamethrin+ PBO were effective in both periods. *A. gambiae* s.l. tested to this insecticide were sensitive (100%). The Kdt_{50} and Kdt_{95} were too early in the second period of May-August 2019, i.e. 18.6 minutes with 95% CI (17.3–19.8) and 31.5 (28.9–35.4) minutes. No effect of Kdt_{50} and Kdt_{95} was observed in anopheles tested with permethrin and DDT during both periods. These anopheles showed very high resistance to these two insecticides with low mortality before and after the ITN mass distribution campaign. The mortality of anopheles exposed to permethrin was 31% in the first period and 36% in the second period, no significant difference was observed.

From **Table 4**, it can be seen that no significant association was observed between the dry and rainy seasons prior to the ITN mass distribution campaign. Microscopy

Période	Insecticides	n	Kdt_{50} (min)	Kdt_{95} (min)	Mortality 24 h(%)	Statut*
Before ITN distribution (September-November 2018)	Deltamethrin 0.05%	100	42.6 (40.7–44.8)	n/a	52	R
	Deltamethrin 0.05% + PBO 5%	100	22.7 (21.5–23.7)	39.7 (37–43.3)	99	S
	Permethrin 0.75%	100	n/a	n/a	31	R
	Permethrin 0.75% + PBO 5%	100	66.6 (61.7–74.2)	n/a	84	R
	Bendiocarb 0.1%	100	27.7 (25.5–29.8)	43.2 (39.1–50.3)	100	S
	DDT 4%	100	n/a	n/a	4	R
After ITN distribution (May-August 2019)	Deltamethrin 0.05%	100	31.5 (30.4–32.5)	51.7 (49.2–54.9)	34	R
	Deltamethrin 0.05% + PBO 5%	100	30.9 (29.5–32.3)	52.1 (48.6–56.8)	100	S
	Permethrin 0.75%	100	n/a	n/a	36	R
	Permethrin 0.75% + PBO 5%	100	67.9 (61.9–77.2)	n/a	97	RP
	Bendiocarb 0.1%	100	18.6 (17.3–19.8)	31.5 (28.9–35.4)	100	S
	DDT 4%	100	n/a	n/a	16	R

**Status: R = resistant S = susceptible PR = probable resistance n/a = no available.*

Table 3.
Mortality of Anopheles gambiae *s.l 24 hours after 60 minutes exposure to insecticides before and after distribution.*

Before ITN distribution						
Seasons	**N**	**%**	**Microscopy**		**OR**	**p-value**
			n (positif)	%		
Dry	62	53.4	35	56.4	1.4(0.6–3,2)	0.36
Rainy	54	46.6	35	64.8		
After ITN distribution						
Dry	44	59.5	28	63.4	0.4(0.1–0.9)	**0.04**
Rainy	30	40.5	12	40		
Total (throughout the period)						
Before	116	61.0	70	60.3	0.8(0.4–1,5)	0.39
After	74	39.0	40	54.0		

Table 4.
Variation in plasmodial indices before and after ITN distribution.

(thick drop) positive cases were in a tie (35 positive cases). The ITN mass distribution campaign had a beneficial effect on reducing the prevalence of malaria cases (malaria index), although no significant association was observed before and after the ITN distribution. After the ITN mass distribution campaign, a significant association was observed between thick drop and the rainy season with p-value = 0.04. Many cases were recorded during the dry season.

During, the second phase (July to December 2018), a very highly significant difference was observed between aggressivity and entomological inoculation rate during the dry season and the rainy season with p˂0.001. A significant difference was observed between density and sporozoite indices in both seasons (p = 0.01).

Comparing the two capture phases, no significant difference was observed between aggressivity, sporozoite index and entomological inoculation rate, respectively with p (0.098 and 0.896) before and after ITN distribution. During the second phase, the season influenced the entomological transmission indices. A highly significant difference was then observed between aggressivity and entomological inoculation rate during the dry and rainy seasons with p<0.001.

2.4 Discussion

2.4.1 Evaluation of the bioefficacy of ITN

Vector control is one of the important components of the global malaria control strategy. It is the main pillar of malaria control aiming to interrupt the transmission of malaria parasites through indoor residual spraying (IRS) or the use of pyrethroid-impregnated fabrics (nets and/or curtains) [7, 30].

Worldwide, pyrethroids are the insecticides of choice for impregnation, as they are highly effective and fast acting, with an irritating effect on mosquitoes and less toxicity to humans [1, 30]. Besides the less effectiveness of insecticides treated ITNs observed in Bandundu, its use as a physical and chemical barriers against mosquito vectors, constituted a repellent with a killing effect on mosquitoes [7, 30]. Resistance of *An. gambiae* s.l. to insecticides is increasingly widespread and reported in the sub-Saharan region. This resistance now affects nearly two-thirds of the countries where transmission persists. It affects all major vector species and all insecticide classes [1–7, 36]. However, evaluations based on the lab reared *An.gambiae* s.l. Kisumu strain show efficacy.

While both interventions are used in the DRC, IRS is carried out on a limited scale by mining companies and a few non-governmental organisation [1–31, 36]. The National Malaria Control Programme (NMCP) adopted mass distribution of ITNs as a malaria control strategy in 2004, as a tool to interrupt malaria transmission [1–19, 20]. Since then, the NMCP has distributed millions of pyrethroid-treated ITNs. However, little data is available on insecticide resistance in Anopheles mosquitoes in the DRC, while the emergence of insecticide resistance may have an impact on the effectiveness of vector control interventions [19, 38]. The aim of this study was therefore to assess the insecticide resistance of mosquitoes and the main entomological indicators associated with malaria transmission before and after ITN distribution in the city of Bandundu.

In our study, *An. gambiae* s.l. susceptible strain Kisumu showed high susceptibility with 98.1 ± 1.2% of mosquitoes shocked after 60 minutes of observation and 24 hours mortality of 100 ± 0% was recorded. The Kdt_{50} and Kdt_{95} were reached very early at 5.9 ± 0.3 minutes and 39.3 ± 4.4 minutes of observation. This indicates the efficacy of ITNs on the susceptible *An. gambiae* s.l. strain according to the WHO deliberation criteria. These observations corroborate those found by Mansiangi and colleagues on the durability of ITNs [47]. Similarly, several studies conducted in the tropics on the evaluation of ITNs with *An. gambiae* s.l. strain Kisumu have shown very good efficacy [26, 27, 48]. However, observations done on wild A. gambiae mosquitoes showed resistance to pyrethroids. Thus, *An. gambiae* s.l. wild strain, 7.9 ± 5.7% were shocked after 60 minutes of observation and the observed mortality was 22.3 ± 11.5% after 24 hours, thus showing a strong resistance. And the Kdt50 and 95 were not reached. In the DRC, several studies report the emergence of Anopheles resistance to common insecticides [12–27, 48]. Anopheles resistance can impact on the efficacy of ITNs [30–37, 49]. This work focused first on the bio-efficacy and compliance with WHO specifications of ITNs distributed by the DRC NMCP in high malaria prevalence areas in Bandundu-city. We compared the bio-efficacy of *An. gambiae* s.l. wild and Kisumu strains.

From this quality control, it appears that none of these nets demonstrated efficacy on local *An. gambiae* s.l. strains according to WHO deliberation criteria (24 hour mortality greater than or equal to 80% of *An. gambiae* s.l. tested and 95% of mosquitoes shocked after 60 minutes of observation). These results are similar to those found by Bamou and colleagues in Yaoundé who, after exposing wild *An. gambiae* s.l., found high resistance [50]. Riveron and colleagues in Kinshasa on the evaluation of the efficacy of newly purchased nets: OlysetNet and Permanet 2.0 with local strains of *An. gambiae* s.l. had revealed low efficacy [27].

Our results are also similar to those found by Ahogni, in Benin [51], Loonen and colleagues in Baraka, DRC [13], Abilio and colleagues in Mozambique [15], and Darriet and colleagues in Côte d'Ivoire [12], who proved the ineffectiveness of new ITNs on wild strains. The presence in the DRC of mosquito populations capable of resisting diagnostic doses of insecticides may account for the reduced efficacy of ITNs.

The results of this study contrast with those found by Kweka and colleagues in Tanzania on the evaluation of PermaNet®3.0 ITNs on An. gambiae s.l. wild strain populations, which showed 98–100% effectiveness [48].

This difference is believed to be due to the mosquito colony used in this study being tolerant to pyrethroids and Permanet 3.0 being impregnated with pyrethroids combined with PBO.

Similarly Bobanga and colleagues in Kinshasa on the bioefficacy of PermaNet 3.0 ITNs on the wild population of vectors, which revealed a 100% mortality [52].

The results obtained by Bobanga et al. with the wild strain of *An. gambiae* s.l. showed low efficacy of treated nets, with mortality ranging from 11 to 66%. This difference in results with the susceptible strain is thought to be due to the different brand of ITNs, Olyset being made of permethrin-impregnated polyethylene [52].

2.4.2 Evaluation of entomological transmission indices

Entomological inoculation rates during ITN distribution in Bandundu town in December 2018 resulted in a decrease in the number of anopheles mosquitoes collected from households by both the pyrethroid spray capture and human landing capture techniques, although the difference was not statically significant. Similarly, no significant difference was found between sporozoite indices, bite rates or entomological inoculation rates (EIR) between the two periods. The risk of infectious bites before net distribution was approximately 0.13 infectious bites per person per night, or 47.2 infectious bites per person per year, compared to 0.08 infectious bites per person per night, or 27.6 infectious bites per person per year after ITN distribution. However, this decrease was not significant.

ITN distribution resulted in a decrease in the number of Anopheles mosquitoes. However, it is difficult to attribute this decrease to ITNs. There was a clear seasonal influence on entomological transmission indices, which were high during the rainy season and low during the dry season. In addition, there is the distribution of two seasons, the rainy season (September-December and April-May) and the dry season (June-August and January-March) which makes it difficult to assess the decrease in entomological indices. A high rate of mosquito bites was recorded outside houses in Bandundu town during the collection campaign, suggesting changes in the behaviour of *An. gambiae* s.l. as reported elsewhere [25, 29]. However, it is difficult to attribute the change in behaviour to the repellent effect of deltamethrin-treated ITNs alone [25, 29]. A habit was observed among the population of staying out late at night to watch TV programmes. This may explain why the peak of anopheline activity was reached between 2 and 3 am.

2.4.3 Evaluation of the parasitological indices of transmission of malaria

The improvement in the epidemiological situation of malaria remains unstable and could even worsen due to the emergence of parasite resistance to the usual and affordable antimalarial drugs.

The deterioration of primary health services, the emergence of insecticide-resistant strains in mosquitoes and the misuse of antimalarial drugs are believed to have contributed to the selection of resistant strains [13–35, 38]. Diagnostic confirmation is crucial because clinical diagnosis is at the root of thousands of erroneous treatments and this leads to economic consequences as well as increased morbidity and mortality due to the delay of specific treatment [6–35, 38]. Reliable diagnosis could thus serve to avoid unnecessary exposure of patients to antimalarial drugs (risk of parasite resistance and economic loss) and allow for timely exploration of other possible pathologies. Thus, the success of the challenge of containing the spread of resistance absolutely implies an efficient diagnosis.

Currently, two modalities are used in the field for the biological diagnosis of malaria: microscopy and rapid tests (RDT). The NMCP has chosen the SD-Bioline test with HRP2, which is distributed free of charge in the country's health facilities via the central office [9, 44, 45].

In this study, the sensitivity (Se) of the SD-Bioline test evaluated in the field was 77%, specificity (Sp) 78%, positive predictive value (PPV) 82%, negative predictive value (NPV) 72% and overall test value (VG) 77%. This can be justified by the fact that Bandundu-ville is an endemic area and the presence of other non-falciparium plasmodial species could be detected in the area. These observations are similar to those made by Muhindo and colleagues in Kinshasa [53].

Similar results were found by Laurent and colleagues in Tanzania in an area of intense malaria transmission. These results varied by age group and disease prevalence [54] and are in contrast to those found by Abeku and colleagues in East Africa, where the difference was related to prevalence [55]. The prevalence of malaria by parasite index was 57.9% by microscopy and 53.6% by RDT. This is justified by the possibility of diagnosing non-falciparum species by microscopy. In Tanzania, the prevalence by microscopy was low (34.3%) and slightly higher by RDT (57.2%) [53].

Pf was the dominant species in 94% of mono-infections and 4.7% of co-infections. This dominant presence of Pf may justify this high prevalence. This plasmodial species is at the root of the severity and complications of malaria infection [56]. These results are consistent with those found in Kano State, Nigeria, with high malaria prevalence (60%) and this prevalence was strongly related to age [57].

Malaria infection was seasonally influenced; thus there was a significant association between malaria infection and the long rainy season (September-October) with a risk of 2.8. Similarly, during the short dry season (January-March), a significant association was observed with a risk of 2.6 [55, 56, 58].

We find that age and fever during collection were strongly correlated with the presence of parasites. Children <5 years of age were at higher risk of infection, with a 6.0-fold risk than adults, followed by children aged 6–12 years with a 3.2-fold risk.

The presence of fever at the time of sampling was 6.4 times more associated with the presence of malaria infection, reflecting the fact that in endemic areas fever is the main sign of malaria. These results corroborate those found by Mokoso and colleagues in Bandundu-city, of the aetiologies associated with fever in this area, 80% are due to malaria [59]. Our results corroborate those found by several authors in endemic areas [54–57, 58].

The inhabitants of the commune of Mayoyo in Bandundu-city were more exposed to infections with a risk of 2.3. This commune is urban-rural and has biotopes favourable to anopheles, as well as high entomological parameters.

In Dielmo, Senegal, an area where pyrethroids were the main insecticides used for malaria control, a rebound in malaria cases was recorded, followed by the development of resistance after multiple distributions of ITNs (**Table 5**) [60]. In another study in Benin, a reduction in the efficacy of ITNs was observed, leading to an increase in malaria cases in an area where An.gambiae is resistant to pyrethroids and where nets are treated with deltamethrin [15, 51].

As shown in **Table 1**, a considerable number of unfed mosquitoes were collected from the houses, which may have played a role in malaria transmission by later feeding. These results therefore probably underestimate the number of bites per person and may have been biased when new ITNs were deployed, resulting in more mosquitoes exiting before they could be collected. In addition, blood-fed mosquitoes were not tested for human blood, although it was assumed that most blood-fed An.

Parameters (Index)	**Phase 1 (July-December 2018) before distribution of ITNs**								
	Dry seasons				**Rainy seasons**				**p-value**
	Index	**Median**	**P25**	**P75**	**Index**	**Median**	**P25**	**P75**	
Density	7.67	0.04	0.02	0.22	15.8	0.15	0.027	0.35	**0.01**
SI	6.03	0	0	9	11.7	0.1	0	22	**0.01**
BR	2.8	0.52	0.52	1.55	9.1	1.81	1.55	2.72	**<0.001**
EIR	0.16	0	0	0	1.22	0.18	0	0.58	**<0.001**
Phase 2 (January-June 2019) after distribution of ITNs									
Density	3.3	0.07	0.03	0.1	2.2	0.16	0.04	0.11	**0.24**
SI	8.8	0	0	0.22	11.3	0.07	0	0.25	**0.04**
BR	2.4	1.55	0.52	2.6	7.6	9.5	6.2	10.4	**<0.001**
EIR	0.2	0	0	0.4	0.9	0.1	0	2.2	**0.001**

d = Relative density (mean numbers of An. gambiae s.l. collected) (Anopheles per house) SI=Sporozoite index (percentage of mosquitoes positive for CSP) BR = Biting rate (A. gambiae s.l. per person per night) EIR = Entomological Inoculation Rate (Number of infectious bites per person per night).

Table 5.
Distribution of entomological transmission indices according to periods.

gambiae s.l. resting indoors would have fed on humans. Thirdly, as mosquito collections for pre- and post-net distribution were carried out in different months of the dry and rainy seasons, seasonal variations cannot be excluded from the interpretation of the collection and bioassay data.

Metelo et al. reported seasonal differences in An. gambiae s.l. populations in Bandundu between the dry and rainy seasons [49]. It should be noted that in many settings, nets are not used immediately upon receipt, but rather after the old nets have been torn and are no longer usable. The use of newly distributed nets in homes was not quantified, although the presence of Dawa Plus nets was observed in most households during the implementation of CHPs and HLCs. Large-scale use of DHS data has shown that ITN use is always associated with reduced malaria transmission, especially when community use is high, however, insecticide resistance may reduce this effect, Ferrari et al. found that sleeping under an ITN the previous night was associated with a reduced risk of Plasmodium infection [61]. In the present study, however, no significant impact on entomological measures of transmission was observed immediately after ITN distribution. In an area where insecticide resistance levels are already high, the distribution of new ITNs no longer has an immediate or strong effect on key entomological measures of malaria transmission. This may be due to increased resistance in the study area, compromising both new nets with a full dose of insecticide, and old nets, which will have lost some of their insecticide. This may also mean that the old nets remained effective for the full 3 years of the net's life expectancy, and therefore the distribution of new nets did not improve control. However, the presence of sporozoite-positive mosquitoes in both periods indicates that a better control measure is needed to reduce transmission in this area.

Resistance to pyrethroids and DDT: With the exception of bendiocarb which caused 100% mortality of Anopheles mosquitoes, the other insecticides tested were ineffective against An. gambiae s.l. collected before and after ITN distribution. An. gambiae s.l. was resistant to pyrethroids (deltamethrin and permethrin) and DDT in both periods. Mortality of Anopheles to insecticides varied according to the period (before and after mass ITN distribution). Mortality was limited to deltamethrin, 52% before the mass distribution and was reduced to 34% afterwards, which reduced the effectiveness of this product. After pre-exposure to PBO, the efficacy of deltamethrin was fully restored during both study periods. For permethrin (31–36%) and DDT (4–16%), Anopheles mosquitoes were also resistant to varying degrees depending on the period (pre-post). It can be observed that after the mass ITN distribution, permethrin and DDT increased their efficacy somewhat. These two molecules have not been used for a decade. This could be explained by the fact that the distributed ITNs were impregnated with deltamethrin, which increased the selective pressure and served as a basis for the emergence of resistance in *An. gambiae* s.l. this resistance poses fundamental and operational problems as the behaviour of the Anopheles is altered, resulting in a significant decrease in the efficacy of these products. The endemicity of malaria and the high number of infected An. gambiae in the city of Bandundu are of concern and must be taken into account.

3. Conclusions

The ITNs deployed in Bandundu-city in 2018 are still effective on A. gambiae sl strain Kisumu but are ineffective on the wild *An. gambiae* s.l. wild strain found in the city. The wild *An. gambiae* s.l. were resistant to both pyrethroids and DDT.

An increase in the sensitivity of *An. gambiae* s.l to pyrethroids was observed after pre-exposure to 5% PBO suggesting the resistance was partly of metabolic origin, i.e. related to P450 mono-oxygenases. The high entological indices in Bandundu-city throughout the year indicate intense malaria transmission. This reflects the ineffectiveness of the vector control strategy which has been based solely on the mass distribution of ITNs for several years. We find that mass distribution of ITNs in Bandundu has not had a significant effect on malaria transmission. Given the intensity of transmission and the levels of resistance observed, it is necessary to consider a new alternative to curb the emergence of resistance and maintain the gains of mass distribution.

Acknowledgements

The research team would like to thank the CREC teams for their support and assistance in setting up our insectarium, in particular Prof Martin AGKOBETO and Dr. Osée RAZZAK. Our sincere thanks to Marianne Sinka of Oxford University for her contribution to the correction of this paper, especially its translation into English.

The thanks also go postum to the late Professor Paul MANSIANGI, the coordinator of this project where death brutally snatched away our affection, eternal felicity to your soul. The field supervisor Ladius MBAYA for his dedication and perfect collaboration.

Contributions of the authors

E.MM, JZ: drafting of the study protocol.

EMM, JZ, BM, VN: coordination of field activities (larval survey and sensitivity testing). EMM, JZ, VN, SN, AM: Coordination of laboratory activities. EMM, JZ, VN, SN database and statistical analysis. E.MM, JZ, JMNK, FA, EHMN, BM: writing of the article and correction. BM editing of the paper.

Conflict of interest

The authors declare no conflict of interest.

Author details

Emery Metelo-Matubi[1,2,3]*, Josue Zanga[3], Victoire Nsabatien[3], Aimé Mbala[2], Solange Ngamukie[3], Fiacre Agossa[4], El Hadji Amadou Niang[5], Jean Maniania-Nguya-Kalenga[6] and Mulenda Basimike[7]

1 National Institute of Biomedical Research, Kinshasa, Democratic Republic of Congo

2 Faculty of Medicine, University of Bandundu, Bandundu-City, Bandundu, Democratic Republic of Congo

3 Laboratory of Bioecology and Vector Control, Department of Environmental Health, School of Public Health of Kinshasa, DR Congo

4 PMI VectorLink Project, Abt Associates, Rockville, MD, USA

5 Laboratoire d'Ecologie Vectorielle and Parasitaire Ecology (LEVP), Cheikh Anta Diop University, Dakar, Senegal

6 International Centre of Insect Physiology and Ecology, Nairobi, Kenya

7 International Consultant, Malaria Control and Its Elimination, Democratic Republic of Congo

*Address all correspondence to: pathymetelo@gmail.com

References

[1] WHO. World Malaria Report 2019. Geneva: World Health Organization; 2019

[2] WHO. World Malaria Report 2021. Geneva: World Health Organization; 2021

[3] WHO. World Malaria Report 2020. Geneva: World Health Organization; 2020

[4] Griffin JT, Bhatt S, Sinka ME, Gething PW, Lynch M, Patouillard E, et al. Potential for reduction of burden and local elimination of malaria by reducing Plasmodium falciparum malaria transmission: A mathematical modelling study. The Lancet Infectious Diseases. 2016;**16**:465-472

[5] Goesch JN, Schwarz NG, Decker ML, Oyakhirome S, Borchert LB, Kombila UD, et al. Socio-economic status is inversely related to bed net use in Gabon. Malaria Journal. 2008;7(1):60

[6] WHO. World Malaria Report 2016. Geneva: World Health Organization; 2016

[7] OMS. Stratégie technique mondiale de lutte contre le paludisme 2016-2030. Geneva: OMS; 2015

[8] OMS. Moustiquaire imprégnée d'insecticide. Manuel à l'intention des responsables des programmes nationaux. Genève: OMS; 2003

[9] PNLP-RDC. Revue à mi-parcours du plan stratégique national 2016-2020 : Défis et perspectives. Programme de lutte contre le paludisme. Kinshasa RD Congo: PNLP-RDC; 2018

[10] PNLP-RDC. Plan stratégique national 2020-2023. Programme de lutte contre le paludisme. Kinshasa RD Congo: PNLP-RDC; 2019

[11] OMS/FRP. La déclaration d'Abuja et le plan d'action. Genève: OMS/FRP; 2003

[12] Darriet F. Moustiquaires imprégnées et résistance des moustiques aux insecticides. Paris: Ed. IRD; Collect. Didactique; 2007. pp. 1-116

[13] Jeanine L, Dery DB, Musaka BZ, Bandibabone JB, Bousema T, et al. Identification of main malaria vectors and their insecticide resistance profile in internally displaced and indigenous communities in Eastern Democratic Republic of the Congo (DRC). Malaria Journal. 2020;**19**:425

[14] Lynd A, Oruni A, Arjen E, Naego LB, Pipini D, et al. Insecticide resistance in Anopheles gambiae from the northern Democratic Republic of Congo, with extreme knockdown resistance (kdr) mutation frequencies revealed by a new diagnostic assay. Malaria Journal. 2018;**17**:412

[15] Abílio AP, Marrune P, Nilsa D, Mbofana F, Muianga P, Kampango A. Bio efficacy of new long lasting insecticide treated bed nets against Anopheles funestus and Anopheles gambiae from central and northern Mozambique. Malaria Journal. 2015;**14**(352):015-0885

[16] Overgaard HJ, Reddy VP, Abaga S, Matias A, Reddy MR, Kulkarni V, et al. Malaria transmission after five years of vector control on Bioko Island, Equatorial Guinea. Parasites Vectors. 2012;**5**:253

[17] Mark JM, Irish SR, Reich Brian J, Marc P, Doctor SM, Mwandagalirwa MK, et al. The links between agriculture, Anopheles mosquitoes, and malaria

risk in children younger than 5 years in the Democratic Republic of the Congo: A population-based, cross-sectional, spatial study. The Lancet Planetary Health. 2018;**2**(2):e74-e82

[18] Basilua Kanza JP, El Fahime E, Alaoui S, Essassi EM, Brooke B, Nkebolo Malafu A, et al. Pyrethroid, DDT and malathion resistance in the malaria vector *Anopheles gambiae* from the Democratic Republic of Congo. Transactions of the Royal Society of Tropical Medicine and Hygiene. 2013;**107**(1):8-14

[19] MICS. Institut national de statistique (INS) RDC. Enquête par grappe à indicateurs multiples, 2017-2018. Kinshasa, République Démocratique du Congo: Rapport de résultats de l'enquête; 2019

[20] EDS-RDC. Institut national de statistique (INS) RDC. Enquête Démographique et de Santé en République Démocratique du Congo 2013-2014. Rapport final des activités du deuxième Enquête Démographique et de Santé (EDS-RDC II). Kinshasa, République Démocratique du Congo. Avril 2014

[21] Bobanga T, Umesumbu SE, Mandoko AS, Nsibu CN, Dotson EB, Ray FB, et al. Presence of species within the *Anopheles gambiae* complex in the Democratic Republic of Congo. Transactions of the Royal Society of Tropical Medicine and Hygiene. 2016;**110**(6):1-3

[22] Rahm U, Vermylen M. Répertoire et répartition des Anophèles de la République Démocratique du Congo. Estratto dalla Rivisita di Malariologia. 1966;**65**:1-3

[23] Sinka ME, Bangs MJ, Manguin S, Coetzee M, Mbogo CM, Hemingway J, et al. The dominant Anopheles vectors of human malaria in Africa, Europe and the Middle East: Occurrence data, distribution maps and bionomic précis. Parasites & Vectors. 2010;**3**:117

[24] Mouchet J, Carnavale P, Coosemans M, Julvez J, Richard-Lenoble D, Sircoulon J. Biodiversité du paludisme dans le monde. Vol. 1. Eurotest Paris: Ed John Libbey; 2004. pp. 12-96

[25] Shah MP, Steinhardt LC, Mwandama D, Mzilahowa T, Gimni JE, et al. The effectiveness of older insecticide-treated bed nets (ITNs) to prevent malaria infection in an area of moderate pyrethroid resistance: Results from a cohort study in Malawi. Malaria Journal. 2020;**19**:24

[26] Watsenga F., Riveron JM, Irving H., Irish SR. High *Plasmodium* infection rate and reduced BeD net efficacy in multiple insecticide-resistant malaria vectors in Kinshasa, Democratic Republic of Congo. The Journal of Infectious Diseases. 2018;**217**(2):320-328

[27] Riveron JM, Watsenga F, Irving H, Irish SR, Wondji CS. High Plasmodium infection rate and reduced bed net efficacy in multiple insecticide-resistant malaria vectors in Kinshasa, Democratic Republic of Congo. The Journal of Infectious Diseases. 2018;**217**(2):320-328

[28] Nardini L, Hunt RH, Dahan-Moss YL, Christie N, Christian RN, Coetzee M, et al. Malaria vectors in the Democratic Republic of the Congo: The mechanisms that confer insecticide resistance in Anopheles gambiae and Anopheles funestus. Malaria Journal. 2017;**16**(1):448

[29] Emery M-M, Bukaka E, Bakambana TL, Situakibanza H, Sangaré I, Mesia G, et al. Détermination des paramètres bioécologiques et entomologiques de l'Anopheles gambiae sl dans la transmission du paludisme à

Bandundu-ville, RD Congo. Pan African Medical Journal. 2015;**22**:108

[30] Lindsay Steve W, Thomas MB, Kleinschmidt I. Threats to the effectiveness of insecticide-treated bednets for malaria control: Thinking beyond insecticide resistance. The Lancet Global Health. 2021;**9**:e1325-e1331

[31] PNLP_RDC. Plan national de gestion de la résistance des vecteurs du Paludisme aux insecticides en République Démocratique du Congo (RDC) 2022-2024. Kinshasa RD Congo: Programme National de Lutte contre le Paludisme; 2021

[32] Kaounga MMGI, Zanga J, Mbuku GB, et al. Insecticide susceptibility of Anopheles gambiae s.l and identification of some resistance mechanisms in Kwilu Province in the Democratic Republic of Congo. Pan African Medical Journal. 2020;**37**:79

[33] DSRP. Unite de pilotage du processus DSRP. Kinshasa, RDC: Monographie de la province de Bandundu, Ministère du plan; 2005

[34] Robertson JL, Russell RM, Preisler HK, Savin E. Bioassays with Arthropods. 2nd ed. Vol. 22. Boca Raton, FL, U.S.A: CRC Press; 2007. p. 199

[35] WHOPES. WHO Recommended Long-Lasting Insecticidal Nets. Geneva: WHOPES; 2014

[36] WHO. Tests Procedures for Insecticide Resistance Monitoring in Malaria Vector Mosquitoes. Vol. 2. Geneva: WHO; 2016. p. 55

[37] Adeogun A, Olojede J, Oduola A, Awolola S. Village-scale evaluation of PermaNet 3: An enhanced efficacy combination long-lasting insecticidal net against resistant population of *Anopheles gambiae s.s*. Malaria Chemotherapy, Control & Elimination. 2012;**1**(1):1-9

[38] WHO. WHO Recommended Long-Lasting Insecticidal Nets. Geneva: WHO; 2012

[39] Pinto J, Williams J. Manuel de Formation à l'Entomologie du Paludisme à l'intention des techniciens en entomologie et lutte anti-vectorielle. U.S.A, Research Triangle Park: RTI International; 2012

[40] WHO. Indoor Residual Spraying: Use of Indoor Residual Spraying for Scaling up Malaria Control and Elimination. Geneva, Switzerland: World Health Organization; 2008

[41] Maureen C. Key to the females of Afrotropical Anopheles mosquitoes (Diptera: Culicidae). Malaria Journal. 2020;**19**:70

[42] Gillies MT, De Meillon B. The Anophelinae of Africa south of the Sahara (Ethiopian Zoogeographical Region). Publication of the south of African institute for Medical Research, Johannesburg. 1968;**2**(54):343

[43] Wirtz RA, Burkot TR. Detection of malarial parasites in mosquitoes. Advances in Disease Vector Research. 1991;**8**:77-106

[44] WHO. Malaria Rapid Diagnostic Test Performance: Results of WHO Product Testing of Malaria RDTs: Round 8 (2016-2018). Geneva: WHO; 2018

[45] WHO/FIND/CDC. Malaria Rapid Diagnostic Test Performance Results of WHO Product Testing of Malaria RDTs: Round 1. Geneva: WHO; 2008

[46] Shillcutt SD, Morel CM, Coleman PG, Mills AJ, Goodman CA. Cost-effectiveness of malaria diagnosis

in Sub-Saharan Africa: The role of rapid diagnostic tests in rural settings with high Plasmodium falciparum transmission. Bulletin of the World Health Organization. 2008;**86**:101-110

[47] Paul M, Umesumbu S, Etewa I, Zandibeni J, Bafwa N, Blaufuss S, et al. Comparing the durability of the long-lasting insecticidal nets DawaPlus ® 2.0 and DuraNet© in northwest Democratic Republic of Congo. Malaria Journal. 2020;**19**:189

[48] Kweka EJ, Tenu F, Magogo F, Mboera LEG. *Anopheles gambiae sensu stricto* aquatic stages development comparison between insectary and semifield structure. Hindawi Publishing Corporation Advances in Zoology. 2015;**2015**:6

[49] Emery M-M, Zanga J, Binene G, Mvuama N, Ngamukie S, Nkey J, et al. The effect of a mass distribution of insecticide-treated nets on insecticide resistance and entomological inoculation rates of *Anopheles gambiae s.l.* in Bandundu City, Democratic Republic of Congo. The Pan African Medical Journal. 2021;**40**:118

[50] Roland B, Kopya E, Nkahe LD, Menze BD, Awono-Ambene P, et al. Increased prevalence of insecticide resistance in Anopheles coluzzii populations in the city of Yaoundé, Cameroon and influence on pyrethroid-only treated bed net efficacy. Parasite. 2021;**28**:8

[51] Ahogni I, Aïkpon R, Ossè R, Dagnon J, Govoetchan R, Attolou R, et al. Field durability of Yorkool®LN nets in the Benin Republic. Advances in Entomology. 2020;**8**:72-92

[52] Bobanga T, Ayieko W, Zanga M, Umesumbu SE, Landela A, Fataki O, et al. Field efficacy and acceptability of PermaNet® 3.0 and OlysetNet® in Kinshasa, Democratic Republic of the Congo. Journal of Vector Borne Diseases. 2013;**50**:206-214

[53] Muhindo H, Ilombe G, Meya R, Lutumba P, Van Geertryders JP. Accuracy of malaria rapid diagnodtic test optimal-TR in Kinshasa, the democratic republic of Congo. Malaria Journal. 2012;**11**:24

[54] Laurent A, Schellenberg J, Kizito S, Ketende SC, Alonso PL, Mshinda H, et al. Performance of HRP-2 based rapid diagnostic test for malaria and its variation with age in an area of intense malaria transmission in southern Tanzania. Malaria Journal. 2010;**9**:294

[55] Abeku TA, Kristan M, Jones C, Beard J, Mueller DH, Okia M, et al. Determinants of the accuracy of rapid diagnostic tests in malaria case management: Evidence from low and moderate transmission settings in the east African highlands. Malaria Journal. 2008;7:202

[56] Gomes AP, Vitorino RR, Costa AP, Gomes EM, Almeida MG, Siqueira-Batista R. Severe Plasmodium falciparum malaria Malária grave por Plasmodium falciparum. Rev Bras Ter Intensiva. 2011;**23**(3):358-369

[57] Dawaki S, Al-Mekhlafi HM, Jamaiah I, Wahib MA, Awatif MA, Sady H, et al. Is Nigeria winning the battle against malaria? Prevalence, risk factors and KAP assessment among Hausa communities in Kano state. Malaria Journal. 2016;**15**:351

[58] Omondi CJ, Onguru D, Kamau L, Nanyingi M, Ong'amo G, Estambale B. Perennial transmission of malaria in the low altitude areas of Baringo County, Kenya. Malaria Journal. 2017;**16**:257

[59] Mukoso F et Situakimbanza H. Etiologies associées à la fièvre dans la ville de Bandundu. In Psychologie et Société nouvelle. CARAS.UNIKIN. Kinshasa, République Démocratique du Congo. 2011;**1**(10):117-122

[60] Nyedzie WA, Doucoure S, Gaudart J, Diagne N, Sarr FD, Faye N, et al. Malaria in Dielmo, a Senegal village: Is its elimination possible after seven years of implementation of long-lasting insecticide-treated nets? PLoS One. 2017;**12**(7):e0179528

[61] Ferrari G, Ntuku HM, Ross A, Schmidlin S, Kalemwa DM, Tshefu AK, et al. Identifying risk factors for plasmodium infection and anaemia in Kinshasa, Democratic Republic of Congo. Malaria Journal. 2016;**15**(1):362

Chapter 12

Mosquito Population Modification for Malaria Control

Rebeca Carballar-Lejarazú, Taylor Tushar, Thai Binh Pham and Anthony James

Abstract

Malaria is a mosquito-borne disease that kills millions of people every year. Existing control tools have been insufficient to eliminate the disease in many endemic regions and additional approaches are needed. Novel vector-control strategies using genetic engineering to create malaria-resistant mosquitoes (population modification) can potentially contribute a new set of tools for mosquito control. Here we review the current mosquito control strategies and the development of transgenic mosquitoes expressing anti-parasite effector genes, highlighting the recent improvements in mosquito genome editing with CRISPR-Cas9 as an efficient and adaptable tool for gene-drive systems to effectively spread these genes into mosquito populations.

Keywords: *Anopheles*, mosquito control, genetic manipulation, CRISPR/Cas9

1. Introduction

1.1 Malaria and mosquito control

Mosquitoes in the genus *Anopheles* transmit to humans the *Plasmodium* parasites that cause malaria. Malaria is one of the most devastating mosquito-borne diseases worldwide, affecting more than 225 million people yearly, especially in sub-Saharan Africa and India [1].

Interventions to control anophelines have been ongoing since Sir Ronald Ross's discovery of the complete malaria transmission cycle in the late nineteenth century. The first large-scale vector control interventions in the early twentieth century relied on management and control of anopheline breeding habitats via manipulation of the environment (**Figure 1**) [2]. However, the discovery and subsequent development of dichloro-diphenyl-trichloroethane (DDT) in the early 1940s led to a new era of vector control after successes with the insecticide by the U.S. Army in World War II and various field trials proved its powerful ability to control malaria [3]. The initial successes with DDT were so great that malaria eradication began to appear feasible to some malariologists, and in 1955, the World Health Assembly launched the Global Malaria Eradication Programme (GMEP) with a goal to assist nations in eradicating malaria by providing technical advice and consolidating the resources needed for large-scale eradication campaigns. The World Health Organization (WHO) Expert Committee

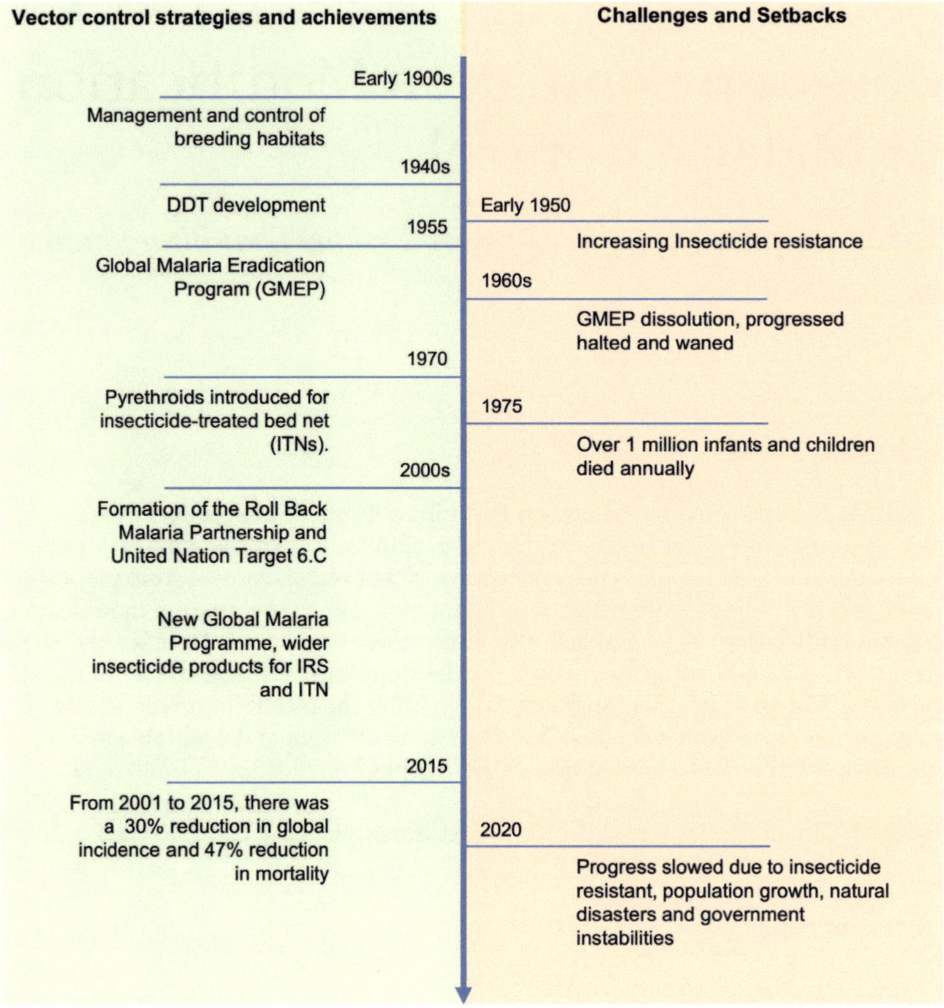

Figure 1.
Timeline of vector-control approaches and outcomes. Important events and timepoints of malaria vector control efforts and progress in the perspective of obstacles and downturns. Although great progress was made through the history of malaria vector control, many natural and artificial challenges have hindered the goal of malaria eradication.

on Malaria was responsible for designing the eradication campaign schedule, which consisted of four distinct phases: preparatory, attack, consolidation, and maintenance. Completion of the eradication schedule was estimated to require 8–10 years [4]. Despite previous observations of insecticide resistance to DDT in Greece in 1951, the attack phase relied almost exclusively on the use of indoor residual spraying (IRS) of this insecticide to reduce adult mosquito populations supplemented by chloroquine to treat infections [5]. Large reductions in malaria case incidence, morbidity and mortality were observed worldwide because of the GMEP campaign and malaria was eliminated in many countries with temperate climates (**Figure 2**) [6–10]. However, progress began to falter by the mid 1960s and some countries participating in the GMEP reverted from the consolidation phase back to the attack phase. Countries such as Sri Lanka, which was an exemplary model for GMEP successes, began to experience

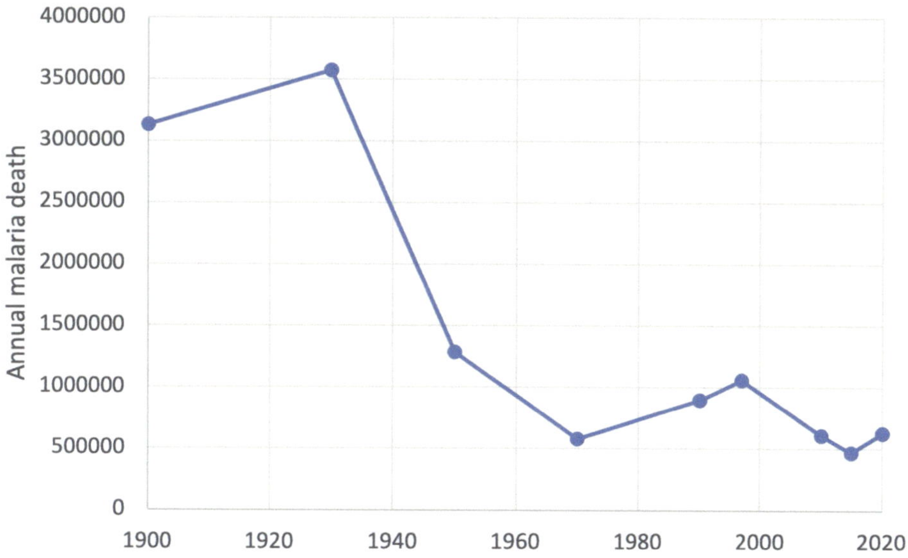

Figure 2.
Global estimated number of malaria deaths. Estimated malaria mortality declined significantly from 1920s to 1970s due to many malaria control efforts countrywide and internationally but slowed from 1970s to 2020. Sources [6–9].

epidemic resurgences of malaria [11]. Additionally, resistance to DDT became widespread throughout the participating countries. By the late 1960s, political and financial support for the GMEP had waned and the aim for eradication within a finite timeline was replaced by the aim of controlling malaria within an indefinite timeline.

Control of malaria after the dissolution of the GMEP devolved to a country-by-country basis. Some nations that had benefited from participation in the GMEP continued to make progress in reducing the burden of malaria. However, most African nations were never included in the GMEP, and without dedicated resources, financial support or personnel trained in vector control techniques, the continent continued to suffer greatly as population growth paralleled an increase in malaria morbidity and mortality. In 1975 the WHO estimated that over one million infants and children were dying annually due to malaria in sub-Saharan Africa [12]. A systemic analysis of global malaria mortality from 1980 to 2010 estimated a peak of malaria deaths occurred in 2004 with over 1.8 million deaths occurring globally [13]. By the beginning of the second millennium, the rapid expansion of disease burden due to the absence of a global strategy and lack of unified political will became soberingly evident in the global malaria mortality rates.

The combination of skyrocketing malaria mortality and philanthropic interests of the world's ultra-wealthy led to a renewed interest and consolidation of financial and political will for advances in malaria control and elimination at the beginning of the second millennium. The formation of the Roll Back Malaria Partnership (RBM) and creation of the United Nations Millennium Development Goals helped to solidify a new global strategy. After years of disparate global malaria control without clearly-defined metrics to track progress, the renewed enthusiasm ushered in a return to specific targets and strategies reminiscent of what was attempted in the 1950s with the GMEP. The new global malaria programme (GMP) had the benefit of additional vector control tools such as a wider variety of insecticide products for IRS and insecticide-treated nets (ITN). The new program also benefited from the historical perspectives of renown malariologists on the causes leading to the failures of the original eradication effort. The UN development goals included Target 6.C with a stated aim "to have halted by 2015 and begun to reverse the incidence of malaria and other major diseases" (UN Millennium goals [14]) and the RBM created a Global Malaria Action Plan, which outlined an overarching strategy and system of support needed to achieve malaria eradication [15]. The enhanced frameworks for combating malaria also were accompanied by increased funding in the formation of the Global Fund to Fight AIDS, Tuberculosis and Malaria and the US President's Malaria Initiative [16]. The renewed efforts and consolidation of strategies and finances in the early 2000s proved successful, and Target 6.C of the development goals was achieved. There was a 30% reduction in global incidence and 47% decline in mortality due to malaria from 2001 to 2015 [1]. Continuing the momentum of the progress made in the early millennium, WHO member states created and adopted a new global technical strategy (GTS) in 2015 and set an ambitious new target for a 90% reduction in global malaria burden by 2030 [17].

The WHO and RBM developed a new framework of strategies and guidelines to meet the ambitious 2030 targets. The first pillar of the WHO's post-2015 GTS called for expansions of access. Firstly, it called for expanded access to vector control using either IRS or long-lasting insecticide treated nets (LLINs) and secondly, it called for expanded access to chemoprevention and treatment, especially in vulnerable groups such as children and pregnant women. The new guidelines also highlighted the importance of generating entomological and epidemiological surveillance data to guide vector control and disease-treatment efforts and advised that accumulation of these data should be considered an intervention in itself. While supporting elements of the post-2015 GTS encouraged advancements in research and new technology, these were secondary to the ramp-up of coverage using existing vector control and treatment technologies. Unfortunately, despite the restructured objectives and continual commitment to malaria elimination by global parties in 2015, progress in reducing malaria morbidity and mortality has slowed or stalled in many mid- to high-transmission countries. The post-2015 GTS set an interim goal of achieving 40% reductions in malaria case incidence and mortality by 2020, however, the case incidence at that time had only decreased by 3% and mortality decreased by 22% compared to 2015 levels [17].

1.2 Current challenges of vector control

Many factors contribute to the decreased rate of reducing malaria incidence and mortality rates. Population growth in malaria-endemic countries has substantially increased the at-risk population. Initial modeling efforts completed during the creation of the post-2015 GTS predicted that with the existing vector control tools and treatment options available, coverage would have to exceed 80% of high-risk populations to reduce the malaria burden [17]. However, growing populations combined with continuing instabilities of governments, natural disasters, conflicts, and epidemics have hampered the ability to reach this needed intervention coverage. As a result, there has been inadequate access to available vector control interventions. It is estimated that only 46% of the population at risk for malaria is protected by an insecticide-treated net and the percent of at-risk population covered by IRS is only 2.4%, a 2.9% decrease when compared to 2010 coverage [1].

In addition to problems of access, the existing vector control interventions face problems of reduced efficacy due to the widespread emergence of insecticide resistance in the major anopheline vectors. Resistance in the form of either target-site insensitivity or metabolomic changes has been observed for all classes of insecticides currently being used to treat bed nets or in IRS campaigns [18]. Cuticular or penetration resistance has also been observed [19], which also reduces the impact of bed nets and IRS campaigns. As of 2020, only eight of the 82 malaria-endemic countries reported no resistance to all classes of insecticides. Resistance to pyrethroids, the only insecticide approved to treat bed nets, is widespread and resistance was reported in just under 70% of the locations that performed WHO approved standardized testing [1]. The varied resistance mechanisms and wide geographical spread of resistance imposes a major threat to the objectives of the GTS, yet no vector control products based on a new class of insecticide have been introduced to global markets since pyrethroids were introduced in the 1970s however, several have been re-purposed for their use in bed-nets and IRS and new formulations are under development with the World Health Organization Pesticide Evaluation Scheme [20, 21]. An additional challenge to current vector control tactics is behavioral resistance of the mosquito vectors. The long-term use of ITN and IRS creates a selective pressure that has been shown to result in behavioral and population compositional changes of malaria-vectoring species over time [22]. Changes in *An. gambiae* spp., the primary vector species of sub-Saharan Africa, to bite earlier in the day and outdoors (exophilic) have been observed [23, 24]. Changes in population structure to favor exophilic and day-biting malaria vectors such as *An. funestus* also have been implicated in areas where residual transmission of malaria occurs despite good ITN or IRS coverage [25].

An increase in access to vector control interventions to above 80% coverage of at-risk populations will likely lead to a reduction in case incidence and mortality but may not result in the desired 90% reduction of malaria burdens due to the challenges presented by resistance. With no new classes of insecticide approved for the control of malaria, widespread insecticide resistance and evidence of behavioral changes perpetuating residual transmission, the limitations of the current GTS vector control initiatives are obvious. New tools and technologies are needed urgently to meet the 2030 targets of the GTS. Ideally, novel vector control strategies should be cost-effective and sustainable as well as implementable and maintainable in a variety of regions irrespective of changes in government stability, conflicts or catastrophes. Population modification using genetic techniques to confer parasite refractoriness in mosquitoes is one such novel strategy that could greatly aid in achieving the ambitious goals of the GMP.

2. Population modification for malaria control

2.1 What is population modification?

Population modification is the concept of incorporating genes or genetic elements in vector species that increase their refractoriness to the pathogens they transmit thereby inhibiting transfer of the pathogens to host species (**Figure 3**). Population modification was first described in the contemporary literature using the term 'population replacement' by Christopher Curtis in 1968 [26]. Due to misinterpretations of population replacement and negative connotations of the term 'modification' related to cultural perspectives on genetically-modified organisms (GMOs), a third term, 'population alteration', also was proposed [27]. The early conceptions of population modification were made prior to the discovery and refinement of current gene-drive technologies, however, the original concept as proposed by Curtis suggested the need for a mechanism to elicit fixation of the favorable genes in a population. The advancements and development of genetic-engineering techniques to inhibit *Plasmodium* spp. have occurred in

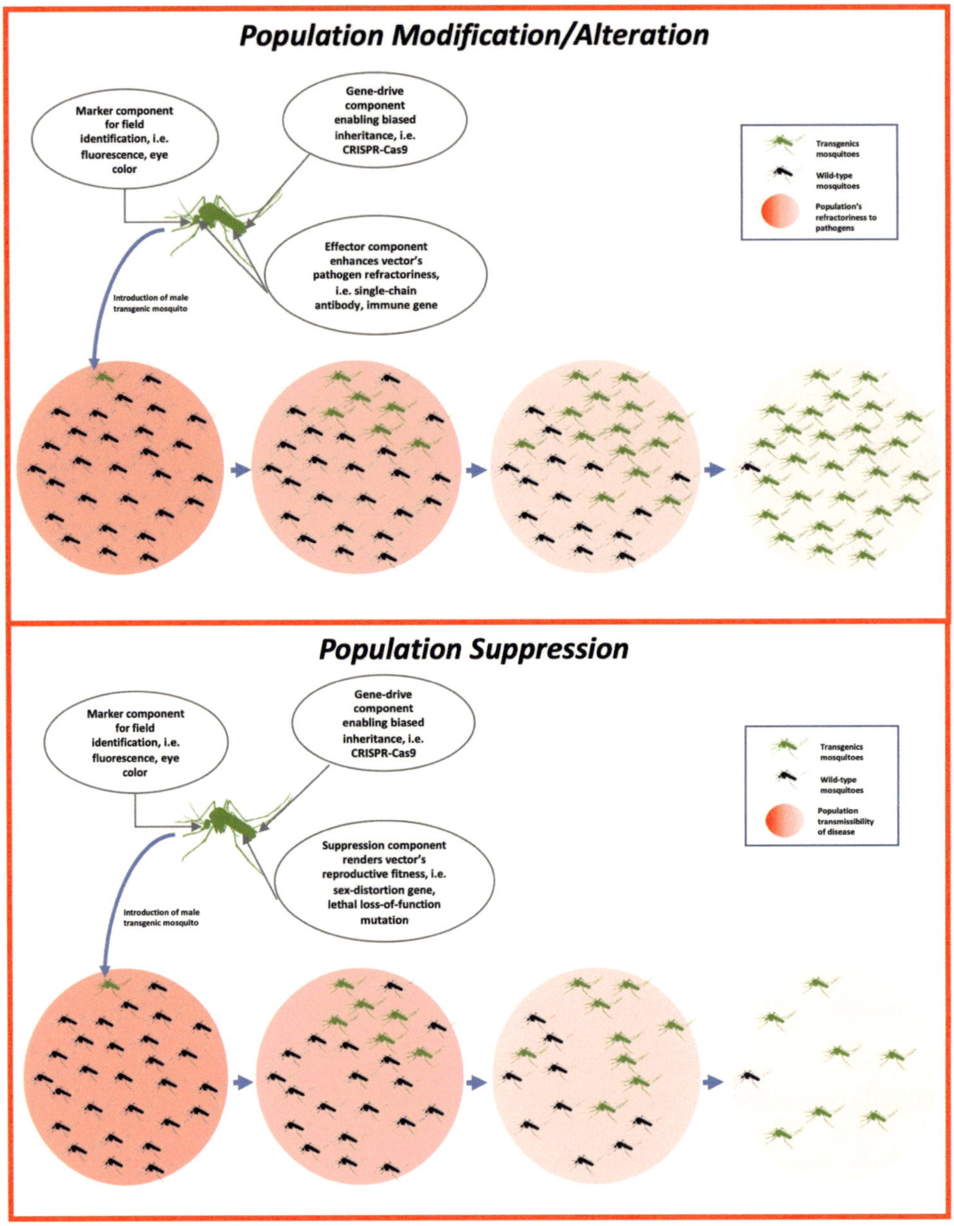

Figure 3.
Outcomes anticipated from genetic control approaches. Vector control strategy utilizes genetic-engineering technology with gene drive via two different approaches, population modification/alteration (top) or population suppression (bottom). In both approaches, the transgenic mosquitoes qualified for releases should carry at least three components: the gene drive system, the marker and the effector or suppression component aiming at reducing the vector competence or the vector population, respectively. The anticipated outcome for the population modification/alteration approach is that the treated population become refractory to pathogen as the effector genes spread into the population; whereas with the population suppression approach the anticipated outcome would be the reduction or elimination of whole population. In both cases, the goal is to break the parasite cycle in the mosquito stages.

parallel with the development of gene-drive technologies and today proof-of-principle concepts for population modification strains exist in both the African malaria vector, *An. gambiae* and the Indo-Pakistani vector, *Anopheles stephensi* (**Table 1**) [28–31].

		AsMCRkh2	Reckh2	AgNosCd-1	AgTP13
Species		*An. stephensi*	*An. stephensi*	*An. gambiae*	*An. gambiae*
Drive system		*vasa*-Cas9	*vasa*-Cas9	*nos*-Cas9	*nos*-Cas9
Target locus		*Kynurenine hydroxylase-white* (kh^{w})	kh^{w}	*Cardinal (cd)*	*cd*
Effector		Cp-1C3, Vg-2A10	None	None	Cp-1C3, Vg-2A10
Drive efficiency	Male	~99%	~99%	~99%	~99%
	Female	65–90%	~56%	~95%	~85–96%
	Maternal effect	Significant	Significant	Mild	Mild
Fitness	Male contribution	Comparable with WT male	Comparable with WT male	mild reduction	Moderate reduction
	Fertility and fecundity	Post Blood meal lethality in homozygotes	Comparable with WT females	Comparable with WT females	Comparable with WT females
Small cage trials	Cage trial ratios, gene drive: wild-type males	1:1, 1:3, 1:10	1:1, 1:3, 1:10	1:1, 1:3, 1:10	1:1, 1:3
	Full introduction result	No	>95% introduction for all ratios	Yes	Yes for 1:1 ratio

Cp, carboxypeptidase gene promoter; Vg, vitellogenin gene promoter; 1C3, 2A10: single-chain antibodies; WT: wild-type.

Table 1.
Proof-of-principle gene-drive systems with and without antimalarial effectors in Anopheles mosquitoes for population modification/alteration strategy.

2.2 Population modification vs. population suppression

Population suppression is an alternative strategy to population modification that utilizes genetic-engineering technologies to reduce vector number and therefore reduce pathogen transmission (**Figure 3**). This can be achieved by diminishing the fitness or distorting sex ratios so that the vector populations reduce in number and eventually go extinct locally. Similar to population modification, proof-of-principle concepts also exist for population suppression in *An. gambiae* [32–34]. The advantages and disadvantages of both population modification and suppression drives are described succinctly in a recent review [35]. One advantage of suppression drives is that they create a rapid reduction in vectorial capacity by immediately having suppressive effects on the targeted mosquito population (reductions in entomological inoculation rate and human biting rate) and thus quickly reducing the basic reproductive rate (R0) of malaria. Another advantage is that suppression drives also will reduce transmission of all possible pathogens vectored by the target species. Unanswered questions that give cause for concern are what happens to the empty ecological niche left by the vector species, and will suppression to extremely low population levels allow re-introduction of wildtype mosquitoes that then transmit the pathogen to a more highly susceptible human population? In contrast, population modification strategies are not likely to have as much of an immediate effect on the vectoral capacity and subsequent R0 as the drive system takes time to introduce the effectors into the population and an R0 < 1 is likely to require a sufficient proportion of the population to carry effector genes [36]. However, population modification strategies do not leave an empty ecological niche and the introduced anti-parasite genes are anticipated to remain stable in a population and this could mitigate the role that re-introduction of infectious wild-type mosquitoes might have in the local population. Population modification is predicted to be sustainable during the control, pre-elimination, elimination, and prevention-of-reintroduction stages of local malaria elimination and thereby provide a cost-effective method for maintaining local elimination [37]. It is expected to be useful in the elimination phase by complementing other strategies that reduce mosquito population sizes. Some potential disadvantages include the potential to select parasites resistant to a single effector mechanism. One strategy to mitigate development of parasite resistance to effectors is by including multiple effector components that target various stages of the parasite development cycle within the mosquito [38]. The effector components used may be exogenous, such as single-chain antibodies (scFvs), endogenous, such as a manipulation of genes associated with mosquito innate immunity or a combination of both [38–41]. A second strategy to mitigate parasite resistance to population modification strains is to reduce the parasite population prior to and during the field release of the modified mosquitoes so that there is less opportunity for resistance to develop due to lower replication rates in the parasite population [42]. Encouragingly, both strategies to mitigate parasite resistance can be combined to provide pathogens with a more insurmountable barrier to developing resistance.

Population modification and population suppression vary in their strengths and weaknesses so a complementary approach that involves the sequential application of both technologies can be proposed (**Figure 4**). This strategy maximizes the benefits of both approaches and lowers their respective hurdles to long-lasting success. The complementary approach includes an initial field release of a population suppression strain that will act to quickly reduce the local population of vectors and their associated population of parasites. When the population structure of native vectors has been sufficiently disrupted by the suppression strategy, the low level of individuals becomes more susceptible to events that may inhibit its ability to persist long term. For example, a re-introduction of wild-type individuals can occur, and these may overwhelm any low levels of remaining drive individuals, or individuals with drive-resistant alleles may build up over time inhibiting future suppression [43]. At this point, when a suppression system has driven the population to levels near extinction, a modification line can be introduced for maximal effect. Allowing a population replacement mosquito line to form the new population of mosquitoes prevents any negative ecological effects that may have occurred due to an empty ecological niche. It also allows the population modification drives to become established in an environment with a minimized risk for resistance to the transgene introduction. The effector genes will be less prone to having pathogen-based resistance develop as the natural pathogen population will have been greatly diminished by the suppression system, and lower pathogen reproduction numbers lower the likelihood of randomly-generated resistance conferring mutations in the pathogens. In the absence of threats from resistance, the only further threat faced by the population modification strain is long-term stability of the effector elements. However, new effector elements can be developed

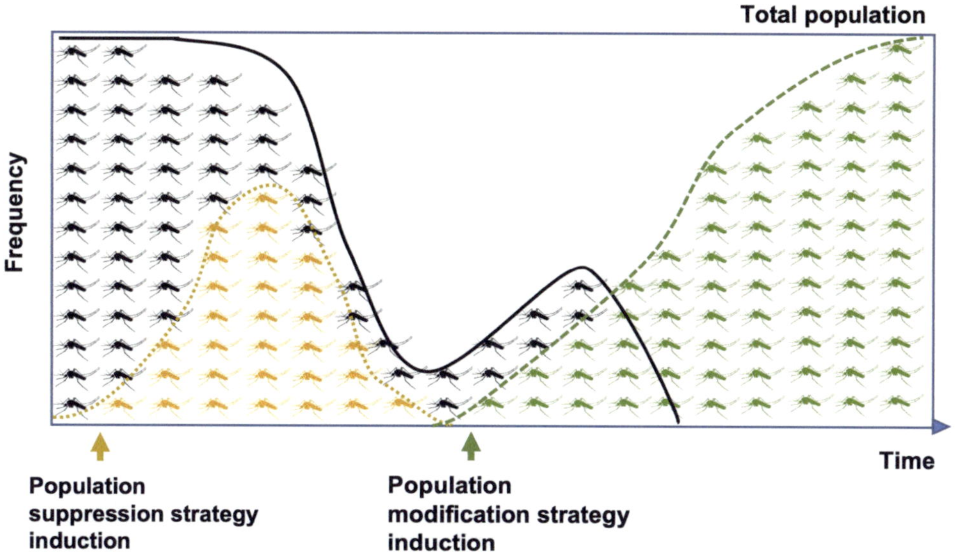

Figure 4.
Vector control with population modification and population suppression complementary approach. Proposed strategy combining sequential releases of mosquitoes with population modification and population suppression drives. The combined approach initiated with releasing population suppression gene-drive mosquitoes, which theoretically reduce the whole mosquito population in the treated area. Follow up with releasing of population modification gene-drive mosquitoes, this strategy ensures avoidance of an empty niche or re-introducing of wild mosquitoes that are susceptible to the malaria parasite. Black: wild-type mosquito; yellow: transgenics mosquitoes with suppression drive; Green: Transgenic mosquitoes with population modification drive.

carefully as the needed window for protection resulting from the complementary approach is likely to be much longer than either approach alone.

3. Engineering refractory mosquitoes

The malaria parasites go through a multi-staged life cycle within their mosquito vectors (**Figure 5**). After the female *Anopheles* mosquito bites an infected human, if ~1000 *Plasmodium* male and female gametocytes are ingested with the blood meal, subsequent fertilization produces as many as 25 diploid zygotes. The zygotes mature to a motile form, the ookinete, that penetrates the mosquito midgut epithelium where only a few (<5) will mature to oocysts. Mitotic and meiotic divisions occur in the oocysts to give rise to several hundred to thousands of haploid sporozoites. The sporozoites (~5000) are released into the hemolymph (the mosquito open circulatory system) within 10–14 days post infection. The sporozoites then travel through the hemolymph to reach and invade the salivary glands and are transmitted as the infectious form of the parasite to a new human host during subsequent bites.

A synthetic approach was used in our laboratory to develop the anti-parasite effector genes and introduce these desired traits into the target genomes to generate the genetically-engineered mosquitoes (GEMs) [37]. This approach has several advantages, for example, the components of a synthetic construct can be relatively small, their functions are more fully known and the site in the mosquito genome where they will be located can be characterized or determined prior to genome integration. A synthetic cassette for population modification has two main components: (1) promoters and (2) antimalarial effector genes.

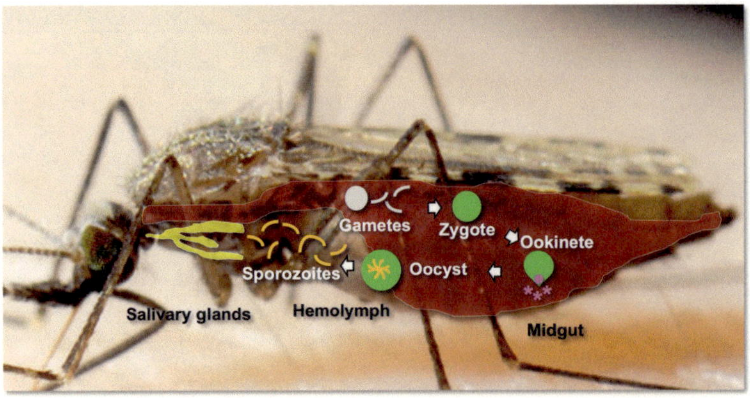

Figure 5.
Malaria developmental pathway and compartments for blocking parasite development. Gametes are ingested with the blood meal. They differentiate, fertile and form a zygote. The zygote develops into a motile form, the ookinete, that then invades the mosquito midgut epithelium. There it develops into an oocyst in which many sporozoites are generated. These burst into the hemolymph and migrate to the salivary glands. From there the sporozoites can be transmitted to a new host during the next blood meal. The midgut compartment allows access to the gametes, zygotes, ookinetes and oocysts. The hemolymph and salivary gland compartments allow access to the sporozoites (image adapted from Isaacs et al. [38]).

3.1 Promoters

Promoters are regulatory DNA sequences that will drive the expression of a transgene (a marker or an antimalarial effector) in mosquitoes. During its development in the mosquito, the malaria parasite occupies three main compartments: midgut lumen, hemocoel and salivary gland lumen (**Figure 5**). Expression of the anti-parasite genes in these compartments is crucial to block their transmission and several tissue-specific promoters have been identified and used in mosquito transgenesis. These include control sequences for a gene encoding a carboxypeptidase, a digestive enzyme, and AgAper1, a peritrophic matrix protein, which are activated in response to a blood meal [44–46]. The vitellogenin-encoding gene promoters drive strong expression in the fat body and hemocoel [47, 48]. A hemocyte-specific hemolectin (hml) gene promoter and three salivary gland-specific promoters, (*Apyrase* [*Apy*], *maltase-like I* [*Mal1*] and *anopheline antiplatelet protein* [*AAPP*] promoter), also have been developed [49–52]. Ubiquitously-expressed gene promoters (*heat-shock protein 70* [*hsp70*], *actin 5C*, and *ubiquitin* and *polyubiquitin*) also could be used to drive expression of the effector genes, however, their generalized expression may impose a higher fitness load in the GEM [53–55]. These gene promoters have been used effectively to drive the expression of genes encoding generally benign fluorescent proteins as dominant markers for transgene presence.

3.2 Antimalarial effector genes

The effector molecules can be classified into four groups depending on their mode of action.

i. Parasite blocking: exogenous molecules that eliminate the parasites such as antimicrobial peptides from the immune system of other insects (gambicin, defensin, cecropin) or other arthropods (scorpine). Natural and synthetic lytic peptides such as angiotensin II, magainins, Shiva-1, Shiva-3 and gomesin have been used to generate refractory *Plasmodium* mosquitoes [56–62].

ii. Interaction with parasites: single-chain monoclonal antibodies (scFvs) that bind to ookinete or sporozoite surface or secreted proteins, such as m2A10 that targets the *P. falciparum* circumsporozoite protein (CSP), m1C3 that binds to the *P. falciparum* chitinase, scFv 4B7 that binds to *P. falciparum* ookinete surface protein Pfs25, and peptides that inhibits mosquito midgut invasion (EPIP- *Plasmodium* enolase-plasminogen interaction peptide) [38, 39, 63].

iii. Interaction with mosquito tissues: molecules that bind putative mosquito receptors in the midgut or salivary glands blocking the ookinete and sporozoite invasion (for example, SM1) and molecules that can modify the properties of the midgut epithelia (mPLA2- phospholipase A2) [64, 65].

iv. Mosquito immune system: manipulation of mosquito immune-related genes can lead to decreased mosquito vectorial competence. Expression of Akt, a key signaling component in the insulin signaling pathway or overexpression of IMD pathway-mediated transcription factor Rel2 can result in refractoriness to the parasite [66, 67].

The identification and characterization of efficient anti-*Plasmodium* effector genes is essential to generate refractory mosquito phenotypes. Expression of these genes may result in GEMs being less competitive than their wild-type counterparts. Ideally, the effector molecules should interfere with parasite transmission without imposing a fitness cost to the mosquito. Furthermore, these genes clearly impose selection pressures on the parasites and the emergence of parasites resistant to the effector molecules could occur. As discussed previously, this may be mitigated by using combinations of multiple anti-*Plasmodium* effector proteins with different modes of action that can overcome the possibility of parasite resistance. Recently, Dong et al. (2020) showed that it is possible to generate a transgenic line (MultiEff) expressing simultaneously five anti-*Plasmodium* effectors (melittin, TP10, shiva1, EPIP, and scorpine) with a significant parasite-blocking effect at the pre-oocyst stage and low fitness cost [68].

4. Spreading transgenes into mosquito populations

Mobile genetic elements called transposons can spread rapidly through populations despite severe costs to the host [69–72]. Their ability to mobilize (excise and insert) led to their being developed as powerful systems for introducing exogenous DNA into several organisms. The adaptation of the P transposable element for transgenesis of the vinegar fly, *Drosophila melanogaster*, was followed 16 years later by the first reliable system for transforming mosquitoes using the *Hermes* elements in the yellow fever mosquito, *Aedes aegypti* [73, 74]. Shortly after this proof-of-principle in mosquitoes, additional systems based on *Hermes, piggyBac, Minos, and mariner Mos1* were demonstrated in both culicine and anopheline species [75–82]. Unfortunately, while transposons could mediate insertion into these genomes at experimentally-useful frequencies, they were not easily remobilized making them impractical as a basis of a gene-drive system to spread transgenes through a mosquito population [83–85].

Other tools and systems for introducing genes into mosquito genomes include site-specific recombinases. These require the presence of an endogenous nucleotide sequence in the genome that is identical to the recombinase target cleavage site, or a mechanism for introducing such a site (called a docking site; [86]) into that genome. This has been achieved using the previously-described transposons. Two recombinases have been used successfully to generate transgenic mosquitoes, the bacteriophage φC31 integrase and Cre/lox recombinase derived from yeast. Their dependence on a precise site for integration of the desired transgene limits their usefulness as the basis of gene-drive systems for spreading transgenes into populations [82, 87–90].

The application of zinc-finger nuclease (ZFNs) and the transcription activator-like effector nucleases (TALENs) for engineering target-site recognition in mosquitoes introduced a major advance for genetic modification in mosquitoes. However, the high cost and low success rate limited their use [91–93]. The application of homing endonucleases nucleases genes (HEGs) for spreading genes into mosquito populations was proposed in 2003 [94] as useful basis for gene drives and in 2011 a successful HEG-based gene drive in *An. gambiae* was reported [95]. The latter required the fortuitous presence of a nuclease target site in the first chromosome (X) of this species.

A major breakthrough for mosquito transgenesis and gene-drive systems was achieved following the discovery and adaptation of the RNA-guided Cas9 nuclease from the bacterial Clustered Regularly Interspaced Short Palindromic Repeats (CRISPR/Cas9) adaptive immune system [96]. This powerful tool simplified the highly-specific genome editing processes and made possible useful gene-drive systems. The Cas9 endonuclease is directed to its genomic target by a single 20 base-pair guide RNA (gRNA) complementary to its DNA target. This gRNA can be designed to target virtually any locus in a chromosome. CRISPR/Cas9 exploits the natural mechanism of cell repair to precisely insert a synthetic construct through homology-directed repair (HDR), a DNA repair system initiated by a double-strand break made at the site of a target location by the Cas9 nuclease [96]. CRISPR/Cas9 has been shown to be an excellent candidate technology for developing gene drive-based strategies to introduce beneficial genes into mosquito populations [28–30]. The properties of the system bias the inheritance of a desired trait, allowing them to quickly increase in frequency and spread through a mosquito population. CRISPR/Cas9 gene drives can efficiently convert pre-meiotic diploid germline cells in hemizygous mosquitoes (carrying one copy of the drive) into homozygotes carrying two copies [28–30]. Recently, the CRISPR/Cas9 technology has been adapted for the development of gene drives in anopheline mosquitoes and shows great promise for rapid introduction of anti-parasite genes into mosquito populations [28–30, 32].

5. CRISPR/Cas9 gene drives for population modification

The recent adaptation of CRISPR/Cas9-based biology to generate gene drives has been proposed to provide a powerful, inexpensive, and easily-implemented solution for malaria control due to the rapid introduction of the antimalarial genes into mosquito populations [37]. To produce the desired epidemiological outcomes of reduced malaria transmission, the drive system and associated effector components must be introduced quickly and efficiently into wild populations. Rapid introduction requires population modification lines to have high rates of drive allele conversion in the germline so that maximally-biased inheritance is achieved. This will result in a remarkable increase in frequency of the gene-drive system in the following generations.

The first CRISPR/Cas9 gene drive for mosquito population modification was described in 2015 for the Indo-Pakistani vector, *An. stephensi* [28]. The AsMCRkh2 gene-drive synthetic cassette used targets the ommochrome biosynthesis pathway involved in development of mosquito eye-color, specifically the locus that encodes the kynurenine hydroxylase (kynurenine monooxygenase) enzyme (referred here as *kynurenine hydroxylase white* [kh^{w}]). Mutations in the gene encoding this enzyme have a recessive white-eye phenotype. Drive efficiency in the AsMCRkh2 line was high with ~99% of progeny from both male and female hemizygous parents inheriting a copy of the drive allele [28]. Despite high initial efficiencies from both male and females, follow-up analyses of these lineages uncovered a return to near Mendelian inheritance in the progeny derived from female hemizygous parents. The diminished drive efficiency in female lineages was later attributed to the accumulation of indel alleles in these offspring (Section 6.2). Drive efficiency experiments in a second-generation *An. stephensi* population modification line, Reckh, resembled the observed efficiencies in the AsMCRkh2 line with ~99% of the progeny from hemizygous male parents inheriting a copy of the drive after two generations of outcrossing to wild-type mosquitoes and only ~56% of progeny from hemizygous female parents inheriting a copy of the drive after two generations of outcrosses [30].

A next-generation gene drive system for *An. gambiae* was developed [29]. The resulting strain, AgNosCd-1, targets the *An. gambiae cardinal* gene ortholog, encoding a protein downstream of the *kh* product in the ommochrome pathway. Mosquitoes with two loss-of function (LOF) alleles at this locus have a red-eye phenotype in subadult stages and newly-emerged adults (**Table 1**). AgNosCd-1 has a high drive efficiency in both male and female lineages (maternal/paternal daughters/sons and grand-daughters/grand-sons). AgNosCd-1 hemizygous males can pass the drive system with ~99% efficiency within their lineages and hemizygous females had only a slightly reduced ~95% drive efficiency within their lineages [29]. The individuals not inheriting a copy of the drive were found to have wild-type alleles as opposed to insertion or deletion (indel) alleles indicating that failures of the drive system were more likely due to Cas9/gRNA complexes not performing cleavage as opposed to cleavages that did not result in HDR [97]. Moreover, the AgNosCd-1 drive efficiency achieved a 98–100% inheritance bias in both males and females and full introduction within six to ten generations following single releases of gene drive males in small laboratory cage trials [29]. Drive efficiency experiments in a second-generation AgNosCd-1 population modification line, AgTP13 (AgNosCd-1 background linked to two anti-parasite effector genes), resulted in similar rates of drive efficiency in hemizygous males and females suggesting no impact of the effector load on the ability of the drive system to facilitate accurate HDR in the germline [31].

6. CRISPR/Cas9 considerations

6.1 Fitness impacts

The fitness load in population modification CRISPR/Cas9 drive lines have been assessed on male and female mosquitoes. An ideal CRISPR/Cas9 drive candidate for population modification would have little-to-no fitness effects resulting from the drive system and its corresponding locus, as it is predicted that the effector components are likely to have some effect on overall fitness [98, 99].

One notable example of a fitness cost was observed in the *An. stephensi* AsMCRkh2 gene drive line following disruption of both copies of the kh^{w} gene. As described, the enzyme encoded by this gene is responsible for generating the precursors for the formation of eye-pigments, but interestingly it also plays an important role in tryptophan metabolism in adult females following a blood meal [100, 101]. AsMCRkh2 individuals containing two LOF alleles resulting from homozygous or heteroallelic combinations of gene-drive construct insertions or Non-Homologous End Joining (NHEJ) alleles produce a white-eye phenotype and show a high lethality and reduced fecundity following a blood meal. Follow up experiments showed that after achieving fixation in multi-generation cage trial experiments, the populations experienced extinction due to the significant fertility and fecundity load on homozygous AsMCRkh2 females [100]. The AsMCRkh2 prototype was later modified to include a re-coded version of the *kh* locus (Reckh) to reduce the previously observed fitness load on females by restoring the function of the *kh* gene and thereby reversing the eye phenotype to wild-type [30]. Homozygous Reckh female adults show no significant differences in fertility and fecundity in comparison to the hemizygous Reckh or wild-type females. The improvements of female fitness translated to the success of the drive system in multi-generational cage trials with >95% of individuals carrying a copy of the drive at the termination of the experiments [30].

In contrast, AgNosCd-1 individuals do not have reduced fitness in most of the fitness parameters evaluated (fertility, fecundity, longevity, larval and pupal development), but a mild reduction in male mating competitiveness was observed [29]. AgNosCd-1 males are slightly less likely to contribute to the next generation than wild-type males, ~2% less likely for hemizygote males and ~8% for homozygote males. Despite these observed reductions in fitness, the power of the drive system was sufficient to negate the effects in subsequent generations and the AgNosCd-1 line achieved fixation in all multi-generation cage trial experiments at different release ratios of homozygous AgNosCd-1 to wild type males [29]. However, the AgTP13 homozygous males were ~22% less likely to contribute to the next generation than wild-type males in competition experiments and have a significantly reduced median lifespan than the hemizygous AgTP13 or the wild-type males. Despite the increased fitness burden in AgTP13 males, there was no increased fitness load on AgTP13 females [31]. Theoretical modeling supports the conclusion that given an appropriate drive mechanism, a gene-drive system could have a significant fitness cost and still be driven through the population [102, 103].

Ideally, GEMs should have no or minimal fitness costs to avoid reducing the effectiveness of the genetic drive mechanism that is used to introduce the synthetic construct into field mosquito populations and to maximize the likelihood of successfully introducing refractory genes into a wild population [98]. Several factors can impact the fitness, including the possible negative effect of the transgene products, insertional position effects (chromatin rearrangement and/or new regulatory element interactions/pressure), inbreeding, and to "leaky (low level constitutive) promoter expression". GEMS can have different degrees of fitness cost and estimates of transgene fitness costs are essential for modeling and planning release strategies. However, it is clear that a robust drive system can compensate for reduced fitness.

6.2 Maternal effects and resistant alleles

The efficacy of population modification mosquito drive lines may be reduced by the presence of naturally-occurring cleavage-resistant allelic variants of the target site in wild populations or by such alleles generated through NHEJ during the Cas9/gRNA targeting and DNA repair processes. The latter may result from double-stranded DNA breaks necessary for drive that are occasionally repaired through NHEJ resulting in insertions or deletions at the target site, making them refractory to the drive system. Both the naturally-occurring and induced allelic variants have been called resistance alleles [104–107]. The latter may arise in the germline and be passed on to subsequent generations or may be generated in somatic cells where they give rise to mosaic phenotypes [28–30]. Resistance alleles in the form of naturally-occurring mutations at the target site can be avoided by careful choice of the gene-drive target locus. Resistance alleles occurring because of NHEJ due to undesired Cas9 activity can be controlled by careful choice of the promoter used to induce Cas9 transcription.

Extensive analysis of suitable target loci must be performed prior to the creation of each proof-of-principle modification drive system. Loci must be chosen, in part, based on the minimization of naturally-present single nucleotide polymorphisms (SNPs) and overall conservation of the target site. Several SNPs in the AgNosCd-1 *cardinal* target site were identified after a screening effort of hundreds of diverse *Anopheles gambiae* s.l. sequences [29]. Interestingly, all these major variants still exhibited Cas9/gRNA-mediated cleavage in assays *in vitro*.

The pathways and frequency of resistance allele formation via undesired activity of the drive system was analyzed extensively for the AgNosCd-1 and AsMCRkh2 lines [29, 97]. Exceptional phenotype individuals (mosaics and LOF phenotypes) have been correlated to undesired Cas9 activity and possess indel mutations that would cause LOF in AgNosCd-1 and AsMCRkh2 lines. However, in contrast to the AgNosCd-1 drive system, the mosaic and LOF phenotypes made up the majority of the offspring (>99%) from AsMCRkh2 mothers [28]. The presence of mosaic and LOF phenotypes from female drive parents has been hypothesized to occur due to a maternal effect. The maternal effect is proposed to result from the accumulation of Cas9/gRNA complexes in the cytoplasm of embryos derived from mothers carrying the drive system, which perform cleavage on the paternally-donated allele during embryonic development. The differences in mosaic and LOF phenotypes observed in the progeny from AgNosCd-1 and AsMCRkh2 hemizygote females supports this hypothesis and this affect is higher in females with two copies (homozygous) of the drive system than those with one (hemizygous) [28, 29, 97]. In addition, the frequencies of such events are higher in the AsMCRkh2 line when compared to AgNosCd-1. These differences may result from the difference in the gene promoters used to express the Cas9 nuclease for each drive system, *vasa* for AsMCRkh2 and *nanos* for AgNosCd-1. Follow up studies showed that the transcripts expressed from the *nanos* promoter are more confined to germline cells than those expressed from the *vasa* promoter [108], which likely results in fewer Cas9/gRNA complexes in the cytoplasm of the former embryos.

As described previously, females homozygous for the drive system had a higher rate of resistance allele formation via maternal effect (~57% with mosaic phenotype and ~6% of progeny with LOF phenotype) than hemizygous females (~20% with mosaic phenotype and ~1% of progeny with LOF phenotype) but mosaic individuals were able to bias inheritance of the drive allele and had similar rates of drive efficiency when compared to AgNosCd-1 hemizygotes with wild-type eye phenotypes suggesting that the indels were primary somatic [29].

Suppression gene drive systems are much less flexible to drive-resistant alleles than population modification gene drive systems. Population modification mosquito lines can tolerate higher rates of drive-resistant alleles than population suppression mosquitoes, however, the former are still susceptible to instability and inability to achieve fixation in a population due to resistance alleles, especially if the drive system and respective cargo are associated with a significant fitness load [109]. Recent work suggests that suppression drive systems that incur a 100% fitness cost (death of females) would require a very low frequency of drive resistant alleles $<5 \times 10^{-7}$ in order to provide a 4–5-year window of protection, as opposed to population modification systems, which would provide a 4–5-year window of protection at a resistance allele frequency of 1%, given that fitness costs of the population modification strain are below 15% [109].

Multiplexed gene drives using additional gRNA target sites are expected to substantially decrease the likelihood of gene-drive resistant allele formation [110]. Practical ways to multiplex Cas9-based gene drives have been demonstrated using post-transcriptional processing of several gRNAs expressed from a single promoter, but these have not yet been applied to mosquitoes [110–113].

6.3 Off-targets

The utility of CRISPR/Cas9 gene-drive systems may be affected by sequence similarity among gRNAs target and off-target sites in the mosquito genomes. Potential off-target sites can be predicted *in silico* by computational algorithms and then confirmed *in vivo* by deep-sequence screening of indels or SNPs by PCR-based assays. The possible impact of unwanted mutations linked to a drive system are higher since the arising mutations will have the potential to persist within the populations. Off-target mutations also can induce a potential fitness load. Efforts to detect Cas9 off-targets in *An. gambiae* gene drive mosquitoes found very few following sequencing of large number of samples containing putative target variants [29]. The detected indels neither increased in frequency nor were detected through multiple generations in long-term cage trials (indicating that they were not heritable) and did not significantly differ in number from variants observed in wild-type individuals [29]. New approaches to increase Cas9 specificity are being developed in other organisms and include the use of highly-specific Cas9 mutant enzymes together with the constant updating of computational algorithms to better predict the possible off-targets, but their applications for gene drive mosquitoes remain unclear [114–119].

6.4 Deployment challenges

The discovery, development, and deployment of CRISPR/Cas9 technologies is challenging due to the lack of an accepted pathway to move them from the laboratory to the field. The WHO released in 2014 the Guidance Framework for testing genetically modified (GM) mosquitoes (WHO Guidance Framework) describing a phased testing pathway and best practices to evaluate GEMs proposed as public health tools [120]. The Framework proposes a pathway to move from physically-confined studies in the laboratory/insectary (Phase 1) to a small-scale confined field-testing (Phase 2) that will lead to a staged open release trial (Phase 3). After successful completion of Phase 3, the national authorities in a malaria-endemic country will be responsible for determining if the tested GEMs can be included as part of their malaria control program and further deployment of the technology (Phase 4) [120]. However, pathways for moving gene-drive population modification mosquitoes to the field will be defined simultaneously with the laboratory work progress. As more CRISPR/Cas9 population modification gene-drive systems and strains are developed, new knowledge is being generated about the impact of introduced anti-parasite genes on the mosquitoes that carry them. Insight into genetic loads and their effects on fitness, generation of drive-resistant individuals as well as selection of resistant parasites and long-term stability of the system will emerge from these studies. The new empirical data generated is critical in the development of a phased pathway for further development and deployment. In 2018, James et al. published a series of recommendations that attempt to envision the development pathway for gene drive mosquitoes (from discovery to deployment) and to inform decision-making by regulators and policymakers [121]. They recognized that it is important to examine both the benefits and risks of this approach. Risk assessment will provide guidance on decision-making and information for the regulatory applications as well as for the development of mitigation plans, while cost-benefit analyses will compare the projected or estimated costs and benefits associated to the intervention. It also was recommended that these analyses be done by external third-party organizations or institutions with no interests in the success of the product and the outcomes of these analyses be made publicly available.

Any decision made to release gene-drive mosquitoes must be made on a case-by-case basis following a comprehensive environmental risk assessment [122], moreover, gene-drive population modification mosquitoes must meet the established Target Product Profile (TPP) criteria of safety and efficacy. A comprehensive draft TPP for gene-drive population modification mosquitoes was published providing the basis for evaluation of whether gene-drive mosquitoes should be made available for use [37]. Population modification TPPs will need to meet the efficacy and safety standards as well as the demands of different regulatory and social contexts. In addition, viable models for the inclusion of end-user and stakeholder involvement and control are absolutely needed before any such system can be brought to the field. We have favored the relationship-based model (RBM), which gives stakeholders and community key roles at the center of the decision-making processes [123]. It is important that open dialog and relationships with the scientists developing the technologies be established and that appropriate capacity-building take place to empower the communities affected by malaria to make informed decisions about the risk and use of the new technologies.

7. Conclusions

Population modification genetic control focuses on targeting the mosquito vector to interrupt the malaria transmission by introducing effector genes into the mosquito genome with the purpose of generating parasite-refractory mosquitoes.

Advances in gene-editing technologies using CRISPR/Cas9 gene drives have made available new possibilities for an efficient introduction of the desired genetic traits into mosquito populations. Gene drives represent a powerful tool to achieve genome editing in a species-specific targeted way with minimal infrastructure, are predicted to be self-sustaining and able to spread anti-parasite effectors to fixation.

Gene-drive systems for population modification of anopheline vector species to prevent transmission of parasites may play a future role in the malaria eradication agenda. Future steps will need to consider how to evaluate gene drives at large scale and evaluate their efficacy and robustness under more realistic ecological settings.

Challenges to such technologies are being addressed by scientists and regulators by development of pathways for their deployment and establishing acceptable efficacy and safety criteria. Importantly, the knowledge transfer process is being addressed in new models for public engagement that will further development, testing and eventual deployment of gene drives for malaria control.

Acknowledgements

Funding was provided by the University of California Irvine Malaria Initiative and 'anonymous donor'. AAJ is a Donald Bren Professor at the University of California, Irvine.

Conflict of interest

The authors declare no conflict of interest.

Author details

Rebeca Carballar-Lejarazú[1*†], Taylor Tushar[1†], Thai Binh Pham[2] and Anthony James[1,2]

1 Department of Microbiology and Molecular Genetics, University of California, Irvine, CA, USA

2 Department of Molecular Biology and Biochemistry, University of California, Irvine, CA, USA

*Address all correspondence to: rcarball@uci.edu

† These authors contribute equally to the preparation of this chapter.

References

[1] World Health Organization. World Malaria Report 2020: 20 Years of Global Progress and Challenges. Geneva: World Health Organization; 2020. Available from: https://www.who.int/publications/i/item/9789240015791

[2] Keiser J, De Castro MC, Maltese MF, Bos R, Tanner M, Singer BH, et al. Effect of irrigation and large dams on the burden of malaria on a global and regional scale. The American Journal of Tropical Medicine and Hygiene. 2005;**72**(4):392-406

[3] Pampana E. A Textbook of Malaria Eradication. 2nd ed. London, New York, Toronto: OXFORD University Press; 1969

[4] Nájera JA, González-Silva M, Alonso PL. Some lessons for the future from the Global Malaria Eradication Programme (1955-1969). PLoS Medicine. 2011;**8**(1):e1000412. DOI: 10.1371/journal.pmed.1000412

[5] Li XH, Kondrashin A, Greenwood B, Lindblade K, Loku Galappaththy G, Alonso P. A historical review of WHO certification of malaria elimination. Trends in Parasitology. 2019;**35**(2):163-171. DOI: 10.1016/j.pt.2018.11.011. Epub 2019 Jan 10

[6] Carter R, Mendis KN. Evolutionary and historical aspects of the burden of malaria. Clinical Microbiology Reviews. 2002;**15**(4):564-594. DOI: 10.1128/CMR.15.4.564-594.2002

[7] World Health Organization. World Malaria Report 2012. Geneva: World Health Organization; 2012. Available from: https://www.who.int/malaria/publications/world_malaria_report_2012/wmr2012_full_report.pdf

[8] World Health Organization. World Malaria Report 2021. Geneva: World Health Organization; 2021. Available from: https://www.who.int/teams/global-malaria-programme/reports/world-malaria-report-2021

[9] World Health Organization. The Global Health Observatory, Estimated Number of Malaria Death [Internet]. World Health Organization; 2022. Available from: https://www.who.int/data/gho/data/indicators/indicator-details/GHO/estimated-number-of-malaria-deaths

[10] Ghebreyesus TA. The malaria eradication challenge. Lancet. 2019;**394**(10203):990-991. DOI: 10.1016/S0140-6736(19)31951-8

[11] Nasir SMI, Amarasekara S, Wickremasinghe R, Fernando D, Udagama P. Prevention of re-establishment of malaria: Historical perspective and future prospects. Malaria Journal. 2020;**19**(1):452. DOI: 10.1186/s12936-020-03527-8

[12] World Health Organization. Information on the world malaria situation. In: Weekly Epidemiological Record. Vol. 52(07). Geneva: World Health Organization; 1977. p. 65. Available from: https://apps.who.int/iris/handle/10665/221226

[13] Murray CJL, Rosenfeld L, Lim S, Andrews K, Foreman K, Haring D, et al. Global malaria mortality between 1980 and 2010: A systematic analysis. The Lancet. 2012;**379**(9814):413-431. DOI: 10.1016/S0140-6736(12)60034-8

[14] Way C. The Millennium Development Goals Report. New York, United Nations:

2015. Available from: https://www.un.org/millenniumgoals/2015_MDG_Report/pdf/MDG%202015%20rev%20(July%201).pdf

[15] Roll Back Malaria. Global Malaria Action Plan For a Malaria-free World. 2008. Available from: https://www.unhcr.org/4afac5629.pdf

[16] Newby G, Bennett A, Larson E, Cotter C, Shretta R, Phillips AA, et al. The path to eradication: A progress report on the malaria-eliminating countries. Lancet. 2016;**387**(10029):1775-1784. DOI: 10.1016/S0140-6736(16)00230-0

[17] World Health Organization. Global Technical Strategy for Malaria 2016-2030, 2021 Update. Geneva: World Health Organization; 2021. Available from: https://www.who.int/publications/i/item/9789240031357

[18] Sougoufara S, Sokhna C, Diagne N, Doucouré S, Sembène PM, Harry M. The implementation of long-lasting insecticidal bed nets has differential effects on the genetic structure of the African malaria vectors in the *Anopheles gambiae* complex in Dielmo, Senegal. Malaria Journal. 2017;**16**(1):337. DOI: 10.1186/s12936-017-1992-8

[19] Riveron J, Tchouakui M, Mugenzi L, Menze B, Chiang MC, Wondji C. Insecticide resistance in malaria vectors: An update at a global scale. In: Manguin S, Dev V, editors. Toward Malaria Elimination—A Leap Forward [Internet]. London: IntechOpen; 2018. DOI: 10.5772/intechopen.78375. Available from: https://www.intechopen.com/chapters/62169

[20] Kupfershmidt K. Pick your poison. Science. 2016;**354**(6309):171-173. DOI: 10.1126/science.354.6309.171

[21] World Health Organization. Report of the twentieth WHOPES working group meeting, WHO/HQ, Geneva, 20-24 March 2017: Review of Interceptor G2LN, DawaPlus 3.0 LN, DawaPlus 4.0 LN, SumiLarv 2 MR, Chlorfenapyr 240 SC. Geneva: World Health Organization; 2017. Available from: https://www.who.int/publications/i/item/who-htm-ntd-whopes-2017.04

[22] Sougoufara S, Ottih EC, Tripet F. The need for new vector control approaches targeting outdoor biting Anopheline malaria vector communities. Parasites & Vectors. 2020;**13**(1):295. DOI: 10.1186/s13071-020-04170-7

[23] Wamae PM, Githeko AK, Otieno GO, Kabiru EW, Duombia SO. Early biting of the *Anopheles gambiae s.s*. and its challenges to vector control using insecticide treated nets in western Kenya highlands. Acta Tropica. 2015;**150**:136-142. DOI: 10.1016/j.actatropica.2015.07.008

[24] Meyer Steiger DB, Ritchie SA, Laurance SG. Mosquito communities and disease risk influenced by land use change and seasonality in the Australian tropics. Parasites & Vectors. 2016;**9**(1):387. DOI: 10.1186/s13071-016-1675-2

[25] Russell TL, Govella NJ, Azizi S, Drakeley CJ, Kachur SP, Killeen GF. Increased proportions of outdoor feeding among residual malaria vector populations following increased use of insecticide-treated nets in rural Tanzania. Malaria Journal. 2011;**10**:80. DOI: 10.1186/1475-2875-10-80

[26] Curtis CF. Possible use of translocations to fix desirable genes in insect pest populations. Nature. 1968;**218**(5139):368-369. DOI: 10.1038/218368a0

[27] Roberts A, Andrade PP, Okumu F, Quemada H, Savadogo M, Singh JA, et al. Results from the workshop "problem formulation for the use of gene drive in mosquitoes". The American Journal of Tropical Medicine and Hygiene. 2017;**96**(3):530-533. DOI: 10.4269/ajtmh.16-0726

[28] Gantz VM, Jasinskiene N, Tatarenkova O, Fazekas A, Macias VM, Bier E, et al. Highly efficient Cas9-mediated gene drive for population modification of the malaria vector mosquito *Anopheles stephensi*. Proceedings of the National Academy of Sciences of the United States of America. 2015;**112**:E6736-E6743. DOI: 10.1073/pnas.1521077112

[29] Carballar-Lejarazú R, Ogaugwu C, Tushar T, Kelsey A, Pham TB, Murphy J, et al. Next-generation gene drive for population modification of the malaria vector mosquito, *Anopheles gambiae*. Proceedings of the National Academy of Sciences of the United States of America. 2020;**117**(37):22805-22814. DOI: 10.1073/pnas.2010214117

[30] Adolfi A, Gantz VM, Jasinskiene N, Lee HF, Hwang K, Terradas G, et al. Efficient population modification gene-drive rescue system in the malaria mosquito *Anopheles stephensi*. Nature Communications. 2020;**11**(1):5553. DOI: 10.1038/s41467-020-19426-0

[31] Carballar-Lejarazú R, Dong YM, Pham TB, Tushar T, Marshall J, Dimopoulos G, et al. An autonomous gene-drive strain for population modification of the African malaria mosquito, *Anopheles gambiae* (in preparation)

[32] Hammond A, Galizi R, Kyrou K, Simoni A, Siniscalchi C, Katsanos D, et al. A CRISPR-Cas9 gene drive system targeting female reproduction in the malaria mosquito vector *Anopheles gambiae*. Nature Biotechnology. 2016;**34**(1):78-83. DOI: 10.1038/nbt.3439

[33] Kyrou K, Hammond AM, Galizi R, Kranjc N, Burt A, Beaghton AK, et al. A CRISPR-Cas9 gene drive targeting doublesex causes complete population suppression in caged *Anopheles gambiae* mosquitoes. Nature Biotechnology. 2018;**36**(11):1062-1066. DOI: 10.1038/nbt.4245

[34] Simoni A, Hammond AM, Beaghton AK, Galizi R, Taxiarchi C, Kyrou K, et al. A male-biased sex-distorter gene drive for the human malaria vector *Anopheles gambiae*. Nature Biotechnology. 2020;**38**(9):1054-1060. DOI: 10.1038/s41587-020-0508-1

[35] Bier E. Gene drives gaining speed. Nature Reviews. Genetics. 2022;**23**:5-22. DOI: 10.1038/s41576-021-00386-0

[36] Eckhoff PA, Wenger EA, Godfray HC, Burt A. Impact of mosquito gene drive on malaria elimination in a computational model with explicit spatial and temporal dynamics. Proceedings of the National Academy of Sciences of the United States of America. 2017;**114**(2):E255-E264. DOI: 10.1073/pnas.1611064114

[37] Carballar-Lejarazú R, James AA. Population modification of Anopheline species to control malaria transmission. Pathogens and Global Health. 2017;**111**(8):424-435. DOI: 10.1080/20477724.2018.1427192

[38] Isaacs AT, Jasinskiene N, Tretiakov M, Thiery I, Zettor A, Bourgouin C, et al. Transgenic *Anopheles stephensi* coexpressing single-chain antibodies resist *plasmodium* falciparum development. Proceedings

of the National Academy of Sciences of the United States of America. 2012;**109**(28):E1922-E1930. DOI: 10.1073/pnas.1207738109

[39] Isaacs AT, Li F, Jasinskiene N, Chen X, Nirmala X, Marinotti O, et al. Engineered resistance to *plasmodium* falciparum development in transgenic *Anopheles stephensi*. PLoS Pathogens. 2011;**7**(4):e1002017. DOI: 10.1371/journal.ppat.1002017

[40] de Lara CM, Coleman J, Beerntsen BT, Myles KM, Olson KE, Rocha E, et al. Virus-expressed, recombinant single-chain antibody blocks sporozoite infection of salivary glands in *Plasmodium gallinaceum*-infected *Aedes aegypti*. The American Journal of Tropical Medicine and Hygiene. 2000;**62**(4):427-433. DOI: 10.4269/ajtmh.2000.62.427

[41] Cirimotich CM, Dong Y, Garver LS, Sim S, Dimopoulos G. Mosquito immune defenses against *Plasmodium* infection. Developmental and Comparative Immunology. 2010;**34**(4):387-395. DOI: 10.1016/j.dci.2009.12.005

[42] Marshall JM, Raban RR, Kandul NP, Edula JR, León TM, Akbari OS. Winning the tug-of-war between effector gene design and pathogen evolution in vector population replacement strategies. Frontiers in Genetics. 2019;**10**:1072. DOI: 10.3389/fgene.2019.01072

[43] Godfray HCJ, North A, Burt A. How driving endonuclease genes can be used to combat pests and disease vectors. BMC Biology. 2017;**15**(1):81. DOI: 10.1186/s12915-017-0420-4

[44] Moreira LA, Edwards MJ, Adhami F, Jasinskiene N, James AA, Jacobs-Lorena M. Robust gut-specific gene expression in transgenic *Aedes aegypti* mosquitoes. Proceedings of the National Academy of Sciences of the United States of America. 2000;**97**(20):10895-10898. DOI: 10.1073/pnas.97.20.10895

[45] Ito J, Ghosh A, Moreira LA, Wimmer EA, Jacobs-Lorena M. Transgenic anopheline mosquitoes impaired in transmission of a malaria parasite. Nature. 2002;**417**(6887):452-455. DOI: 10.1038/417452a

[46] Abraham EG, Donnelly-Doman M, Fujioka H, Ghosh A, Moreira L, Jacobs-Lorena M. Driving midgut-specific expression and secretion of a foreign protein in transgenic mosquitoes with AgAper1 regulatory elements. Insect Molecular Biology. 2005;**14**(3):271-279. DOI: 10.1111/j.1365-2583.2004.00557.x

[47] Kokoza V, Ahmed A, Cho WL, Jasinskiene N, James AA, Raikhel A. Engineering blood meal-activated systemic immunity in the yellow fever mosquito, *Aedes aegypti*. Proceedings of the National Academy of Sciences of the United States of America. 2000;**97**(16):9144-9149. DOI: 10.1073/pnas.160258197

[48] Chen X, Zhang Y, Zheng X, Wang CM. Robust and regulatory expression of defensin A gene driven by vitellogenin promoter in transgenic *Anopheles stephensi*. Chinese Science Bulletin. 2007;**52**:1964-1969. DOI: 10.1007/s11434-007-0292-z

[49] Pondeville E, Puchot N, Parvy JP, Carissimo G, Poidevin M, Waterhouse RM, et al. Hemocyte-targeted gene expression in the female malaria mosquito using the hemolectin promoter from drosophila. Insect Biochemistry and Molecular Biology. 2020;**120**:103339. DOI: 10.1016/j.ibmb.2020.103339

[50] Coates CJ, Jasinskiene N, Pott GB, James AA. Promoter-directed expression

of recombinant fire-fly luciferase in the salivary glands of Hermes-transformed *Aedes aegypti*. Gene. 1999;**226**(2):317-325. DOI: 10.1016/s0378-1119(98)00557-5

[51] Lombardo F, Nolan T, Lycett G, Lanfrancotti A, Stich N, Catteruccia F, et al. An *Anopheles gambiae* salivary gland promoter analysis in *Drosophila melanogaster* and *Anopheles stephensi*. Insect Molecular Biology. 2005;**14**(2):207-216. DOI: 10.1111/j.1365-2583.2004.00549.x

[52] Yoshida S, Watanabe H. Robust salivary gland-specific transgene expression in *Anopheles stephensi* mosquito. Insect Molecular Biology. 2006;**15**(4):403-410. DOI: 10.1111/j.1365-2583.2006.00645.x

[53] Carpenetti TL, Aryan A, Myles KM, Adelman ZN. Robust heat-inducible gene expression by two endogenous hsp70-derived promoters in transgenic *Aedes aegypti*. Insect Molecular Biology. 2012;**21**(1):97-106. DOI: 10.1111/j.1365-2583.2011.01116.x

[54] Pinkerton AC, Michel K, O'Brochta DA, Atkinson PW. Green fluorescent protein as a genetic marker in transgenic *Aedes aegypti*. Insect Molecular Biology. 2000;**9**(1):1-10. DOI: 10.1046/j.1365-2583.2000.00133.x

[55] Anderson MA, Gross TL, Myles KM, Adelman ZN. Validation of novel promoter sequences derived from two endogenous ubiquitin genes in transgenic *Aedes aegypti*. Insect Molecular Biology. 2010;**19**(4):441-449. DOI: 10.1111/j.1365-2583.2010.01005.x

[56] Kokoza V, Ahmed A, Woon Shin S, Okafor N, Zou Z, Raikhel AS. Blocking of *Plasmodium* transmission by cooperative action of Cecropin A and Defensin A in transgenic *Aedes aegypti* mosquitoes. Proceedings of the National Academy of Sciences of the United States of America. 2010;**107**(18):8111-8116. DOI: 10.1073/pnas.1003056107

[57] Vizioli J, Bulet P, Hoffmann JA, Kafatos FC, Müller HM, Dimopoulos G. Gambicin: A novel immune responsive antimicrobial peptide from the malaria vector *Anopheles gambiae*. Proceedings of the National Academy of Sciences of the United States of America. 2001;**98**(22):12630-12635. DOI: 10.1073/pnas.221466798

[58] Conde R, Zamudio FZ, Rodríguez MH, Possani LD. Scorpine, an anti-malaria and anti-bacterial agent purified from scorpion venom. FEBS Letters. 2000;**471**(2-3):165-168. DOI: 10.1016/s0014-5793(00)01384-3

[59] Maciel C, de Oliveira Junior VX, Fázio MA, Nacif-Pimenta R, Miranda A, Pimenta PF, et al. Anti-*Plasmodium* activity of angiotensin II and related synthetic peptides. PLoS One. 2008;**3**(9):e3296. DOI: 10.1371/journal.pone.0003296

[60] Gwadz RW, Kaslow D, Lee JY, Maloy WL, Zasloff M, Miller LH. Effects of magainins and cecropins on the sporogonic development of malaria parasites in mosquitoes. Infection and Immunity. 1989;**57**(9):2628-2633. DOI: 10.1128/iai.57.9.2628-2633.1989

[61] Possani LD, Zurita M, Delepierre M, Hernández FH, Rodríguez MH. From noxiustoxin to Shiva-3, a peptide toxic to the sporogonic development of *Plasmodium berghei*. Toxicon. 1998;**36**(11):1683-1692. DOI: 10.1016/s0041-0101(98)00161-5

[62] Moreira CK, Rodrigues FG, Ghosh A, Varotti Fde P, Miranda A, Daffre S, et al. Effect of the antimicrobial peptide gomesin against different life stages of *Plasmodium* spp. Experimental

Parasitology. 2007;**116**(4):346-353. DOI: 10.1016/j.exppara.2007.01.022

[63] Ghosh AK, Coppens I, Gårdsvoll H, Ploug M, Jacobs-Lorena M. *Plasmodium* ookinetes coopt mammalian plasminogen to invade the mosquito midgut. Proceedings of the National Academy of Sciences of the United States of America. 2011;**108**(41):17153-17158. DOI: 10.1073/pnas.1103657108

[64] Ghosh AK, Ribolla PE, Jacobs-Lorena M. Targeting *Plasmodium* ligands on mosquito salivary glands and midgut with a phage display peptide library. Proceedings of the National Academy of Sciences of the United States of America. 2001;**98**(23):13278-13281. DOI: 10.1073/pnas.241491198

[65] Moreira LA, Ito J, Ghosh A, Devenport M, Zieler H, Abraham EG, et al. Bee venom phospholipase inhibits malaria parasite development in transgenic mosquitoes. The Journal of Biological Chemistry. 2002;**277**(43):40839-40843. DOI: 10.1074/jbc.M206647200

[66] Corby-Harris V, Drexler A, Watkins de Jong L, Antonova Y, Pakpour N, Ziegler R, et al. Activation of Akt signaling reduces the prevalence and intensity of malaria parasite infection and lifespan in *Anopheles stephensi* mosquitoes. PLoS Pathogens. 2010;**6**(7):e1001003. DOI: 10.1371/journal.ppat.1001003

[67] Dong Y, Das S, Cirimotich C, Souza-Neto JA, McLean KJ, Dimopoulos G. Engineered anopheles immunity to *Plasmodium* infection. PLoS Pathogens. 2011;**7**(12):e1002458. DOI: 10.1371/journal.ppat.1002458

[68] Dong Y, Simões ML, Dimopoulos G. Versatile transgenic multistage effector-gene combinations for *Plasmodium* falciparum suppression in *Anopheles*. Science Advances. 2020;**6**(20):eaay5898. DOI: 10.1126/sciadv.aay5898

[69] McClintock B. In: Moore JA, editor. The Discovery and Characterization of Transposable Elements. The C ollected Papers of Barbara McClintock. New York: Garland Publishing; 1987. pp. vii-xi

[70] Engels WR. Invasions of P elements. Genetics. 1997;**145**(1):11-15. DOI: 10.1093/genetics/145.1.11

[71] Charlesworth B, Sniegowski P, Stephan W. The evolutionary dynamics of repetitive DNA in eukaryotes. Nature. 1994;**371**:215-220. DOI: 10.1038/371215a0

[72] Mackay T. Transposable element-induced fitness mutations in *Drosophila melanogaster*. Genetical Research. 1986;**48**(2):77-87

[73] Rubin GM, Spradling AC. Genetic transformation of *Drosophila* with transposable element vectors. Science. 1982;**218**(4570):348-353. DOI: 10.1126/science.6289436

[74] Jasinskiene N, Coates CJ, Benedict MQ, Cornel AJ, Rafferty CS, James AA, et al. Stable transformation of the yellow fever mosquito, *Aedes aegypti*, with the Hermes element from the housefly. Proceedings of the National Academy of Sciences of the United States of America. 1998;**95**(7):3743-3747. DOI: 10.1073/pnas.95.7.3743

[75] Allen ML, O'Brochta DA, Atkinson PW, Levesque CS. Stable, germ-line transformation of *Culex quinquefasciatus* (Diptera: Culicidae). Journal of Medical Entomology. 2001;**38**(5):701-710. DOI: 10.1603/0022-2585-38.5.701

[76] Grossman GL, Rafferty CS, Clayton JR, Stevens TK, Mukabayire O,

Benedict MQ. Germline transformation of the malaria vector, *Anopheles gambiae*, with the *piggyBac* transposable element. Insect Molecular Biology. 2001;**10**(6):597-604. DOI: 10.1046/j.0962-1075.2001.00299.x

[77] Rodrigues FG, Oliveira SB, Rocha BC, Moreira LA. Germline transformation of *Aedes fluviatilis* (Diptera:Culicidae) with the *piggyBac* transposable element. Memórias do Instituto Oswaldo Cruz. 2006;**101**(7):755-757. DOI: 10.1590/s0074-02762006000700008

[78] Nolan T, Bower TM, Brown AE, Crisanti A, Catteruccia F. *piggyBac*-mediated germline transformation of the malaria mosquito *Anopheles stephensi* using the red fluorescent protein dsRED as a selectable marker. The Journal of Biological Chemistry. 2002;**277**(11):8759-8762. DOI: 10.1074/jbc.C100766200

[79] Perera OP, Harrell RA II, Handler AM. Germ-line transformation of the South American malaria vector, Anopheles albimanus, with a *piggyBac*/EGFP transposon vector is routine and highly efficient. Insect Molecular Biology. 2002;**11**(4):291-297. DOI: 10.1046/j.1365-2583.2002.00336.x

[80] Catteruccia F, Nolan T, Loukeris TG, Blass C, Savakis C, Kafatos FC, et al. Stable germline transformation of the malaria mosquito *Anopheles stephensi*. Nature. 2000;**405**(6789):959-962. DOI: 10.1038/35016096

[81] Coates CJ, Jasinskiene N, Miyashiro L, James AA. Mariner transposition and transformation of the yellow fever mosquito, *Aedes aegypti*. Proceedings of the National Academy of Sciences of the United States of America. 1998;**95**(7): 3748-3751. DOI: 10.1073/pnas.95.7.3748

[82] Labbé GM, Nimmo DD, Alphey L. *piggyBac*- and *PhiC31*-mediated genetic transformation of the Asian tiger mosquito, *Aedes albopictus* (Skuse). PLOS Neglected Tropical Diseases. 2010;**4**(8):e788. DOI: 10.1371/journal.pntd.0000788

[83] Kidwell MG, Ribeiro JM. Can transposable elements be used to drive disease refractoriness genes into vector populations? Parasitology Today. 1992;**8**(10):325-329. DOI: 10.1016/0169-4758(92)90065-a

[84] O'Brochta DA, Sethuraman N, Wilson R, Hice RH, Pinkerton AC, Levesque CS, et al. Gene vector and transposable element behavior in mosquitoes. The Journal of Experimental Biology. 2003;**206**(Pt 21):3823-3834. DOI: 10.1242/jeb.00638

[85] Macias VM, Jimenez AJ, Burini-Kojin B, Pledger D, Jasinskiene N, Phong CH, et al. Nanos-driven expression of *piggyBac* transposase induces mobilization of a synthetic autonomous transposon in the malaria vector mosquito, *Anopheles stephensi*. Insect Biochemistry and Molecular Biology. 2017;**87**:81-89. DOI: 10.1016/j.ibmb.2017.06.014

[86] Morris AC, Schaub TL, James AA. FLP-mediated recombination in the vector mosquito, *Aedes aegypti*. Nucleic Acids Research. 1991;**19**(21):5895-5900. DOI: 10.1093/nar/19.21.5895

[87] Nimmo DD, Alphey L, Meredith JM, Eggleston P. High efficiency site-specific genetic engineering of the mosquito genome. Insect Molecular Biology. 2006;**15**(2):129-136. DOI: 10.1111/j.1365-2583.2006.00615.x

[88] Meredith JM, Basu S, Nimmo DD, Larget-Thiery I, Warr EL, Underhill A, et al. Site-specific integration and expression of an anti-malarial gene in transgenic

Anopheles gambiae significantly reduces *Plasmodium* infections. PLoS One. 2011;**6**(1):e14587. DOI: 10.1371/journal.pone.0014587

[89] Volohonsky G, Terenzi O, Soichot J, Naujoks DA, Nolan T, Windbichler N, et al. Tools for *Anopheles gambiae* Transgenesis. G3 (Bethesda). 2015;**5**(6):1151-1163. DOI: 10.1534/g3.115.016808

[90] Jasinskiene N, Coates CJ, Ashikyan A, James AA. High efficiency, site-specific excision of a marker gene by the phage P1 cre-loxP system in the yellow fever mosquito, *Aedes aegypti*. Nucleic Acids Research. 2003;**31**(22):e147. DOI: 10.1093/nar/gng148

[91] Aryan A, Anderson MA, Myles KM, Adelman ZN. Germline excision of transgenes in *Aedes aegypti* by homing endonucleases. Scientific Reports. 2013;**3**:1603. DOI: 10.1038/srep01603

[92] Smidler AL, Terenzi O, Soichot J, Levashina EA, Marois E. Targeted mutagenesis in the malaria mosquito using TALE nucleases. PLoS One. 2013;**8**(8):e74511. DOI: 10.1371/journal.pone.0074511

[93] DeGennaro M, McBride CS, Seeholzer L, Nakagawa T, Dennis EJ, Goldman C, et al. *Orco* mutant mosquitoes lose strong preference for humans and are not repelled by volatile DEET. Nature. 2013;**498**(7455):487-491. DOI: 10.1038/nature12206

[94] Burt A. Site-specific selfish genes as tools for the control and genetic engineering of natural populations. Proceedings of the Biological Society. 2003;**270**(1518):921-928

[95] Windbichler N, Menichelli M, Papathanos PA, Thyme SB, Li H, Ulge UY, et al. A synthetic homing endonuclease-based gene drive system in the human malaria mosquito. Nature. 2011;**473**(7346):212-215. DOI: 10.1038/nature09937

[96] Jinek M, Chylinski K, Fonfara I, Hauer M, Doudna JA, Charpentier E. A programmable dual-RNA-guided DNA endonuclease in adaptive bacterial immunity. Science. 2012;**337**(6096):816-821. DOI: 10.1126/science.1225829

[97] Carballar-Lejarazú R, Tushar T, Pham TB, James AA. Cas9-mediated maternal-effect and derived resistance alleles in a gene-drive strain of the African malaria vector mosquito, Anopheles gambiae. Genetics. 2022 Apr 7:iyac055. DOI: 10.1093/genetics/iyac055. Epub ahead of print. PMID: 35389492

[98] Marrelli MT, Moreira CK, Kelly D, Alphey L, Jacobs-Lorena M. Mosquito transgenesis: What is the fitness cost? Trends in Parasitology. 2006;**22**(5):197-202. DOI: 10.1016/j.pt.2006.03.004

[99] Riehle MA, Srinivasan P, Moreira CK, Jacobs-Lorena M. Towards genetic manipulation of wild mosquito populations to combat malaria: Advances and challenges. The Journal of Experimental Biology. 2003;**206**(Pt 21):3809-3816. DOI: 10.1242/jeb.00609

[100] Pham TB, Phong CH, Bennett JB, Hwang K, Jasinskiene N, Parker K, et al. Experimental population modification of the malaria vector mosquito, *Anopheles stephensi*. PLOS Genetics. 2019;**15**:e1008440. DOI: 10.1371/journal.pgen.1008440

[101] Bottino-Rojas V, Ferreira-Almeida I, Nunes R, Feng XC, Pham TB, Kelsey A, et al. Beyond the eye: Kynurenine pathway impairment causes midgut homeostasis dysfunction and survival and reproductive costs in blood-feeding mosquitoes. Insect Biochemistry

and Molecular Biology. 2022;**142**:103720. DOI: 10.1016/j.ibmb.2022.103720

[102] Ribeiro JM, Kidwell MG. Transposable elements as population drive mechanisms: Specification of critical parameter values. Journal of Medical Entomology. 1994;**31**(1):10-16. DOI: 10.1093/jmedent/31.1.10

[103] Boëte C, Koella JC. A theoretical approach to predicting the success of genetic manipulation of malaria mosquitoes in malaria control. Malaria Journal. 2002;**1**:3. DOI: 10.1186/1475-2875-1-3

[104] Champer J, Reeves R, Oh SY, Liu C, Liu J, Clark AG, et al. Novel CRISPR/Cas9 gene drive constructs reveal insights into mechanisms of resistance allele formation and drive efficiency in genetically diverse populations. PLoS Genetics. 2017;**13**(7):e1006796. DOI: 10.1371/journal.pgen.1006796

[105] Unckless RL, Clark AG, Messer PW. Evolution of resistance against CRISPR/Cas9 gene drive. Genetics. 2017;**205**(2):827-841. DOI: 10.1534/genetics.116.197285

[106] Drury DW, Dapper AL, Siniard DJ, Zentner GE, Wade MJ. CRISPR/Cas9 gene drives in genetically variable and nonrandomly mating wild populations. Science Advances. 2017;**3**(5):e1601910. DOI: 10.1126/sciadv.1601910

[107] Noble C, Olejarz J, Esvelt KM, Church GM, Nowak MA. Evolutionary dynamics of CRISPR gene drives. Science Advances. 2017;**3**(4):e1601964. DOI: 10.1126/sciadv.1601964

[108] Terradas G, Hermann A, James AA, McGinnis W, Bier E. High-resolution in situ analysis of Cas9 germline transcript distributions in gene-drive Anopheles mosquitoes. G3 (Bethesda). 2021:jkab369. DOI: 10.1093/g3journal/jkab369

[109] Lanzaro GC, Sánchez CHM, Collier TC, Marshall JM, James AA. Population modification strategies for malaria vector control are uniquely resilient to observed levels of gene drive resistance alleles. Bioessays. 2021;**43**(8):e2000282. DOI: 10.1002/bies.202000282

[110] Marshall JM, Buchman A, Sánchez CHM, Akbari OS. Overcoming evolved resistance to population-suppressing homing-based gene drives. Scientific Reports. 2017;**7**(1):3776. DOI: 10.1038/s41598-017-02744-7

[111] Gao Y, Zhao Y. Self-processing of ribozyme-flanked RNAs into guide RNAs in vitro and in vivo for CRISPR-mediated genome editing. Journal of Integrative Plant Biology. 2014;**56**(4):343-349. DOI: 10.1111/jipb.12152

[112] Port F, Bullock SL. Augmenting CRISPR applications in *Drosophila* with tRNA-flanked sgRNAs. Nature Methods. 2016;**13**(10):852-854. DOI: 10.1038/nmeth.3972

[113] Champer J, Liu J, Oh SY, Reeves R, Luthra A, Oakes N, et al. Reducing resistance allele formation in CRISPR gene drive. Proceedings of the National Academy of Sciences of the United States of America. 2018;**115**(21):5522-5527. DOI: 10.1073/pnas.1720354115

[114] Zetsche B, Gootenberg JS, AbudayyehOO,SlaymakerIM,MakarovaKS, Essletzbichler P, et al. Cpf1 is a single RNA-guided endonuclease of a class 2 CRISPR-Cas system. Cell. 2015;**163**(3):759-771. DOI: 10.1016/j.cell.2015.09.038

[115] Kleinstiver BP, Pattanayak V, Prew MS, Tsai SQ, Nguyen NT, Zheng Z, et al. High-fidelity CRISPR-Cas9 nucleases with no detectable genome-wide off-target effects. Nature. 2016;**529**(7587):490-495. DOI: 10.1038/nature16526

[116] Slaymaker IM, Gao L, Zetsche B, Scott DA, Yan WX, Zhang F. Rationally engineered Cas9 nucleases with improved specificity. Science. 2016;**351**(6268):84-88. DOI: 10.1126/science.aad5227

[117] Ran FA, Hsu PD, Lin CY, Gootenberg JS, Konermann S, Trevino AE, et al. Double nicking by RNA-guided CRISPR Cas9 for enhanced genome editing specificity. Cell. 2013;**154**(6):1380-1389. DOI: 10.1016/j.cell.2013.08.021

[118] Pattanayak V, Lin S, Guilinger JP, Ma E, Doudna JA, Liu DR. High-throughput profiling of off-target DNA cleavage reveals RNA-programmed Cas9 nuclease specificity. Nature Biotechnology. 2013;**31**(9):839-843. DOI: 10.1038/nbt.2673

[119] Fu Y, Sander JD, Reyon D, Cascio VM, Joung JK. Improving CRISPR-Cas nuclease specificity using truncated guide RNAs. Nature Biotechnology. 2014;**32**(3):279-284. DOI: 10.1038/nbt.2808

[120] World Health Organization. Guidance Framework for Testing Genetically Modified Mosquitoes. 2nd ed. Geneva: World Health Organization; 2021. Licence: CC BY-NC-SA 3.0 IGO, 2014. Available from: Guidance framework for testing of genetically modified mosquitoes, second edition (who.int)

[121] James S, Collins FH, Welkhoff PA, Emerson C, Godfray HCJ, Gottlieb M, et al. Pathway to deployment of gene drive mosquitoes as a potential biocontrol tool for elimination of malaria in sub-Saharan Africa: Recommendations of a scientific working group. American Journal of Tropical Medicine and Hygiene. 2018;**98**(6_Suppl):1-49. DOI: 10.4269/ajtmh.18-0083

[122] Australian Academy of Science. Synthetic Gene Drives in Australia: Implications of Emerging Technologies. Australian Academy of Science; 2017. Available from: https://www.science.org.au/files/userfiles/support/documents/gene-drives-discussion-paper-june2017.pdf

[123] Kormos A, Lanzaro G, Bier E, Dimopoulos G, Marshall J, Pinto J, et al. Application of the relationship-based model to community and regulatory engagement for field trials of genetically-engineered mosquitoes for malaria control. The American Journal of Tropical Medicine and Hygiene. 2021;**104**:805-811

Chapter 13

Bacterial Silver Nanoparticles: Method, Mechanism of Synthesis and Application in Mosquito Control

Jeyaraj John Wilson, Thangamariyappan Harimuralikrishnaa, Ponnirul Ponmanickam and Muthumadasamy Ponseetha Lakshmi

Abstract

Silver nanoparticles (AgNPs) received tremendous attention due to their fascinated applications. Extensive research reports are available on the physical, chemical, and biological synthesis of colloidal Ag NPs. Research on biological systems mediated silver nanoparticle synthesis is essential to explore more applications. Microbial synthesis has been recognized as an eco-friendly and influential source among biological sources. Therefore, the bacteria are often considered an exciting reducer for silver and gold nanoparticles fabrication. Further, the synthesized nanoparticles incorporated different biological agents from what we need as bio reducing agents. The cell membrane of microorganisms plays a crucial role in the endogenous synthesis of nanoparticles. The cell membrane interacts electronically with the charged metal ions because it is charged. Enzymes inside the cell membrane biodegrade metal ions into nanoparticles, which eventually propagate through the cell membrane in small volumes. The fabricated silver nanoparticles were characterized by different spectroscopy techniques, to reveal the structural and functional properties. The synthesized nanoparticle reacts against many pathogens and insects and is used in medical fields. One of the pesticide industry's significant applications is mosquito larvicidal application. This chapter dealt with the microbial-mediated synthesis of silver nanoparticles, characterization, and mosquito larvicidal applications.

Keywords: bacteria, silver nanoparticle synthesis, mosquito larvicidal activity, intracellular and extracellular synthesis

1. Introduction

Nanotechnology can regulate and manipulate objects at the individual level of atoms and particles. Physicist Richard Feynman previously envisioned the hypothetical utilization of nanotechnology in 1959, and indeed, the term "Nanotechnology" was coined by Norino Taniguchi. When a parameter is stated as a measure of 10^{-9} meters of SI units, it is called "nano" [1].

Dimensionality, shape, composition, homogeneity, and aggregation are used to classify nanoparticles. The shape and syllable structure of nanoparticles plays a significant role in their function and harmful impacts on the environment and people. Nanoparticles can be classified into one, two, and three-dimensional nanoparticles. One-dimensional nanoparticle includes thin flicks used in electronics and sensor devices. Two-dimensional nanoparticles are high in carbon nanotubes absorption capacity and constancy. Three-dimensional nanoparticles are dendrimer quantum points. On top of that, morphology may be the basis of nanoparticles flat, spherical, and crystal in structure. They may be in a single form or the arrangement of compounds. Nanoparticles can be supplementary classified oxide nanoparticles, sulfide nanoparticles, and magnet nanoparticles [2, 3].

Various physical, chemical, and biological strategies are generally utilized to synthesize nanoparticles. Integrated nanoparticles are considered unfavorable due to high capital cost, energy requirements, anaerobic conditions, utilization of toxicity generation of furnaces, and harmful waste. Nanoparticles are less biodegradable, and utilizing toxic chemicals for synthesis, and the absence of sustainability have restricted their utilization in medical applications. Therefore, the development of ecologically safe, economical, and biological compatibility events for the assembly of nanoparticles is preferred. The fabrication of nanoparticles by natural resources is economical and alternate for physical and chemical methods. The latest advances were made in developing nanotechnology collection of Nano-sized particles. These nanoparticles are considered building blocks for developing optoelectronic electronics and numerous biochemical and chemical sensors [2, 4].

Development of ecologically safe, economical, and biological compatibility procedures for the assembly of nanoparticles is preferred. The synthesis of nanoparticles by biological means is low-priced. For the fabrication of nanoparticles, biological synthesis, including microbes, has been exploited worldwide. Bacteria, fungi, and yeasts are chosen for synthesis due to their rapid growth rate, easy cultivation, and ability to grow ambient temperature, pH, and pressure environments. Because of their adaptation to a toxic metal environment, eco-friendly microorganisms have the inherent ability to integrate nanoparticles by following the reduction mechanism through internal and external-external routes. Microbes trap metal ions from the location and convert them into the basic form using their enzymes [2].

Nanomedicine utilizes nanoscale structures to diagnose, treat, and prevent diseases in improving human health. Nanomaterials are comparable to cellular elements, including nano quantity proteins; thus, they can target chosen sites without contacting other cellular machinery. Now scientists aim to integrate the modernity of nanomedicine with conventional molecular tools and biotechnology to develop advanced therapies for the treatment of disease and tissues repair, novel drug delivery systems, rapid and ultrasensitive analytic tools such as biosensors, biopharmaceuticals, surgical aids compatible biomaterials [2, 5].

Arthropods are extremely dangerous vectors of pathogens and parasites, which may hit epidemics or pandemics in the increasing world population of humans and animals [6]. Among them, mosquitoes (Diptera: Culicidae) represent a huge threat for millions of people worldwide, vectoring important diseases, including malaria, dengue, yellow fever, filariasis, Japanese encephalitis and Zika virus [7]. Furthermore, Culicidae transmits key pathogens and parasites that dogs and horses are very susceptible to, including dog heartworm, West Nile virus, and Eastern equine encephalitis [8, 9]. Unfortunately, no treatment is available for most of the arboviruses vectored by mosquitoes, with special reference to dengue. A promising interface between nanotechnology and arthropod control recently opened new routes to manage vector and pest populations [10].

Now the researcher is strongly promoting the development of nano-based insecticides. Nanobiotechnology is a new discipline in nanosciences that emerged from the interface between nanotechnology and biotechnology. This crossbreeding performance is green and environmentally friendly, biocompatible, inexpensive, and a great alternative to traditional chemical approaches in the pest control industry [11]. Among the bio-based insecticides, microbial insecticides are essential for improving the toxicity of mosquito larvae, causing less harm to non-target species, and reducing environmental risks. Therefore, microbially mediated nano metallic synthesis has proven to be an environmentally friendly and efficient source, and bacteria have been reported to be effective reducing agents in synthesizing silver and gold nanoparticles (NPs). In this synthesis method, several metabolites of microorganisms can be used, which simultaneously promote the reduction and stabilization of nanoparticles and the adhesion and formation of a layer of biomolecules on their surface, the corona, which increases their biocompatibility. In this context, the current work was aimed to study the method, mechanism of synthesize of silver nanoparticles using bacteria, characterize the silver nanoparticles and assess its larvicidal effectiveness against mosquito vectors.

2. Synthesis of silver nanoparticle

The specific mechanism for synthesizing nanoparticles using biological agents has not yet been developed, as diverse biological agents react inversely with metal ions. The composition of nanoparticles contains different biological molecules. In addition, the mechanism for intracellular and extracellular synthesis of nanoparticles differs in other biological agents (**Figure 1**). The cell wall of microorganisms plays a vital role in the endogenous synthesis of nanoparticles. The cell wall interacts electronically with the positively charged metal ions as it is negatively charged. Enzymes inside the cell wall biodegrade metal ions into nanoparticles, which eventually propagate through the cell wall in small volumes [12].

2.1 Biosynthesis of metal nanoparticles using bacteria

Many reports proved that bacteria is an excellent organic apparatus for the fabrication of metal nanoparticles—for instance, Streptomyces sp. M25 was isolated from a soil sample of Western Ghats and is used to synthesize silver nanoparticles [13]. The bacterial sample was inoculated into 100 ml of YEM broth and incubated in the rotary shaker for 5 days. 10 g bacterial mass was mixed with the 100 ml 1 Mm AgNO3. The reaction mixture was kept in a rotary shaker for 24 h. The color change is the primary confirmation of the synthesis of Ag NPs. The same solution was centrifuged, and the Ag NP was collected from the supernatant. The reaction mixer was further subjected to spectrometric UV-VIS spectrophotometer, Transmission electron microscopy, X-ray diffraction (XRD), and further characterization. The result showed that the size of the Ag NPs is 10-35 nm [13].

Bacillus safensis LAU 13 is the gram-positive spore-forming bacteria isolated from the waste dumpsite, and it was used for the biosynthesis of silver nanoparticles using

Extracellular synthesis of nanoparticles	Intracellular synthesis of nanoparticles
Secretion of reductase by microorganisms in the external environment ⇩	Metal ions (positive charge) attached to the microbial cell wall (negative charge) ⇩
Reduction of metal ions by the enzyme ⇩	Reduction of metal ions by the enzyme present in the cell surface ⇩
Fabrication of nanoparticles from cell-free media	Formation of nanocluster in the microbial cell wall

Figure 1.
Schematic flow diagram for intracellular and extracellular synthesis of nanomaterials.

the supernatant of *B. safensis* LAU 13. 1 mM of $AgNO_3$ was diluted into the 40 ml of distilled water and add 1 ml of the supernatant of *B. safensis* LAU 13. The synthesized silver nanoparticle is spherical shaped, having a size of 5–95 nm, and it is confirmed by UV-VIS spectrophotometer, Fourier transform infrared spectroscopy, and Transmission electron microscope. Bio synthesized silver nanoparticles were used for bioassay against first instar Anopheles larvae in 10–100 μg/ml [14].

2.2 Mechanism of bacterial silver nanoparticle synthesis

All the bacteria cannot reduce the metal ions. The capability of the reduction mechanism depends upon the bacterial defense mechanism. If the bacteria are exposed to the metal environment, metal ions like Ag + enter the cell and bind to the bacterial DNA. Silver particles have a positive charge, and DNA is contrarily charged. It changed the nature of DNA, resulting in a loss of structure and replication ability. Ag + binds with protein, especially thiol-containing proteins, and inhibits the function of proteins. The reductase enzyme of bacteria reacts metal (active Ag + – inactive Ag0) into inactive and is not lead to cell death. Most of the reductase enzymes are NADPH dependent, and bacteria can have or secrete this cofactor NADH dependent enzyme. The quantity of reductase enzymes varies between microorganisms. Extracellular and intracellular reductions do the defense mechanism. Extracellular means the bacteria can release the reductase enzyme to the external environment and reduce the metal ions. Intracellular implies the removal of metal ions by reductase that takes place inside the cell. If the bacteria do not have a reductase mechanism, they will die [12].

2.3 Method for intracellular synthesis of silver nanoparticles

Prepare the pure bacterial seed culture in 100 ml nutrient broth and incubate it on a rotary shaker (150 rpm) for 24 hours.

1. After incubation, centrifuge the cell suspension and separate the bacterial pellet.

2. Suspend the pellet into the 100 ml distilled water. Then add 1 mM silver nitrate into the pellet suspension.

3. Incubate pellet suspension overnight at 60°C, pH 10.

4. The silver nanoparticle will deposit on the bacterial cell. Whitethorn changes the color of suspension (white to dark brown) (**Figure 2**).

2.4 Separation of nanoparticles

The synthesized nanoparticles are separated from reaction mixture by adapting the following method [12, 15]:

Solution 1: 0.9% NaCl.

Solution 2: NaCl 0.5 M + Sucrose 0.5 M (equal volume of each solution).

Solution 3: NaCl [17.5 g/L] + KCL [0.74 g/L] + $MgSO_4 . 7H_2O$ [12.3 g/L] + Tris HCL [0.15 g/L].

pH = 7.5[Salt solution]

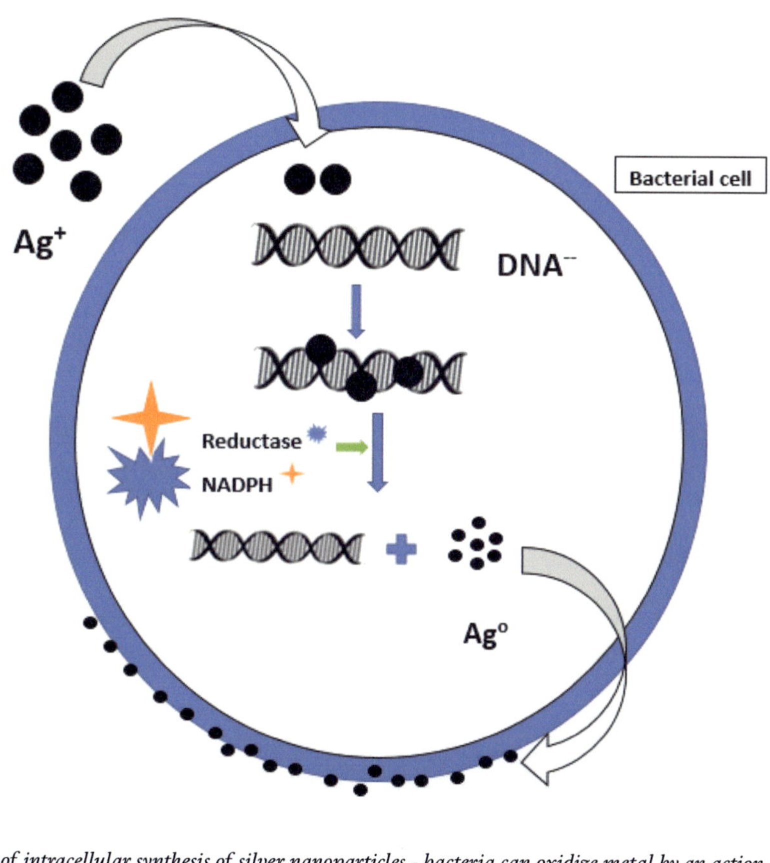

Figure 2.
Mechanism of intracellular synthesis of silver nanoparticles - bacteria can oxidize metal by an action of reductase enzyme (direct mechanism of gaining electrons from reduced minerals). The redacted Nano metal ions are attached to the surface of the bacterial cell wall.

1. Centrifuge the bacterial suspension holding nanoparticle at 4000–9000 rpm for 10 minutes.

2. Suspend the pellet using solution 1 (equal volume of the pellet) and centrifuge at 4000–9000 rpm for 10 minutes. Repeat the step three times in order to remove the unwanted materials.

3. Homogenize the bacterial pellet by mortar with 20 mg Egg White Lysozyme and solution 2 (equal volume of the pellet) and centrifuged at 12000 rpm for 10 minutes.

4. Transfer the pellet to an enormous container, add solution three and incubate this mixture at room temperature for 18 hours.

2.5 Nanoparticle purification

1. Centrifuge the lysate at 12000 rpm and discard the supernatant (salt solution).

2. Suspend the pellet into the distilled water and wash twice at 5000–8000 rpm. Separated nanoparticles suspend into milli-Q water.

3. Separated nanoparticles purified by gel electrophoresis and column chromatography [2, 12, 15].

2.6 Extracellular synthesis of silver nanoparticles

1. Prepare 100 ml of seed culture in nutrient broth and incubate at 37°C for 72 hrs.

2. After incubation, centrifuge the broth culture at 5000-8000 rpm for 15 minutes.

3. Discard the pellet and transfer the supernatant into a new flask. Add the 1 mM silver nitrate and set pH 10.

4. Incubate this mixture overnight at 60°C. Centrifuge the culture supernatant at 7000 rpm and discard the supernatant.

5. Suspend the pellet into distilled water and wash two times at 5000 rpm.

6. Purified nanoparticles are again suspended into milli-Q water for further use [14] (**Figure 3**).

2.7 The optimum condition for the synthesis

One of the most critical factors in bacteria-mediated Ag NP synthesis is a high pH. In the presence of silver ions, high pH catalyzes the opening of monosaccharide rings to open chain aldehyde forms, which then undergo oxidation to the appropriate carboxylic acid while simultaneously reducing silver ions to Ag NPs. Reductases of oxidoreductase enzymes are also activated by high pH [16]. Some bacterial proteins are involved in the synthesis of silver nanoparticles. It binds the thiol region at alkaline conditions (there is no need for agitation). In addition, alkaline ions are very much required for the reduction of metal ions. Under the alkaline state, it enhances the enzyme activity to do a reduction

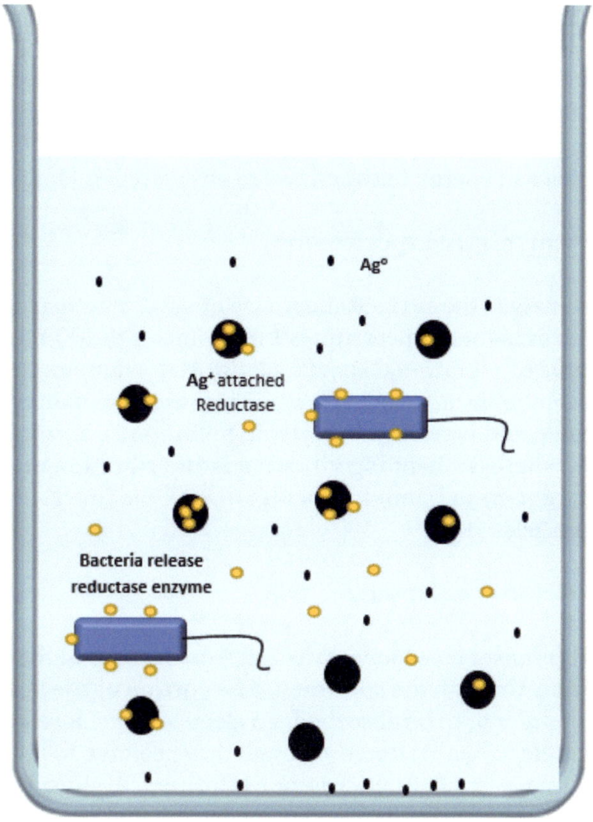

Figure 3.
Mechanism of extracellular synthesis of silver nanoparticles - the bacteria can release the metabolite or type of reductase enzyme to the environment. It oxidizes the metal to an inactive form.

mechanism. In acidic conditions, it will take up to 4 days for silver nanoparticle synthesis. In alkaline conditions, the nanoparticle will be synthesized within 4 hours [12].

The high temperature will increase the dynamics of ions and the formation of more nucleation regions due to the obtainability of OH ions and the conversion of silver metal to the silver nanoparticle. At 60°C, nanoparticles are redacted up to 2–15 nm; in acidic conditions (50 nm), size is not reduced [12].

3. Characterization of silver nanoparticle

Once the synthesis procedure is completed, it is necessary to characterize the nanoparticles to know their structure, size, purity, and efficacy by studying their physiochemical properties, size, shape, surface area, and homogeneity. UV- visible spectroscopy, FTIR, TEM, SEM-EDAX, X-ray diffraction (XRD), and atomic force microscopy (AFM) are the tools used to characterize the synthesized nanoparticles [17].

3.1 UV: visible spectroscopy

UV-visible spectroscopy is a primary tool to analyze the availability of nanoparticles in the reaction mixture at 200–500 nm. It is based on the transition of electrons from one molecular orbital to another due to the absorption of electromagnetic radiation of UV and visible regions. It is the type of absorption spectroscopy when electromagnetic radiation interacts with matter, and the incident light can be reflected off, absorbed by, or transmitted through a sample. Electromagnetic radiation is absorbed by atoms or molecules, transitioning from lower energy to an excited state. Then the energy matched the difference in energy between two energy samples [18].

3.2 Fourier transform infrared spectroscopy

FTIR is used to analyze the surface chemistry of silver nanoparticles. The range that covers the electromagnetic spectrum is 1 micrometer to 100 micrometers. This spectroscopy is a type of vibrational spectroscopy. At the temperature above absolute zero, the bonds within molecules will vibrate. There are two main types of bond vibrations - stretching and bending. A stretching vibration occurs along the line of the chemical bond, whereas a bending vibration is any vibration that does not occur along the line of the chemical bond. It provides that all the functional groups are present in silver nanoparticles [18].

3.3 Transmission electron microscope

In the TEM, a condenser lens focuses the electron beam onto the specimen, transmitting electrons through the specimen. The portion of the beam absorbed by the specimen is minimal; to be absorbed, an electron must lose all its energy to the specimen. Some electrons scattered through the specimen focus on forming an image, like how an image in a light microscope is formed. A phosphorescent screen, a photographic plate, or a high-resolution camera can be used to view the image [18].

3.4 Scanning electron microscope

The scanning electron microscope views the surface nature of specimens. The sample is fixed, dried, and coated with a thin layer of heavy metal, such as gold or silver, scanned with a very narrow beam of electrons. Molecules in the specimen are excited, and they release secondary electrons. Molecules in the specimen are excited, and they release secondary electrons captured by a detector, generating an image of the specimen's surface. The resolving power of scanning electron microscopes, limited by the thickness of the metal coating, is only about 10 nm; they produce three-dimensional in SEM [18].

3.5 Atomic force microscopy (AFM)

Atomic force microscopy (AFM) offers ultra-high resolution in particle size measurement by physically scanning samples at the sub-micron level with an atomic probe tip. Based on forces between the tip and the sample surface, the instrument generates a topographical map of the sample [15]. Depending on the qualities of the sample, it is usually scanned in contact or non-contact mode. In contact mode, the topographical map is created by tapping the probe across the sample surface, while in the non-contact method, the probe hovers over the conducting surface. The ability to image non-conducting samples without special treatment is AFM's main advantage, allow ing imaging of delicate biological and polymeric nano and microstructures. The most accurate description of size and size distribution is provided by AFM, which does not require any mathematical treatment. Furthermore, the AFM technique provides a realistic picture of particle size, which aids in understanding the impact of diverse biological circumstances [19].

3.6 X-ray diffraction

XRD is one of the most common analytical techniques for phase identification and crystalline structure determination in solid-state materials. To determine the structure of a molecule, X-rays focused on constrictive use of destructive interference caused by scattering radiation from a single crystal's regular and repeating lattice [19].

4. Nanotechnology in mosquito control

The life of mosquitoes is intertwined with human life, and they have been a significant factor in human society for many years. Although they have been recognized as criminals for hundreds of years, their nuisance has not diminished. We have been suffering from the effects of mosquitoes since the beginning of humankind. These cause hundreds or more diseases against the human race. Millions of people have died as a result. Although, the elimination of mosquitoes is octagonal. Even though various countries have implemented many health promotion programs against mosquitoes, it is still a significant problem globally. Mosquitoes transmit dangerous diseases known to humans, such as malaria, yellow fever, dengue, encephalitis, filariasis. More than 3500 species have been recorded worldwide across five continents. Mosquito-borne diseases, such as malaria, arboviruses, and filariasis, and their vectors are present worldwide [20].

Mosquitoes are severe vectors of critical human parasites and microbes. *Culex quinquefasciatus* is a domestic mosquito that thrives close to human activities and habitation. West Nile virus, St. Louis encephalitis, and lymphatic filariasis are among the pathogens *Cx. quinquefasciatus* can transmit to humans and animals. *Cx. quinquefasciatus* can transmit pathogens such as avian malaria and zoonotic dirofilariasis to livestock, birds, domestic and wild animal species, resulting in loss of productivity and death. *Cx. quinquefasciatus* is also a nuisance because its bites can cause local dermatitis or acute systemic allergic reactions in many people [21].

There is no aquatic habitat anywhere; it does not lend itself to being a breeding ground in the world for mosquitoes. They are temporary and permanent colonial, very dirty and clean, big and small waters, even the most miniature accumulation buckets filled with water, flower vases, tires, hoof, etc., possible sources of prints and leaf axes. Flood mosquitoes in temporarily flooded areas, rivers, or lakes with water fluctuation *Aedes vexans* or *Ochlerotatus sticticus* formed in large numbers and within a range of miles. They can become a significant nuisance even in places far away from their breeding grounds.

Many methods are used to control the mosquitoes, but they have disadvantages; chemical control was one of the most widely used conventional methods for mosquito control [20]. Since chemical pesticides are relatively inexpensive, they usually produce immediate control. Generally, the chemical control is carried out by the indoor residual spraying of insecticides such as DDT, organophosphates, chlorpyrifos-methyl, fenthion, fenitrothion, malathion, pirimiphos-methyl, temephos, carbamates bendiocarb, propoxur, pyrethroids alpha-cypermethrin, bifenthrin, cyfluthrin, cypermethrin, deltamethrin, etofenprox, lambda-cyhalothrin, permethrin, hexachlorocyclohexane, benzene hexachloride, malathion, and synthetic pyrethroid. However, the development of resistance against these chemicals in various mosquito populations has been reported [20]. Therefore, biological control can provide a practical and environmentally friendly approach that can be used as an alternative to reduce the number of mosquitoes. Microbially mediated AgNPs are powerful tools for combating mosquitoes and agricultural insects [20].

Marimuthu et al. [22] reported that synthesized metal nanoparticles derived from *B. thuringiensis* showed remarkable larvicidal activity against *A. subpictus* and *A. aegypti*. Similarly, AgNPs obtained from *B. thuringiensis* (Bt) and *F. oxysporumculture* filtrate showed strong larvicidal activity against *A. aegypti*, *A. stephensi* and *C. quinquefasciatus* mosquitoes [23]. In addition, several studies have reported that the bacterial strains of *L. monocytogenes*, *B. subtilius*, and *S. anulatus*-mediated AgNPs showed larvicidal activity [24]. The *Pseudomonas aeruginosa* synthesized Ag NPs were treated against *Cx.quinquefasciatus* and showed a higher susceptibility to the synthesized AgNPs and showed that 100% mortality was observed after 1 hour of incubation [25].

4.1 Procedure for studying Larvicidal activity of silver nanoparticle

4.1.1 Stock solution

1. 20 ml (solvent) + 200 mg (nanoparticle) = 1000 ppm.

2. 2 ml of stock solution is serially diluted in 18 ml of solvent (working solution) = 100 ppm.

4.1.2 Procedure

1. The fourth instar of mosquito larvae is taken in a 250 ml container. Each container has 200 ml distilled water and 10 mosquito larvae. It makes up of three replicates.

2. Add the silver nanoparticle to 1 ppm–100 ppm concentration. Furthermore, monitor the larval behavior in 24 hrs – 48 hrs. Twenty-four hours of fasting mosquito larvae were used in the test, and the control organism was fed two times per day.

3. The action of silver nanoparticle mosquito larval behavior will be changed activity like slow swimming, stand in a single place, larval color was changed, damage the body parts and last mortality.

4. The mortality will be observed and tabulated [26].

4.2 Mechanism of actions of nanoparticles on mosquitoes

Surprisingly, despite a mass of information on their toxicity against specific pests and vectors, exact information on nanoparticles' potential mode of action against insects is limited. This information is crucial for predicting the toxicological effects of using nanoparticles as insecticides in the actual world. Silver nanoparticle cytotoxicity and genotoxicity mechanisms have been extensively studied, as their toxicity in biological models is strongly influenced by their size, shape, and charge [27].

According to accepted theory, the toxicity of several nanoparticles is considered to be achieved by causing oxidative stress in arthropod tissues [28]. Furthermore, nanoparticle penetration through the exoskeleton may increase their toxicity. The nanoscale material then binds to sulfur from proteins or phosphorus from DNA in the intracellular space, causing organelles and enzymes to denature rapidly. As a result of the decreased membrane permeability and disturbance in the proton motive force, cellular function and cell death may be lost. The green-capped nano-Ag significantly reduced total protein levels. It also reduced the activities of acetylcholinesterase and - α and ß-carboxylesterase [28].

5. Conclusion

The efficacy of green-fabricated nanoparticles is promising, and this excited much research groups worldwide, opening new ways to manage arthropod pests and vectors. However, while some researchers have tried to clarify how silica, alumina, silver, gold, titania, and graphene nanoparticles act as toxins against arthropods, our knowledge in this research field is still scarce.

Green fabrication processes rely on selected compounds to rule out the insecticidal impacts of botanicals and microbial products used as reducing and capping agents. This allows us to avoid hard-to-reproduce results due to tested green reducing agents [29].

Finally, more effort is necessary to validate the proposed nano pesticides in field conditions while simultaneously monitoring their stability, environmental fate, and sublethal effects on non-target organisms, focusing on genotoxicity and acceptable physiological and behavioral modifications. It is essential to understand the various mechanisms leading to chronic toxicity of nanoparticles invertebrates, focusing on humans.

Acknowledgements

The authors are grateful to the Management Ayya Nadar Janaki Ammal College and the Principal for providing well-equipped research facilities during this work.

Conflict of interest

"The authors declare no conflict of interest."

Author details

Jeyaraj John Wilson[1*], Thangamariyappan Harimuralikrishnaa[1],
Ponnirul Ponmanickam[1,2] and Muthumadasamy Ponseetha Lakshmi[1]

1 Department of Microbiology, Ayya Nadar Janaki Ammal College (Autonomous), Sivakasi, Tamil Nadu, India

2 Department of Zoology, Ayya Nadar Janaki Ammal College (Autonomous), Sivakasi, Tamil Nadu, India

*Address all correspondence to: jjwilson333@gmail.com

References

[1] Samer B, Muhammad A, Tiziano T, Marco C, Flavio R. The History of nanoscience and Nanotechnology: From Chemical–Physical Applications to Nanomedicine. Molecules. 2020;**25**(112):1-15

[2] Fariq A, Khan T, Yasmin A. Microbial synthesis of nanoparticles and their potential applications in biomedicine. Journal of Applied Biomedicine. 2017;**15**(4):241-248

[3] Pal SL, Jana U, Manna PK, Mohanta GP, Manavalan R. Nanoparticle: an overview of preparation and characterization. J. Appl. Pharmaceut. Sci. 2011;**1**:228-234

[4] Ahmed S, Ikram S. Biosynthesis of gold nanoparticles: A green approach. J. Photochem. Photobiol. 2016;**161**:141-153

[5] Karunaratne DN. Nanotechnology in medicine. J. Natl. Sci. Found. Sri. 2010;**35**:149-152

[6] Benelli G. Plant-mediated biosynthesis of nanoparticles as an emerging tool against mosquitoes of medical and veterinary importance: A review. Parasitol. Res. 2016a;**115**:23-34

[7] Saxena SK, Elahi A, Gadugu S, Prasad AK. Zika virus outbreak: An overview of the experimental therapeutics and treatment. Virus Dis. 2016;**27**:111-115

[8] WHO. Handbook for Integrated Vector Management. Geneva: World Health Organization; 2012

[9] Mehlhorn H, editor. Encyclopedia of Parasitology. fourth ed. New York: Springer; 2015. p. 893

[10] Benelli G, Lukehart CM. Special issue: Applications of green synthesized nanoparticles in pharmacology, parasitology and entomology. J Clust Sci. 2017;**28**:1-2

[11] Hassan HH, Aldujaili NH. Characterization and optimization of Ag NPs biosynthesis by *Klebsiella pneumoniae* HHHS1 isolated from silver rich environment. Biochemical and Cellular Archives. 2018;**18**(2):2533-2546

[12] Rai M, Duran N. Metal Nanoparticles in Microbiology, first Ed. Springer, Berlin, Heidelberg. 2011, 17-35 and 177-195

[13] Balagurunathan TSR. Mosquito larvicidal activity of silver nanoparticles synthesized using actinobacterium, *Streptomyces* sp. M25 against *Anopheles subpictus*, *Culex quinquefasciatus,* and *Aedes aegypti*. Journal of Parasitic Diseases. 2015;**39**(4):677-684

[14] Lateef A, Ojo SA, Akinwale AS, Azeez L, Gueguim-kana EB, Beukes LS. Biogenic synthesis of silver nanoparticles using cell-free extract of *Bacillus safensis* LAU 13: antimicrobial, free radical scavenging, and larvicidal activities. Biologia. 2015;**70**:1295-1306

[15] Salunke BK, Sawant SS, Beom SL, Kim S. Microorganisms as efficient biosystem for the synthesis of metal nanoparticles: Current scenario and future possibilities. World Journal of Microbiology and Biotechnology. 2016;**32**(5):1-16

[16] Singh R, Utkarsha U, Shedbalkar SAW, Balu AC. Bacteriagenic silver nanoparticles: synthesis, mechanism, and applications. Appl Microbiol Biotechnol. 2015;**99**: 4579-4593

[17] Kalaimurugan D, Vivekanandhan P, Sivasankar P, Durairaj K, Senthilkumar P, Shivakumar MS, et al. Larvicidal activity of silver nanoparticles synthesized by *Pseudomonas fluorescens* YPS3 isolated from the Eastern Ghats of India. Journal of Cluster Science. 2019;**30**(1):225-233

[18] Kumar P. Fundamentals and Techniques of Biophysics and Molecular Biology. 3rd ed. New Delhi, India: Pathfinder Publications; 2020

[19] Pandey P, Dahiya M. A Brief review on inorganic nanoparticles. Journal of Critical Reviews. 2016;**3**(3):18-26

[20] Becker N, Petric D, Zgomba M, Boase C, Madon MB, Dahl C, et al. Mosquitoes and Their Control. second ed. Berlin, Heidelberg: Springer; 2010

[21] Sutthanont N, Attrapadung S, Nuchprayoon S. larvicidal activity of synthesized silver nanoparticles from *Curcuma zedoaria* essential oil against *Culex quinquefasciatus*. Insects. 2019;**10**:1-11

[22] Marimuthu S, Rahuman AA, Kirthi AV, Santhoshkumar T, Jayaseelan C, Rajakumar G. Eco-friendly microbial route to synthesize cobalt nanoparticles using *Bacillus thuringiensis* against malaria and dengue vectors. Parasitol Res. 2013;**112**(12):4105-4112

[23] Banu AN, Balasubramanian C, Moorthi PV. Biosynthesis of silver nanoparticles using *Bacillus thuringiensis* against dengue vector, *Aedes aegypti* (Diptera:Culicidae). Parasitology Research. 2014;**113**(1):311-316

[24] Shankar S, Rai A, Ankamwar B. Biological synthesis of triangular gold nanoprisms. Nature Mater. 2004;**3**:482-488

[25] Rajesh P, Sabah S. Biosynthesis of silver nanoparticles for mosquito control. British J. Medi. and Health Res. 2017;**4**:2394-2967

[26] World Health Organization. Guidelines for laboratory and field testing of mosquito larvicides. World Health Organization; 2005

[27] Benelli G. Mode of action of nanoparticles against insects. Environmental Science and Pollution Research. 2018;**25**(13):12329-12341

[28] Benelli G. Green synthesized nanoparticles in the fight against mosquito-borne diseases and cancer—a brief review. Enzyme Microbial Technol. 2016b;**95**:58-68

[29] Heng MY, Tan SN, Yong JWH, Ong ES. Emerging green technologies for the chemical standardization of botanicals and herbal preparations. TrAC Trends Anal Chem. 2013;**50**:1-10

Chapter 14

Role of CRISPR Technology in Gene Editing of Emerging and Re-emerging Vector Borne Disease

Kaushal Kumar Mahto, Pooja Prasad, Mohan Kumar, Harshita Dubey and Amar Ranjan

Abstract

Vector borne diseases are rampant across the world. Due to spread and establishment of vector species in different geographical areas, vector adaptation and resistance towards many insecticides the only option left is vector control for various vector borne diseases. Recent advancement in the field of genome editing have provided a variety of tools like, CRISPR, a novel genome editing techniques which can be applied for the control and prevention of many deadly diseases like dengue, chikungunya, filariasis, Japanese encephalitis and Zika. The present chapter is aimed to discuss the recent advancement in genome editing tools such as, their application, challenges, and limitations in vector control. Additionally, this chapter would potentially be advantageous to understand the hurdles, knowledge gaps in eliminating vector borne disease.

Keywords: CRISPR, gene editing, vector borne disease, insecticide, resistance

1. Introduction

Vector-borne disease account for more than 17% of all infectious diseases, affecting approximately 700,000 people each year and dengue alone accounts for more than 3.9 billion people in 129 countries [1]. Mosquitoes are becoming increasingly resistant to insecticides and antimalarial drugs, necessitating the development of new methods to combat the disease as the gap between frequent outbreaks has been decreasing now. Children are very prone to malaria and children under the age of five account for the majority of fatalities. To combat vector borne diseases scientific communities have been working for decades and have successfully developed several techniques like sterile insect technique (SIT), precision-guided sterile insect technique (PgSIT), Zink Finger (ZFN), transcription activator-like effector nuclease (TALEN) and clustered regularly interspaced short palindromic repeats (CRISPER). CRISPR is a novel gene editing technique in the scientific community developed by Emmanuelle Charpentier of France and Jennifer A. Doudna of the United States who were awarded the Nobel Prize 2020 in the field of chemistry for discovering the CRISPR/Cas9 genetic scissors. CRISPER technique was initially introduced by Ishino et al. in the year 1987 [2] and

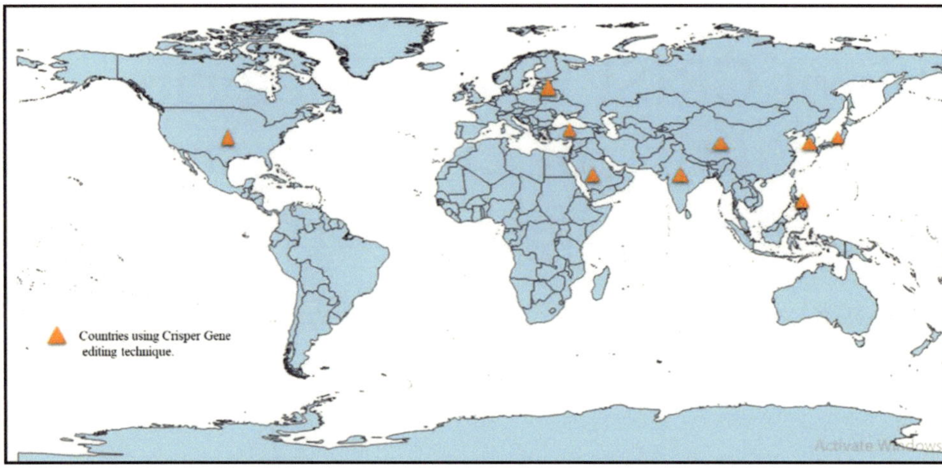

Figure 1.
Countries using crisper as gene editing tool in different areas.

Mosquito vector species	Disease	Distribution	Burden	Vaccine availability	Intervention	References
Aedes	Chikungunya, Zika, dengue lymphatic filariasis, Rift Valley fever, yellow fever	Central and South America, Asia, Africa, South Eastern United State	390 million (DEN), Avr 106,000 (CHK, ZK), Approx. 200,000 (YF), 859 million (LF)	NO	DEET, IR3535 or icaridin, elimination of breeding site	[6]
Anopheles	Lymphatic filariasis, malaria	Countrywide	859 million (LF), 241 million (Malaria)	Malaria (yes)	LLINs, ITNs, IRS	[7, 8]
Culex	Japanese encephalitis, lymphatic filariasis, West Nile fever	Middle East Europe, Asia, Japan, China, India	3 billion (JE), 859 million (LF)	Only JE (Yes)	Mosquito repellents, vaporizers	[8, 9]
Mansonia	Brugian filariasis, yellow fever	South East Asia Australia	App. 200,000 (YF)	No	Repellents, elimination of breeding site	[6]

Table 1.
Showing mosquito borne disease and their distribution, burden and intervention.

has been widely used in genome editing in mosquito species for a number of years [3–5]. CRISPER-Cas9 based genome editing has emerged as one pf the most effective, diverse, and adaptive technique for gene editing.

Countries like Saudi Arabia, Turkey, Korea, Philippines, India, USA, Europe, China, and Japan are using crisper technique for combating much vector borne disease (**Figure 1**). Based on the burden of mosquito vector associated disease across various geographical areas there is an immediate requirement of advancement in these techniques (**Table 1**).

2. Brief history of CRISPER

Ishino and his colleagues identified CRISPER for the first time in *E. coli* in 1987, with a 1664-nucleotide sequence [2]. From 1993 until 2005, it was extensively discovered. CRISPER function were established in 2007 following the discovery of genes proximal to the CRISPER locus in 2002 and foreign viral DNA sequences in CRISPER space in 2005. CRISPER was discovered by two laboratories at the same time in 2013 to become the most powerful gene editing technique known (**Figure 2**).

Arbo viral diseases such as dengue, chikungunya, Zika and malaria are a major public health problem across the world. To counteract the spread of mosquito-borne disease, researchers transformed CRISPER/Cas 9 into extremely effective "gene

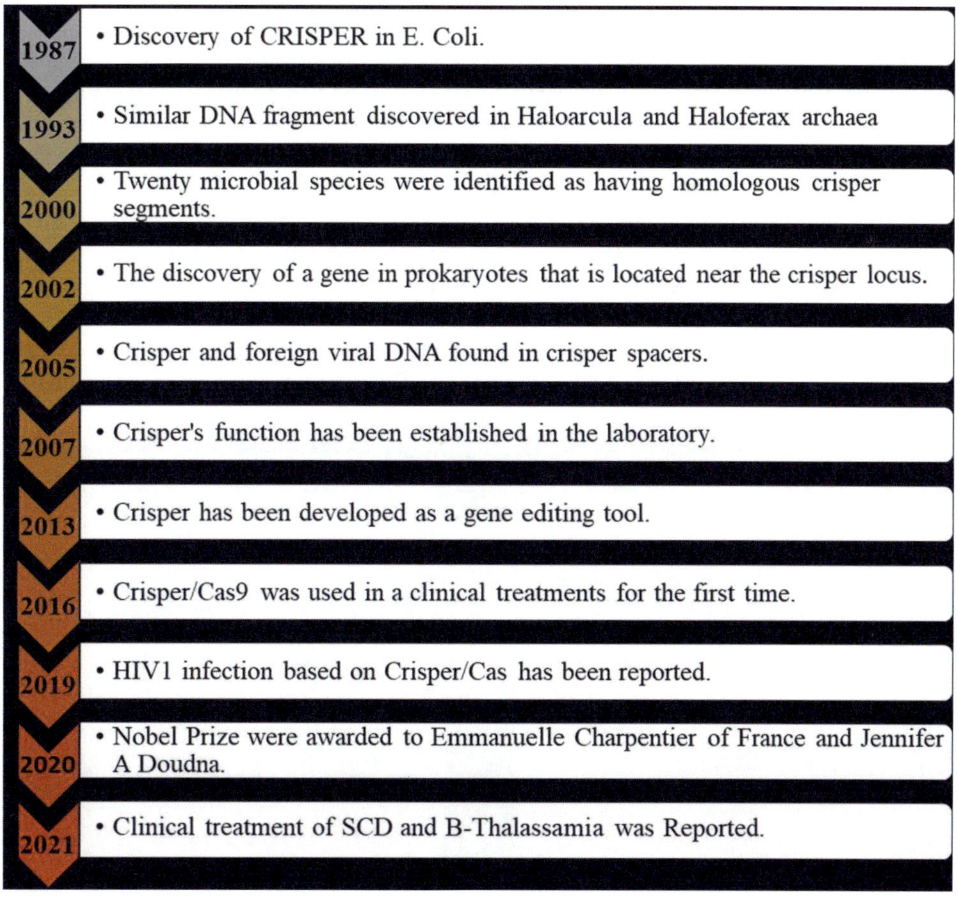
1987
• Discovery of CRISPER in E. Coli.
1993
• Similar DNA fragment discovered in Haloarcula and Haloferax archaea
2000
• Twenty microbial species were identified as having homologous crisper segments.
2002
• The discovery of a gene in prokaryotes that is located near the crisper locus.
2005
• Crisper and foreign viral DNA found in crisper spacers.
2007
• Crisper's function has been established in the laboratory.
2013
• Crisper has been developed as a gene editing tool.
2016
• Crisper/Cas9 was used in a clinical treatments for the first time.
2019
• HIV1 infection based on Crisper/Cas has been reported.
2020
• Nobel Prize were awarded to Emmanuelle Charpentier of France and Jennifer A Doudna.
2021
• Clinical treatment of SCD and B-Thalassamia was Reported.

Figure 2.
Flow chart showing history and discovery of CRISPER/Cas technique.

drive" systems capable of spreading disease resistance genes across whole populations. Researchers packaged disease resistance genes, CRISPER, gRNA, and Cas9 components into a single DNA construct to produce a gene drive [10]. After insertion, the gene drive replicates autonomously into both parental chromosomes and is inherited by around 99.5% of progeny. Advances in gene drive technology promises urgent alternatives for disease control. Two approaches for controlling arbo-viral diseases for controlling arbo-viral disease using gene-edited mosquitoes have recently gained significant attention. The first approach is "Population Replacement" where the wild mosquito population, which carry or transmits the pathogen, is replaced by the normal ones. The principle of gene drive underlies this strategy. Gene drive makes use of an inheritance quirk to pass on a trait to more than half of a mosquito's offspring allowing it to spread rapidly over a population. Another strategy is "Population Suppression" which involves the reduction of mosquito population, resulting in less mosquito genic condition and fever mosquito capable of transmitting pathogens.

3. Gene drive

Gene drive are selfish genetic tools that can be re-designed to invade a population and they hold tremendous potential for the control of mosquitoes that transmit disease [10]. Targeting the mosquito vector in order to interrupt transmission has been the mainstay of successful malaria control programs over to interrupt transmission has been the mainstay of successful malaria control programs over the years. Gene drives represents a powerful tool to achieve this in a targeted way that is species-specific, requires minimal infrastructure and is self-sustaining (**Figure 3**). Moreover, if successful, the benefits of this type of intervention would be available to all, regardless of differential access to healthcare.

Several CRISPER/Cas9 based clinical therapies have been described in the last 3 years. Many clinical trials have been completed in recent years, with some results reported; including the CRISPER/Cas9 based clinical treatment of acquired immunodeficiency syndrome (AIDS) [10], sickle cell disease (SCD) [11], thalassemia and various cancer [12, 13]. Emmanuelle Charpentier and Jennifer Doudna

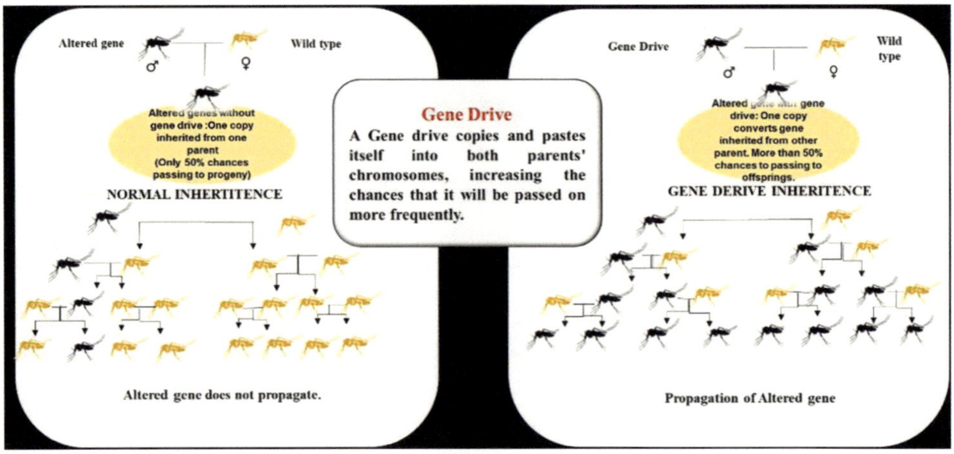

Figure 3.
Propagation of altered gene through gene drive mechanism.

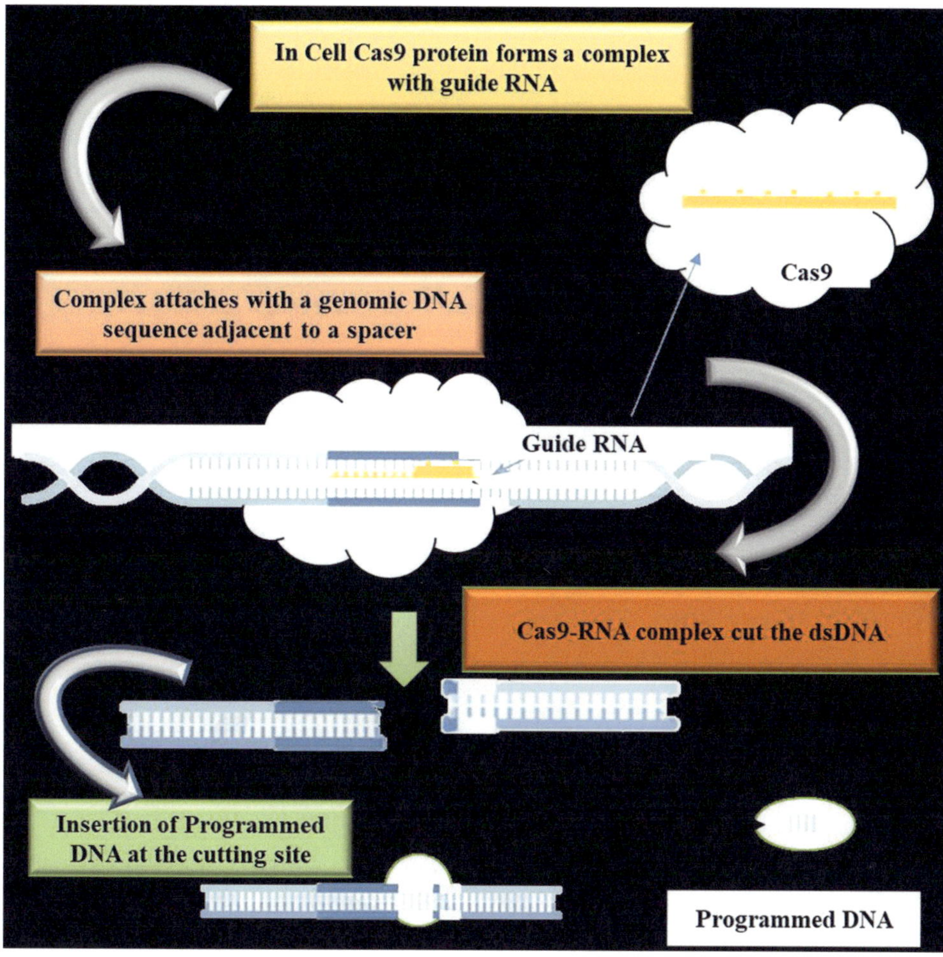

Figure 4.
Mechanism of Crisper/Cas9.

were given the Nobel Prize in 2020 in recognition of their accomplishment using CRISPER/Cas9 technology. The mechanism behind Crisper technique is shown in **Figure 4**. CRISPER gene editing tool in mosquito species mainly *Aedes aegypti*, *Anopheles stephensi*, *Anopheles gambiae* with target site and its application are shown is **Tables 2** and **3**.

3.1 How crisper work?

A detailed description of each technique is given below:

3.2 Sterile insect technique (SIT)

SIT is a proven ecologically safe method of controlling wild populations. Since the 1950s, SITs have been employed to manage insect pests in the United States and across the world. SIT is a species-specific, non-polluting insect management approach that depends on the release of a large number of sterile insect [21–23]. Throughout

Mosquito species	Genome editing tool	Targeted genes	Application	Reference
Ae. aegypti	CRISPR/Cas9	ECFP	Functional genomics	[14]
Ae. aegypti	CRISPR/Cas9	Nix	Conversion of females into harmless males	[15]
Ae. aegypti	CRISPR/Cas9	Aaeg-wtrw	Site-specific mutations	[16]
Ae. aegypti	CRISPR/Cas9	Kmo, loqs, r2d2, ku70, lig4 and nix genes	Transgenic strains and gene drive	[17]
An. stephensi	CRISPR/Cas9	M1C3 and m2A10	*P. falciparum* resistance strains	[18]
An. gambiae	CRISPR/Cas9	AGAP005958, AGAP007280 and AGAP011377	*An. gambiae* population suppression	[19]
An. gambiae	CRISPR/Cas9	X-linked rDNA sequence	Sex-distortion in *An. gambiae*	[20]

ECFP, enhanced cyan fluorescent protein; Nix, male-determining factor gene; Aaeg-wtrw, Ae. aegypti water witch locus; kmo, kynurenine 3-monoxygenase; loqs, loquacious; r2d2, r2d2 protein; ku70, ku heterodimer protein gene; lig4, ligase4; m1C3 and m2A10, anti-parasite effector genes; AGAP005958, AGAP007280 and AGAP011377, An. gambiae female-fertility genes.

Table 2.
Crisper gene editing tool with target site and its application.

the twentieth century, large-scale vector control initiative effectively reduced disease transmission levels to zero or near zero levels over areas. Countries which were close to elimination of malaria and yellow fever, include Cuba, Panama, Brazil and in Pan America [46–49] and Singapore (very low level of dengue incidence) [50–52].

Sterile insect technique involves following steps:

- Mass production of mosquitoes.
- Separation and sterilization of males.
- Mass release of male mosquito by drone, jeep, helicopter, etc.
- Sterile male compete with wild males to mate with wild females.
- Production of infertile egg.

SIT may be a preferable method of reducing mosquito populations in places where the use of insecticides is not practical, is not accepted by the community, or where pesticide resistance has diminished insecticide efficacy (**Figure 5**).

3.3 Precision-guided sterile insect technique (PgSIT)

A revolutionary scalable genetic control technology uses a CRISPR-based technique to design deployable mosquitoes capable of population suppression (41). Males do not transmit diseases; hence, the strategy is to release an increasing number of sterile males. Mosquito populations can be reduced without the use of toxic chemicals and pesticides. It affects genes associated with male fertility (resulting in sterile progeny)

	SIT	(HEGs)	(ZFN)	TALEN	PgIT	Crisper
Origin and biological basis	The method was first employed to remove screw-worms in 1950.	Prior to 1970, yeast group I introns with greater than Mendelian inheritance proportions were identified.	Zinc-binding first fused for site-specific DNA cleavage in 1996	TALE proteins discovered in *Xanthomonas* species 2009 and conjugated to FokI endonuclease	Changes genes associated with male fertility (resulting in sterile progeny) and female flight in *Aedes aegypti*	*S. pyogenes* destruction and memory of parasitic nucleic acid
Initial use for genome modification	*Cochliomyia* (1954)	*E. coli* (1998)	*Xenopus laevis* (2001)	*S. cerevisiae* (2010)	*D. melanogaster*	Human cell lines (2012)
Year used in mosquitoes	1955	2011	2013	2013	2013	2015
Mechanism	Rearing of mosquito followed by separation of males and sterilize them and releasing of irradiated males to mate with wild females resulting infertile egg.	Endonuclease encoded by HEG detects and cleaves genomic DNA, allowing a gene cassette to be integrated by cell HDR machinery.	ZFN domain recognizes and bind to a sequence of nucleotide triplets, and crate a dsDNA breaks in backbone.	TALE domains recognize and bind to a sequence of nucleotides, and cut DNA backbone, together creating a double-stranded break.	Strategy is to release an increasing number of sterile males based on SIT.	Cas 9 protein make complex with guide RNA and binds to genomic DNA and produce a double stranded and with insertion of programmed DNA.
Gene drive	No	Yes	No	No	Yes	Yes
Benefits	• Produced offspring's were infertile	• Insertion into a known site • High efficiency	• First gene editing technique for reverse genetics. • Site-specific editing.	• Site-specific editing • Efficient mutagenesis.	• Production of infertile male. • Flightless female	• Site-specific highly efficient for mutagenesis and as a drive.

	SIT	(HEGs)	(ZFN)	TALEN	PgIT	Crisper
Drawback	• Mass rearing and irradiation require precision processes. • Radiation can reduce male mating fitness	• Requires pre-existing target-sites. • Re-engineering of the HEG, or transgenesis for insertion of target sites.	• Expensive, requires in vitro optimization	• Requires protein engineering	• Radiation can reduce male mating fitness	• Drive mechanism generates drive-resistant alleles
References	[21–23]	[24–29]	[30–34]	[35–40]	[41]	[2, 42–47]

Table 3.
Showing a brief comparison of Crisper and other gene editing techniques.

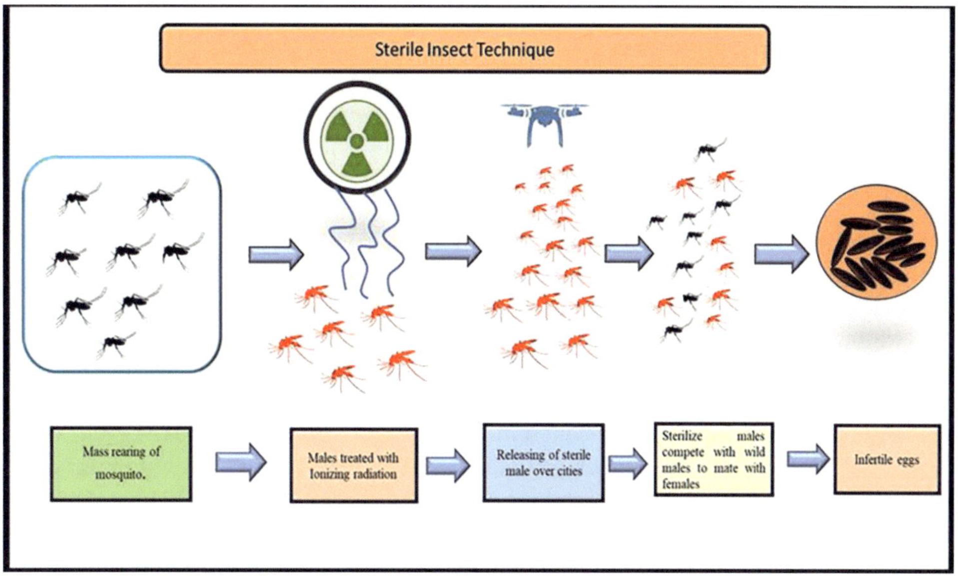

Figure 5.
Showing application of sterile insect technique.

and female flight in *Aedes aegypti*, the mosquito species responsible for the transmission of illnesses such as dengue fever, chikungunya, and Zika.

PgSIT is based on a dominant genetic technique that permits simultaneous sexing and sterilization, allowing eggs to be released into the environment while assuring only sterile adult males emerge. The system is self-limiting and is not expected to persist or spread in the environment, which are two safety factors that should allow this technology to be accepted. PgSIT eggs can be delivered to a place threatened by mosquito-borne disease or generated at an on-site laboratory that can manufacture the eggs for nearby deployment. Once the PgSIT eggs are released into the wild, infertile PgSIT males will develop and eventually mate with females, reducing the natural population as desired.

3.4 Zink Finger (ZFN)

A few researchers have used ZFN to custom-edit the genomes of vector mosquitoes. Zinc-finger domains identify the shapes of nucleotide triplets in the major groove of a DNA double-helix and may be engineered to recognize a specific 18-nucleotide sequence, allowing a large number of protein effectors to be recruited to a specific place in the genome [53–55]. Zinc-finger domains are conjugated to a FokI type II restriction endonuclease and designed in pairs to recognize sequences flanking a target-site, resulting in a double-stranded break at a particular genomic locus [37, 55].

Inspite of the high cost and the low success rate of a ZFN, it was still being used by most laboratories for biological studies. For example, DeGennaro et al. [32] investigated the involvement of the odorant receptor coreceptor (orco) gene and the odorant receptor pathway in host identification and susceptibility to the chemical repellent N,N-diethyl-meta-toluamide (DEET) in *Aedes aegypti* [35]. The developed ZFN was injected into embryos of *Aedes aegypti* in this experiment. When compared to the wild type, the orco mutants developed in this work had lower spontaneous activity and odor-evoked responses. In the absence of CO_2, orco mutant mosquitoes did not respond to human odor.

In an another set of experiment McMeniman et al. injected ZFNs into pre-blastoderm stage embryos to mutate the *Aedes aegypti* gustatory receptors (AaegGr3) gene, a subunit of the heteromeric CO_2 receptor, and found that the Gr3 mutant lacked electrophysiological and behavioral responses to CO_2 [54].

3.5 Transcription activator-like effector nuclease (TALEN)

Finally, in 2010, a low-cost technology that could be developed in-house made targeted mutagenesis available to molecular biology laboratories: transcription activator-like effector (TALE) nucleases, or TALENs. TALENs, like ZFNs, are modular, can be encoded on a plasmid via cloning, and are relatively efficient [31]. Finally, the recognition of each nucleotide on a DNA target was encoded in the 12th and 13th amino acids of each 34 amino-acid repeat; a peptide stretch of 18 or 19 repeats could be engineered to recognize any nucleotide sequence and could induce site-specific DNA cleavage when conjugate to the FokI domain [30, 35, 56]. Smidler et al. reported the targeted disruption of the thioester containing protein1 (TEP1) gene using TALEN in *Anopheles gambiae* mosquitos, which transmit malaria. TEP1 has been identified as an immunity gene in *An. gambiae* against plasmodium infection [57]. The induced mutations lowered protein synthesis, and the resulting TEP1 mutants were more vulnerable to *Plasmodium berghei* infections. In addition to the previously described ZFN, TALEN has been employed as a powerful genome editing technique to alter the targeted genes in disease-causing mosquitoes. Gene-editing in *Ae. aegypti* and *An. stephensi* using ZFNs and TALENs were reported in 2013 [32, 33, 57]. As there is a less difficulty to construct TALENs in the lab, therefore, TALENs were more accessible than previous gene-editing approaches. However, the timing of TALEN development was almost concurrent with the leveraging of CRISPR/Cas9 biology for gene-editing, meaning that TALENs usefulness was short-lived.

3.6 Meganucleases

Usefulness HEs, also known as meganucleases, can cleave double-stranded DNA at specific recognition site of 14–40 bp in length [58]. HEG-induced dsDNA break and activate the cell's recombination repair system, which uses the HEG-containing homologous chromosome as a template for repair. As a result, in a process known as 'homing' the HEG is copied to the broken chromosome. HEGs spread through populations by using this transmission distortion mechanism [59]. In *An. gambiae*, HEs have recently been proposed as a method of genetic sterilization or sex-ratio distortion [58, 59].

4. Ethical issues

CRISPR/Cas9 offers a wide range of uses and enormous life-changing potential, but it will take decades to develop. The proper use of biotechnology necessitates meticulous planning and strict control, both of which are far from reality. Altering a gene might have unforeseeable and unfavorable repercussions in the genetically edited species, as well as in other species, and can result in the emergence of new and undiscovered animal and human disease. CRISPR/Cas9 has a wide range of potential immediate public health benefits: it can be used to treat vector borne disease, but there are, nevertheless, significant dangers. Gene editing should be implemented with caution and followed by more research. Gene editing techniques have the potential to diminish biodiversity and harm ecosystems. The UNESCO Declaration on Bioethics and Human Rights recognizes humans as essential members of the ecosystem. How and under what conditions do we have the authority to alter biological beings, and how far do we have that authority? Is it possible to foresee the effects of modifying or removing a particular animal species from its ecosystem? Is there a method to limit the negative consequences as well? The variety of prospective uses for gene drive technology (particularly the manufacturing of bioweapons) and their consequences in this predicted situation are certainly unexpected. Besides this, there are environmental concerns; for example, what will be the impact on predatory fish and insects that consume mosquito larvae, is still under debate. Therefore, in order to environment interest, it should be thoroughly investigated.

5. Discussion

Insects are a highly diversified group that inhabits many biological niches, has specific habitat adaptations, and performs diverse behaviors. CRISPR system is a very successful tool for precision genome editing in the mosquito compared to the relatively low throughput and high cost of ZFN- and TALEN-mediated mutagenesis. Precision genome engineering in mosquitos holds a lot of potential for studying the genetic basis of behavior and developing genetic strategies to control vector populations [56]. The development of new CRISPR tools and platforms for molecular diagnostics has the potential to revolutionize health care and enhance global epidemiological management. SIT approach has various limitations, adopting innovative methods like PgSIT to control mosquito-borne diseases is a suitable way to implement population control measures.

6. Conclusion

CRISPER technology is a new approach in the field of vector-transmitted disease that is causing dispute among government, non-government, and policymakers. Scientists all around the world, however, have the opportunity to implement this technology for the benefit of society, notably for the control of the vector mosquitoes. However, it is more crucial to adhere to all the rule and regulations and take stringent biosafety precautions to avoid unintended and unwanted outcomes from genome editing. Existing vector control strategies are unprepared to deal with arboviral disease's exceptional development and reemergence. The tremendous successes in localized eradication, as well as the final inability to eradicate malaria globally, aroused interest in genetic methods to mosquito control. In contrast to several application of Crisper technique it might be disused and scientific discussion around CRISPR is crucial. Despite the risks, CRISPR represents a tremendous potential for humanity, and the precise gene editing will bring in a bright future.

Acknowledgements

Authors are gratefully acknowledging ICMR-National Institute of Malaria Research, New Delhi, India, for providing the suitable environment facilities that help us to draft the proposed study.

Conflict of interest

The authors declare that they have no known competing financial interests or personal ties that would seem to have influenced the work presented in this study.

Author details

Kaushal Kumar Mahto[1,2*], Pooja Prasad[1,3], Mohan Kumar[2,4], Harshita Dubey[4] and Amar Ranjan[4]

1 ICMR-National Institute of Malaria Research, New Delhi, India

2 School of Computational and Integrative Sciences, Jawaharlal Nehru University, New Delhi, India

3 Department of Zoology, D.S.B. Campus, Kumaun University, Nainital, Uttarakhand, India

4 All India Institute of Medical Sciences, New Delhi, India

*Address all correspondence to: kausha63_sit@jnu.ac.in

References

[1] WHO [Internet]. 2020. Available from: https://www.who.int/news-room/fact-sheets/detail/vector-borne-diseases [Accessed: 18 January 2022]

[2] Ishino H, Shinagawa K, Makino M, Amemura AN. Nucleotide sequence of the IAP gene, responsible for alkaline phosphatase isozyme conversion in *Escherichia coli*, and identification of the gene product. Journal of Bacteriology. 1987;**169**:5429-5433

[3] Gantz VM, Jasinskiene N, Tatarrenkova O, Fazekas A, Macias VM, Bier E, et al. Highly efficient Cas9-mediated gene drive for population modification of the malaria vector mosquito *Anopheles stephensi*. Proceedings of the National Academy of Sciences of the United States of America. 2015;**112**:E6736-E6743

[4] Hammond A, Galizi R, Kyrou K, Simoni A, Siniscalchi C, Katsanos D, et al. A CRISPER-Cas9 gene drive system targeting female reproduction in the malaria mosquito vector *Anopheles gambiae*. Nature Biotechnology. 2016;**34**: 78-83

[5] Galizi R, Hammond A, Kyrou K, Taxiarchi C, Bernardini F, O'Loughlin SM, et al. A CRISPER-Cas9 sex-ratio distortion system for genetic control. Scientific Reports. 2016;**6**:31139

[6] Scitable by Nature Education [Internet] 2020. Available from: https://www.nature.com/scitable/topicpage/dengue-transmission-22399758/ [Accessed: 18 January 2022]

[7] WHO [Internet]. 2020. Available from: https://www.who.int/news-room/fact-sheets/detail/malaria [Accessed: 18 January 2022]

[8] WHO [Internet]. 2020. Available from: https://www.who.int/news-room/fact-sheets/detail/lymphatic-filariasis [Accessed: 18 January 2022]

[9] WHO [Internet]. 2020. Available from: https://www.who.int/news-room/fact-sheets/detail/japanese-encephalitis [Accessed: 18 January 2022]

[10] Xu L, Wang J, Liu Y, Xie L, Su B, Mou D, et al. CRISPR-edited stem cells in a patient with HIV and acute lymphocytic leukemia. New England Journal of Medicine. 2019;**381**:1240-1247

[11] Frangoul H, Altshuler D, Cappellni MD, Chen YS, Domm J, Eustace BK, et al. CRISPER-Cas9 gene editing for sickle cell disease and β-thalassemia. New England Journal of Medicine. 2021;**384**:252-260

[12] Stadtmauer EA, Fraietta JA, Davis MM, Cohen AD, Weber KL, Lancaster E, et al. CRISPER-engineered T cells in patients with refractory cancer. Science. 2020;**367**(6481):eaba7365

[13] Lu Y, Xue J, Deng T, Zhou X, Yu K, Deng L, et al. Safety and feasibility of CRISPER-edited T cells in patients with refractory non-small-cell lung cancer. Nature Medicine. 2020;**26**:732-740

[14] Gaj T, Gersbach CA, Barbas CF. ZFN, TALEN, and CRISPR/Cas-based methods for genome engineering. Trends in Biotechnology. 2013;**31**:397-405

[15] Ledford H. CRISPR, the disruptor. Nature. 2015;**522**:20-24

[16] Vogel GUK. Researcher receives permission to edit genes in human embryos. Science News. Available from: http://www.sciencemag.

org/news/2016/02/uk-researcher-receivespermission-edit-genes-human-embryos [Accessed: 22 September 2016]

[17] DeFrancesco L. Move over ZFNs. Nature Biotechnology. 2012;**29**:681-684

[18] Alphey L. Can CRISPR-Cas9 gene drives curb malaria? Nature Biotechnology. 2016;**34**:149-150

[19] Wickramasinghe PD, Silva GN, Silva Gunawardene YI, Dassanayake RS. Advances in *Aedes* mosquito vector control strategies using CRISPER/Cas9. In: Genetically Modified and Other Innovative Vector Control Technologies. Singapore: Springer; 2021. pp. 67-87

[20] Paulraj MG, Ignacimuthu S, Reegan AD. Gene silencing and gene drive in dengue vector control: A review. Indian Journal of Natural Products and Resources. 2016;**7**:1-8

[21] Hsu PD, Scott DA, Weinstein JA, Ran FA, Konermann S, Agarwala V, et al. DNA targeting specificity of RNA-guided Cas9 nucleases. Nature Biotechnology. 2013;**31**:827-832

[22] Knipling E. Agriculture Handbook No. 512: The Basic Principle of Insect Population suppression and Management. Washington, DC: USDA; 1979

[23] Knippling E. Role of parasitoid augmentation and sterile insect technique for area-wide management of agriculture insect pest. Journal of Agriculture Entomology. 1998;**15**:273-301

[24] Krafsur E. Sterile insect technique for suppressing and eradicating insect population: 55 years and counting. Journal of Agriculture Entomology. 1998;**15**:303-317

[25] Burt A. Site-specific selfish genes as tools for the control and genetic engineering of natural populations. Proceedings of the Royal Society of London Series B: Biological Science. 2003;**270**:921-928

[26] Windbichler N, Menichelli M, Papathanos PA, Thyme SB, Li H, Ulge UY, et al. A synthetic homing endonuclease-based gene drive system in the human malaria mosquito. Nature. 2011;**473**:212-215

[27] Aryan A, Anderson MA, Myles KM, Adelman ZN. Germline excision of transgene in *Aedes aegypti* by homing endonuclease. Scientific Reports. 2013;**3**: 1603

[28] Sellem CH, Belcour L. Intron open reading frames as mobile elements and evolution of a group I intron. Molecular Biology and Evolution. 1997;**14**:518-526

[29] Bernadini F, Galizi R, Menichelli M, Papathanos PA, Dritsou V, Marois E, et al. Site-specific genetic engineering of the Anopheles gambiae Y chromosome. Proceedings of the National Academy of Science. 2014;**111**:7600-7605

[30] Kim YG, Cha J, Chandrasegaran S. Hybrid restriction enzyme: Zinc finger fusion to Fok I cleavage domain. Proceedings of the National Academy of Science. 1996;**93**:1156-1160

[31] Beerli RR, Barbas CF. Engineering polydactyl zinc-finger transcription factors. Nature Biotechnology. 2002;**20**:135-141

[32] DeGennaro M, McBride CS, Seeholzer L, Nakagawa T, Dennis EJ, Goldman C, et al. orco mutant mosquitoes lose strong preference for human and are not repelled by volatile DEET. Nature. 2013;**498**:487-491

[33] McMeniman CJ, Corfas RA, Matthews BJ, Ritchie SA, Vosshall LB.

Multimodal integration of carbon dioxide and other sensory cues drives mosquito attraction to human. Cell. 2014;**27**:1060-1071

[34] Liesch J, Bellani LL, Vosshall LB. Functional and genetic characterization of neuropeptide Y-like receptors in *Aedes aegypti*. PLOS Neglected Tropical Disease. 2013;**7**:e2486

[35] Christian M, Cermak T, Doyle EL, Schmidt C, Zhang F, Hummel A, et al. Targeting DNA double-strand breaks with TAL effector nuclease. Genetics. 2010;**186**:757-761

[36] Moscou MJ, Bogdanove AJ. A simple cipher governs DNA recognition by TAL effectors. Science. 2009;**11**:1501

[37] Smidler AL, Terenzi O, Soichot J, Levashina EA, Marois E. Targeted mutagenesis in the malaria mosquito using TALE nuclease. PLoS One. 2013;**8**:e74511

[38] Basu S, Aryan A, Overcash JM, Samuel GH, Anderson MA, Dahlem TJ, et al. Silencing of end-joining repair for efficient site-specific gene insertion after TALEN/CRISPER mutagenesis in *Aedes aegypti*. Proceedings of the National Academy of Science. 2015;**112**:4038-4043

[39] Bibikova M, Beumer K, Trautman JK, Carroll D. Enhancing gene targeting with designed zinc finger nucleases. Science. 2003;**300**:764

[40] Aryan A, Anderson MA, Myles KM, Adelman ZN. TALEN based gene disruption in the dengue vector *Aedes aegypti*. PLoS One. 2013;**8**:e60082

[41] Kandul NP, Liu J, Sanchez CHM, Wu SL, Marshall JM, Akbari OS. Transforming insect population control with precision guided sterile males with demonstration in flies. Nature Communication. 2019;**8**:1-2

[42] Jinek M, Chylinski K, Fonfara I, Hauer M, Doudna JA, Charpentier E. A programmable dual-RNA-guided DNA endonuclease in adaptive bacterial immunity. Science. 2011;**337**:816-821

[43] Gantz VM, Jasinskiene N, Tatarenkova O, Fazekas A, Macias VM, Bier E, et al. Highly efficient Cas9 mediated gene drive for population modification of the malaria vector mosquito *Anopheles stephensi*. Proceedings of the National Academy of Sciences. 2015;**112**:E6736-E6743

[44] Li M, Akbari OS, White BJ. Highly efficient site specific mutagenesis in malaria mosquitoes using CRISPER. G3 (Bethesda). 2017;**8**:653-658

[45] Deveau H, Garneau JE, Moineau S. CRISPER/Cas system and its role in phase-bacteria interactions. Annual Review of Microbiology. 2010;**64**:475-493

[46] Li M, Bui M, Yang T, Bowman CS, White BJ, Akbari OS. Germline Cas9 expression yields efficient genome engineering in a major worldwide disease vector, *Aedes aegypti*. Proceedings of the National Academy of Science. 2017;**114**:E10540-9

[47] Soper FL, Wilson DB. Anopheles Gambiae in Brazil, 1930 to 1940. Rockefeller Foundation; 1943

[48] Soper FL. The elimination of urban yellow fever in the Americas through the eradication of *Aedes aegypti*. American Journal of Public Health and the Nation's Health. 1963;**53**:7-16

[49] Kouri GP, Guzman MG, Bravo JR. Hemorrhagic dengue in Cuba: History of an epidemic. Bulletin of the Pan American Health Organization (PAHO). 1986;**20**:24-30

[50] Egger JR, Ooi EE, Kelly DW, Woolhouse ME, Davis CR, Coleman PG.

Reconstructing historical changes in the force of infection of dengue fever in Singapore: Implication for surveillance and control. Bulletin of the World Health Organization. 2008;**86**:187-196

[51] Li M, Yang T, Bui M, Gamez S, Wise T, Kandul NP, et al. Suppressing mosquito population with precision guided sterile males. Nature Communications. 2021;**12**:1-0

[52] Liu Q, Segal DJ, Ghiara JB, Barbas CF. Design of polydactyl zinc-finger proteins for unique addressing within complex genomes. Proceedings of the National Academy of Sciences. 1997;**94**:5525-5530

[53] Miller JC, Holmes MC, Wang J, Guschin DY, Lee YL, Rupniewski I, et al. An improved zinc finger nuclease architecture for highly specific genome editing. Nature Biotechnology. 2007;**25**:778-785

[54] Boch J, Scholze H, Schornack S, Landgarf A, Hahn S, Lahaye T, et al. Breaking the ode of DNA binding specificity of TAL-type III effectors. Science. 2009;**326**:1509-1512

[55] Moscou MJ, Bogdanove AJ. A simpler ciphor governs DNA recognition by TAL effectors. Science. 2009;**336**:1501

[56] Alphey L. Genetic control of mosquitoes. Annual Review of Entomology. 2014;**59**:205-224

[57] Miller JC, Tan S, Qiao G, Barlow KA, Wang J, Xia DF, et al. A TALE nuclease architecture for efficient genome editing. Nature Biotechnology. 2011;**29**:143-148

[58] Windbichler N, Papathanos PA, Ctteruccia F, Ranson H, Burt A, Crisanti A. Homing endonuclease mediated gene targeting in *Anopheles gambiae* cell and embryos. Nucleic Acid Research. 2007;**35**:5922-5933

[59] Windbichler N, Papathanos PA, Crisanti A. Targeting the X chromosome during spermatogenesis induces Y chromosome transmission ratio distortion and early dominant embryo lethality in Anopheles gambiae. PLOS Genetics. 2008;**4**:e1000291